Your Designer Diet

Your Designer Diet

How to stay on any diet for the rest of your life

Todd Hoff

Possibility Outpost, Inc.
Los Gatos, CA

For updates and more references, please visit *http://YourDesignerDiet.com*

Publisher's Cataloging-in-Publication data

Hoff, Todd.
   Your designer diet : how to stay on any diet for the rest of your life /
Todd Hoff.
   p. cm.
   ISBN 978-0-9797071-0-0
1. Weight loss. 2. Weight loss--Psychological aspects. 3. Reducing diets.
4. Nutrition. 5. Health. I. Title.

RM222.2 H573 2007
613.7 21--dc22

Table of Contents

Disclaimer

Your Designer Diet **Does Not Provide Medical Advice.** All content in this book is the opinion or information of its author. This book is not a substitute for medical advice. Always contact your own doctor or other professional health care provider if you have a question concerning your or your family's health.

RELIANCE ON ANY INFORMATION IN THIS BOOK IS AT YOUR OWN RISK. THE AUTHOR AND PUBLISHER ARE NOT RESPONSIBLE OR LIABLE FOR ANY ADVICE, COURSE OF TREATMENT, DIAGNOSIS, DRUG AND DEVICE APPLICATION OR OTHER INFORMATION, SERVICES, OR PRODUCTS THAT YOU OBTAIN FROM THIS BOOK.

Introduction

I am so disappointed in myself for letting myself go yet again. Over the last 20 years, I have gained and lost literally hundreds of pounds. Wouldn't you think I could control my weight by now?—Anonymous

I could have written this. It's me and my life 100%. And if you are reading this book, it's probably your life too.

If you are overweight, I know you are hurting. You are probably embarrassed and ashamed. You are probably at a complete loss to explain how you let your life get so far out of control.

I hate that you keep gaining weight and you don't understand why. I hate that you think gaining weight is all your fault. I hate that you blame yourself and you feel bad that you can't keep the weight off. It's a horrible and preventable downward spiral of depression.

You need to know that your weight problems are not all your fault. You can control your weight once you learn how to work with your nature as a human, your nature as an individual, and the nature of the world you live in. You can find your own strengths and use them to keep your weight off. You don't have to feel bad about yourself and your life anymore.

Through research and experimentation, I created a new weight loss method that helped me lose over 100 pounds, keep the weight off, and control my diabetes. My goal is to share the wonder of what I've learned with you, someone who has probably experienced a lot of the same difficulties I have.

I passionately believe this method, called the Designer Diet, will work for you too. One reason diets fail is they are one-size-fits all. They tell everyone to do exactly the same thing. But you are unique and your life is unique. How can a one-size-fits-all diet possibly keep up with your crazy life?

The Designer Diet is based on the idea of creating and designing the perfect diet just for you and your life. No single problem causes you to be overweight so there is no single solution either. You need a way of controlling your weight that changes as you change, adjusts to your unique individual nature, and takes advantage of your strengths while sidestepping your weaknesses. That's exactly what you learn how to do in the Designer Diet.

Using a simple step-by-step process, the Designer Diet teaches you how to control your weight by paying attention to your life, reacting quickly to reverse any weight gain, trying different strategies to help you eat less and exercise more, creating an encouraging environment, and learning which strategies work best for you. The result is that you continually improve your diet and that's what finally empowers you to lose weight and keep it off for the rest of your life.

Following your Designer Diet is a lot like hiring a world famous designer to create your dream wardrobe. Your new, expertly tailored clothes fit your body perfectly and the style always shows you at your absolute best. The Designer Diet helps you to do the same for your diet. Why use a one-size-fits-all off the rack diet when you can design a diet especially for you?

The Designer Diet goes way beyond simply hiring a designer. Designers hand you clothes and tell you what looks good on you. With the Designer Diet, you learn how to become your own world famous designer for your own diet. You need to be the designer when developing your diet. The Designer Diet teaches you a process to discover what works for you. No more will you have to rely on others to keep your weight under control.

▌ How is the Designer Diet Different?

The world may not need another diet book, but this isn't your typical diet book. It has a fresh, unique and hopeful approach. If you are tired of the same old thing and the never-ending fads and scams, this book is for you. This book is different from all the other diet books in three major ways.

The **first major difference** is that it focuses on controlling your weight by teaching **how to stay on a diet** rather than what to eat. There are enough books in the universe telling you what to eat. This book is a **diet helper,** not another diet. It works alongside your current diet, helping you stay on your own diet, whatever diet you have chosen. What to eat is always your choice.

The **second major difference** is the use of diet threats as a means of understanding why staying on a diet is so hard. A lot of the advice in the diet world is no different from easily ignored marketing slogans. The threats are surprising and put into words the feelings we all have that staying on a diet and losing weight are really, really hard.

The **third major difference** is that this book focuses on developing positive skills, called **strategies,** which you can apply immediately to your daily life. In this book we won't just talk about eating less and exercising more, you'll **learn exactly how** to really eat less and exercise more.

The result is control. You'll put yourself back in control of your weight. Does this sound a little different from the normal diet book? Does it sound like something that might work for you?

How this Book is Organized

This book is organized into three sections:

1. The purpose of the first chapter—*Why is Losing Weight So Hard?*—is to help free you from old ways of thinking about your weight that haven't worked. You need a fresh perspective, a new start. This chapter makes the case that much of what you know about your weight problem is misguided and that once you understand the real causes of your struggles, you can control your weight for the rest of your life. You are not what society says you are. You are not weak, lazy, and undisciplined. Being overweight is not all your fault. You are an amazingly capable world class survival machine. Unfortunately, in our modern world, that puts you at a high risk for being overweight. You can control your weight once you understand your true nature as a human and as an individual.

2. The second chapter—*The 10 Designer Principles for Controlling Your Weight*—presents the big picture of how to control your weight using the Designer Diet. You'll learn about the Designer Way, the Designer Mind, and many other powerful weight control principles.

3. The rest of the book presents all the threats and strategies needed to implement the process described in the 10 Designer Principles. Understanding the threats against your diet and how to use the strategies to defeat them are how you'll put yourself back in control of your weight.

To control your weight, you don't have to become someone different from who you are right now. You don't have to become someone better either. To control your weight, you simply need to become the best at being you. That means learning who you are, making friends with yourself, taking an interest in yourself, and being gentle with yourself. In that process, guided by the Designer Diet, you'll learn all you need to know to control your weight.

There's no better time to start controlling your weight than now. There's no time in the future when you'll be better prepared or more "together." Start with who you are now and where you are at in your life. That's good enough. That's all you need. You can make it work.

▌ Two Ways to Read this Book

The way I imagine you reading this book is by **browsing around** and reading the subjects that **look interesting** to you. This book is organized to make sense if you read it straight through or just by picking a random page. You can read it either way. **Whatever works** for you.

All the Threats and Strategies are Numbered and have Summaries

To make browsing easy, the book is divided into chapters that group related threats and strategies into common themes. For easy reference, each threat and strategy is assigned a unique number.

A threat or strategy can be as small as one line, one paragraph or many pages in length. Each entry begins with a short summary of the essential take-home message of the threat or strategy. You should be able to learn the key points of the book by just reading the summaries.

Accessing the Additional Strategies

Unfortunately, books can only be so large. The publisher wouldn't let me include all the strategies I wanted to. Rather than cut the number of strategies, I decided to put all of them on our website so you can read them at your convenience. Ninety-nine strategies are covered in this book, but there are over 150 on our website *(http://YourDesignerDiet.com)*. Don't think the strategies on the website aren't good ones. They are great! Here are just a few:

❖ **Understanding Taste.** You learn about your amazing sense of taste. Even the best wine experts in the world can't tell the difference between red and white wine and you'll learn why. You'll also learn how to tell if you're a supertaster or a nontaster. Supertasters are thinner so it's good to know which you are.

❖ **Learn How to Taste the Big 5: Wine, Chocolate, Beer, Cheese, and Coffee.** There's a lot of food out there for you to have fun with.

Each of these foods can provide a lifetime of wonderful eating experiences.

❖ **Create Your Senior Safe Zone.** This chapter gives many strategies helping seniors keep themselves healthy. You'll meet my grandma and read one of my favorite strategies, *Think Fierce*, which talks about how those who age well are the ones who don't buy into negative attitudes about aging.

To read these strategies and many more please visit our web site at *http:// YourDesignerDiet.com.*

▌ When You Get Stuck

There may come a time when you get stuck. You will have gained weight. You will have fallen off your diet and you will be looking for what to do next. When that time comes, I hope you can just open up this book to any page and find something, any little thought or idea, that will help you over the bad patch you are having. That's what I truly hope.

Maybe this book will interest you, maybe it won't. I hope it does. If you aren't interested, I appreciate all your time and consideration. If you are interested, please continue reading on. I am confident you can find some of your own answers in this book too.

Chapter 1

Why is Losing Weight So Hard?

've had problems with weight my entire life. I was the pudgy kid who was always last in PE class. And like Rudolf the Red-Nosed Reindeer, I was never picked to join in any reindeer games. You know the type. You may even be the type. We play comic relief in every painful coming of age movie.

Or maybe you've been thin most of your life and only recently has weight become a problem. If so, welcome to the club. And it's a big club. It's projected that in the not too distant future, the majority of people in the world will be overweight.

Whatever road you've traveled to become overweight, maybe you've asked yourself the same question that has haunted and tormented me all these years: why is losing weight so incredibly hard for me?

In my long and difficult struggles with my weight I've thought about this question a lot. And I mean a lot. I tried to understand how I could be so overweight when in my own mind I never thought of myself as the kind of person who would be overweight. It didn't make any sense. I didn't make any sense.

I was driven to try and find an answer. And I think I know the answer now. That's why I wrote this book. I've figured out a process to control weight. A process that's helped me lose over 100 pounds, keep the weight off, and control my diabetes. And there's an excellent chance something I've learned through my years of research and experimentation could help you control your weight too.

But this whole book starts with a frustratingly simple question: why do so many otherwise accomplished people continually fail to lose weight? This perplexing question is what I call the **Oprah Paradox.**

▌ The Oprah Paradox—You're More Like Oprah than You Think

Oprah Winfrey is a billionaire. She runs many businesses. She manages hundreds of people. She has hosted a daily talk show since 1986. And she is a well respected role model and inspiration to millions. Over the years we've all witnessed Oprah's painfully public weight battles. Yet by almost every measure she is more disciplined and more accomplished than most of us even dream of becoming.

If, as many people think, being overweight is simply a lack of discipline, then how can Oprah be overweight? It's not possible. Reaching Oprah's level of success requires almost unimaginable levels of discipline and dedication, yet even she finds it hard to maintain her weight. This is the Oprah Paradox.

I have to think Oprah has thoughts like this in her own mind. She has to wonder with all that she has accomplished, why can't she keep the weight off. Perhaps you have the same thoughts about yourself too. But please consider this...

People who run billion dollar corporations are overweight. People who run countries are overweight. People who make revolutionary scientific discoveries are overweight. People who create and carry out the most intricate plans are overweight. Are all these people suddenly weak when it comes to food?

Let's take a look at your life. Do you get up and go to work? Are you competent at your job? Did you make it through school? Have you experienced and overcome tragedy in your life? Do you manage a mortgage or rent? Are you raising a family? Are your kids clothed, fed and going to school? Are you saving a little for retirement? Have you maintained a long term relationship? Did you stop yourself from hitting that jerk who cut in front of you in the grocery line the other day?

You probably answered "yes" to at least a few of these questions. So, if you look at your life you will find overwhelming evidence that you are a capable and competent person. Although you may not be perfect, all the stuff you do in your life is actually quite remarkable. Think about this a bit. Don't take it for granted. Think about all your amazing abilities and accomplishments.

You don't sound like a weak person to me. Just the opposite. Yet we are supposed to accept that in the area of food, people suddenly break down and turn into incompetent weak-willed wretches who couldn't put a fork down to save their lives. I don't think so.

There must be more to overeating than weakness. Think how amazingly disciplined, strong, and capable you are in most every other aspect of your life. The fact that you have problems with food means that deeper issues must hide under the surface. The fact that the majority of people in the world will have weight problems points to a deeper problem than mere human weakness. Being overweight is not easily explained as simply a breakdown in willpower or discipline.

So please keep the following ideas in the back of your mind as you read on: maybe, just maybe, discipline and willpower aren't the real issues behind being overweight; maybe, just maybe, something deeper and more profound is going on and once you understand what that is you can start controlling your weight.

▌ Just Eat Less and Exercise More—Gee, Thanks

Thin people often used to tell me, in that tone thin people have when they are about to reveal the secret of losing weight, "Hey, **just eat less and exercise more.** It's that simple."

Gee, how helpful. I've never thought of that. Thanks for sharing. Losing weight has never been just that simple for me! Has it ever been that simple for you? I didn't think so.

On the surface, that old favorite recipe of "eat less and exercise more" can't be argued against. If you can "eat less and exercise more" you will lose weight. But there's more to the story.

A thin person telling you to "eat less and exercise more" is a lot like world class sprinters telling you to just "run faster" if you want to be like them. You see, Olympic sprinters have more fast-twitch muscle fibers than your average person. These just happen to be the type of muscle fibers you need to run faster. If you want to be a sprinter having more fast-twitch fibers is a good plan. But you can't plan it—your muscle fiber allowance is part of your genetic gift. It's something you are born with.

Olympic sprinters work amazingly hard, but they couldn't be world class if they didn't have the right genes. The same can be said for world class swimmers, weight lifters, and marathon runners. Almost every sport has an optimal body type.

You and I can become faster, but it's not likely we could we ever be world class. But each of us could become as fast as it is possible for us to become by working hard, by working smart, and by creating an encouraging environment.

Now ask yourself this: what if being thin is like being a world class sprinter? What if people who are naturally thin are that way because their genes make it easier for them to eat less and exercise more? If that were true, then we could figure out what caused the genetically less gifted to have such a hard time eating less and exercising more. And once we understood the causes of the problems we could then figure out how to fix them.

That's exactly what this book does. It explores the causes of why losing weight is so hard and then uses that information to figure out how you can control your weight. You may not be able to become a world class sprinter, but you can learn how to be as lean and strong as possible, given who you are and where you are in your life.

▌ Society is Wrong About You

My repeated weight loss failures made me doubt myself. I've had a few accomplishments in my life. Nothing major, certainly not like Oprah, but I am no slacker either. That probably describes most of us.

In our search for someone to blame for our weight problems, many of us have at one time or another fallen into the popular, yet wrong answer of telling ourselves: I am weak. I am a bad person. If I was only stronger and better and had more willpower, then I'd be thin.

This is what society thinks about us overweight people. This is what we overweight people are told over and over again. We are bad. We are weak. We are unworthy.

Hogwash! There's more to being overweight than personal weakness. After reading this book, you too will understand:

> *Society is wrong about you. You are not weak. You are not bad. You are not unworthy. You can lose weight once you really understand why Mother Nature has purposefully made losing weight so hard for you. With this knowledge, you can then create your personal plan for losing weight and staying on your diet for the rest of your life.*

▌ Being Overweight is Not All Your Fault

Here is a **secret** you probably already suspect and intuitively know down deep in your heart: your hunger is real. Your hunger is not a figment of your imagination and this means being overweight isn't entirely your fault.

"you just burned 100 calories walking up five flights of stairs so let's eat an apple now to get those calories back." And **you don't select foods based on the nutrients you need** either. Your body tries to make you eat a variety of foods so you'll get all the nutrients you need.

Many people have a hard time understanding that it's hard for you to lose weight because they think **everyone is the same.** Not so. Your genetics, environment, and strengths and weaknesses are different than anyone else. We may all look similar on the outside, but everyone is different in so many ways. All these differences impact how easy or hard it is for you to control your weight.

When I think of all the threats and misconceptions, I am left with the feeling of **amazement.** Who would have dreamed the world of weight loss was so bizarre? We humans are more complicated than I ever imagined. This means you can't explain someone's obesity by saying they are lazy and have no willpower. After reading about the threats, you'll probably think to yourself, **"Ah, that's why losing weight and staying on a diet are so hard!"**

▌ How Do You Defeat the Threats?

You defeat the threats using the **strategies** presented in this book and by applying the Designer Way **principles.** Strategies are how you overcome the threats. If you can find ways of preventing slip-ups then you can control your weight. That's what the strategies help you do, prevent the slip-ups caused by the threats. The principles are powerful ideas for helping you make the best use of the strategies. We'll talk a lot more about threats, strategies, and principles in later chapters.

Considering all the forces trying to spin your diet out of control, you do a pretty job good of controlling your weight. You really do. Don't be so surprised! But to do even better, you can't depend on motivation.

▌ Motivation is Not Enough

Some say you'll lose weight if you are really motivated, no matter what. People do lose weight, so motivation can work in the short run, but most people gain the weight right back. Think about how many people, through motivation alone, will never slip-up once in their entire life, once in a year, once in a week, or even once a day? Answer honestly now.

Very few people can sustain enough motivation to stay on a diet every waking moment of their lives. That's not a knock on people. Very few people have the motivation and discipline to become world class athletes either.

That's why the strategies in this book do not assume constant motivation and total control for success. You must learn how to control your weight without depending on motivation. Motivation is not enough because of the immense power food has over you.

▒ Food is Different from Everything Else—Food Has Power

We've talked about how people who show incredible discipline in every other area of their life somehow fail when it comes to food. What makes food so different?

Food is different for a reason that should be obvious, but was still surprising to me: **food is the most important thing in your life, because food is essential to survival.**

Get lost in the woods for a few weeks and you won't worry about sex, your stock portfolio, or how you look. You'll worry about food and how to get more of it. Food is almost all you'll think about.

Tasty food reaches deep into your brain and makes you want to eat with a real and true hunger. Food has power. The unlimited quantities of fatty high-calorie and sugary foods available in our modern world are a constant threat to make us slip up and gain weight. If you are prone to obesity, you will often find yourself eating more than you want and exercising less than you think you should.

Eating isn't something you decide to do. Eating is a powerful drive. Eating is raw survival and your brain wants you to survive above all else.

The Problem: You May be Playing the Wrong Diet Game

For a moment, let's think of your diet as a kind of game. What I have found in my research is that **you are probably playing the wrong diet game.** It's likely you are playing the **lose weight game** instead of the **stay on a diet game,** while your body plays a completely different game called the **survival game.**

Most People Won't Win the Lose Weight Game

Most of us have been playing the **lose weight** game without much success. I know that every time I lost weight it always found me again!

This is why the **lose weight** game isn't the one you need to play. **Up to 95% of all dieters gain back every pound they lose.** And 65% of all Americans are overweight and the trend is up, especially for children.

You Need to Play the Stay on a Diet Game

A recent study showed **most diets are about equally effective** at losing weight. The problem is most people can't stay on their diet. **Dieting is not enough** as Dr. James O. Hill, director for the Center for Human Nutrition said, "The popular plans only help you with weight loss. They don't help you with keeping it off, and that's where the real issue is."

Not playing the **stay on a diet** game prevents you from maintaining your weight loss goals. It is so hard because your body is playing the toughest game of all: the **survival** game.

Your Body is Playing the Survival Game

Everything difficult about controlling your weight makes complete sense once you understand the life humans lived 25,000 years ago.

In our prosperous modern world, survival is not the game most of us are playing, but your body doesn't know that. Your body still drives you to eat like a famine might lurk right around the corner—though it's far more likely there's a fast food joint.

I had always thought of my drive to eat as something unreal. I had always thought wanting to eat was just a figment of my imagination, something I made up, like a bad dream. I had always thought my drive to eat was a weakness of my own character, something I should be able to overcome.

But what I learned in my research is that eating has a real purpose other than making me fat. There's a bigger picture I wasn't seeing. I had never truly understood the deeper purpose of eating before.

Finding Food is Job #1 for Your Brain

We humans are excellent at gaining weight. It takes a lot of training to become a world class sprinter, yet most people can become overweight with absolutely no training at all! It's a natural skill we have.

The problem is, your rational mind isn't totally in charge of natural skills. No one has a calorie calculator constantly running in their head. After eating a handful of berries, you don't say, "I just consumed 100 calories, I need 1,900 more calories today or I'll starve." That's not how it works. Your brain tells you you're hungry and then you eat.

You don't have "drink water" or "go to the bathroom" calculators either. These too are basic and ancient survival drives.

So, the drive to eat isn't under your direct control. Can you imagine if it was? Think about all the tasks you are supposed to remember to do. How many times have you forgotten to take out the garbage, pay the bills, or pick up a gallon of milk on the way home from work? Nothing really bad happens if you forget any of these. Forgetting to eat means death. That's why eating has to be a drive.

Your brain cleverly anticipates what you need to do now, so you won't have problems in the future. And your feelings of hunger are how you know what you're supposed to do: eat. **The number one job of your brain is to find food and eat, so you can survive.**

Mother Nature made us into highly skilled weight gaining machines so we could survive a hostile world. She developed dozens of ways to get you hungry enough that you'll get off your butt and risk death to get enough food to eat. It's only after you have enough food that you will survive long enough to make babies and ensure your genes survive into another generation. Wise old **Mother Nature wants her children to reproduce and survive.**

Scientific research has found that we **modern humans are in an epic struggle with our ancient hunter-gatherer selves.** We are losing an unconscious and hidden war with our bodies . We are ancient, highly tuned survival machines thrust into a modern world of plenty where every instinct drives us to obesity. We simply don't fit the modern world.

This mismatch happens because nowadays very little exercise is needed to earn a living, and tasty, high-calorie food is available anywhere, anytime, in unlimited quantities. Yet we are built to **survive a world of scarcity and high activity.** How could the result be anything other than a stunning rise of obesity throughout the world?

The ease with which we currently survive in our modern Land of Plenty has had an interesting effect: we no longer value our bodies' survival skills. We now hate our survival super powers. When food is always available, it's easy to be lulled into a false sense of security, thinking of food as optional and our urges to eat a nuisance. But your brain doesn't listen. It keeps paying attention to food, like it always has.

A short story might help you understand the situation a little better...

▌ The Land of Plenty—A Surprisingly True Tale

Once upon a time, Hero was told by a playful Genie that he would be stranded on a desert island. The Genie would grant Hero one wish.

Hero's first wish was not to be stranded at all but the Genie said that was against the rules, so try again, smarty pants.

Then Hero boldly wished to be genetically engineered to have the best chance of surviving on the desert island. What genetic changes did the Genie give Hero?

First, Hero was given the ability to efficiently store fat. Your standard desert island doesn't have a lot of food available so making the best use of limited food supplies is top priority. No calorie can go to waste.

Second, Hero was given the ability to eat as much food as became available for the rare times when generous food supplies could be found. No food can go to waste.

Third, Hero was given the ability to just rest and relax until work became necessary. There's no reason to burn precious calories for nothing.

The Genie was very generous. There's no limit to the weight Hero can gain. Hero's fat cells can bank as many calories as are available for later withdrawal when food becomes scarce.

Does this sound like a useful set of genetic mutations? It should. Hero has an excellent chance of surviving under very difficult conditions. What more could you want?

How about rescue...

After many successful years of survival a miracle happened—Hero was rescued and taken to the legendary Land of Plenty. There, delicious foods are free for the taking and are available everywhere you look.

What happened to Hero in the Land of Plenty? Hero gained more and more weight. All the genetic changes that helped Hero survive on the desert island now worked against Hero in the Land of Plenty.

Sadly, the people of the Land of Plenty looked down on Hero because they thought Hero was lazy. Hero couldn't find a mate. And Hero's once excellent health began to fail.

Hero tried telling people about the Genie and how beautifully he'd survived on the desert island, but the people in the Land of Plenty just laughed and turned away.

Hero tried everything to lose weight but he was created for a different environment and nothing worked for long. Then one fine day, he stumbled across a book called *Your Designer Diet*. This book helped Hero so much! It understood the problems he faced in the Land of Plenty. Using *Your Designer Diet*, he was able to create an environment that helped him lose weight and keep it off. Finally, Hero found a way of living in a world he was never meant to live in.

As our tale draws to an end, please consider this: until modern times, nearly everyone lived on a desert island, now most of us live in the Land of Plenty.

What is really amazing is that even more people aren't overweight given our **modern toxic weight environment.** Earning a living now requires almost no exercise. Cheap, tasty, high-caloric food is available everywhere in near unlimited quantities. These forces taken together are why we are seeing an epidemic of obesity. In later chapters, we'll talk in more detail about how our modern environment makes it so easy to gain weight.

▌ My Adventures in the Land of Plenty

Usually, addicts have to hit rock bottom before they make a genuine change in their lives. It's called finding a **point of clarity,** a moment when you realize you can't go on the way you have been.

My point of clarity happened one day at our veterinarian's office. Our dog, Stout, had to go in for some medical tests. Part of the routine is to weigh Stout on a platform scale that looks like it can handle some pretty big animals. For some time, I had been too heavy to weigh myself on a normal scale. I got the idea that I could weigh myself on the vet's scale.

After everyone had left, I took my shoes off. You know how much weight shoes can add. I took a deep breath, hesitated a moment, and then I stepped on the scale: **365.** The scale read 365.

"Oh my God," I thought. "How did that ever happen?" I had no idea I had gained so much weight. No wonder really, I had avoided looking in the mirror for so long I made it easy not to notice. When I look at old photos from that time, I still can't believe how big I was.

That was my bottom. I knew I had to do something, but what?

I started slowly making changes in my life. By developing and using the strategies in this book, I was able to lose over 100 pounds and keep the weight off.

Now, I'm about 255 pounds. Isn't that still a lot? It's a bit more than I would like, but I am naturally a big offensive lineman type of guy, so it's not as bad as you might fear. I think I can maintain this weight, so I am pretty happy with it.

Whoops, I am Diabetic

Then I found out I had Type II diabetes. Tragically, a lot of people these days are hearing the same life-altering diagnosis from their doctor.

Having been overweight most of my life, I was, ironically, losing weight way before my diabetes diagnosis. I just wasn't in time.

By researching my family history, I discovered that I am genetically inclined to get diabetes, but my obesity probably had a hand in triggering its early onset. Now I am at a greater risk of heart attack and a number of other health problems like going blind, having a leg amputated, or suffering a stroke. Oh joy.

It turns out losing weight is one of the most important parts of a treatment plan for diabetes.

This is good news and bad news. It is bad news because losing weight is hard. We all know that. But it is good news because losing weight is something most of us can do, even if it doesn't seem like it right now.

And now that I have diabetes, it's even more important that I keep my weight off. How I am going to do that? By using the strategies in this book, I have been able to keep my diabetes and my weight under control. And I plan to keep it that way.

I am confident I will be able to stick to my diet. I won't stick to my diet because I am strong, no, **I will stick to my diet despite being weak.** How to stick to your diet even though you are prone to obesity is the **true secret of this book.**

How the Strategies Have Worked for Me

I remember one instance with vivid, sparkling clarity where the strategy of Joyful Eating, an important innovation of this book, gave me the courage to stay on my diet. More than that, Joyful Eating gave me hope that my life would still have pleasure and that life was ultimately still worth living.

After I was diagnosed with diabetes, I immediately changed my diet and started exercising more regularly. Rather quickly, my blood sugar numbers were whipped into shape. It all worked as planned. Perfectly. My blood tests showed I was making great progress. Great news, don't you think?

Yes, it was great news. But I was living in a closed bubble of diabetes-inspired fear. My goal was to tackle the diabetes head-on and defeat it soundly. Most of my meals were fixed at home. I never went out to eat at a restaurant at all. I never cheated, not even once. At work I ignored every slice of left-over pizza. And I drove by every donut shop, even that one I love that makes the best donuts in the whole world.

One night I had this weird dream. In my dream I walked into a grocery store and all of the food had poison signs on their label. In my dream while ordering dinner at a restaurant, all the items on the menu had little **poison** signs next to them. In my dream I walked the streets. If I saw anyone eating I would see a floating poison sign in front of their food.

It doesn't take Sigmund Freud to understand: food had become a poison to me. Food wasn't something I enjoyed anymore, but something I was afraid of. Food was something that would kill me. Obviously not a good long term situation.

It was then time for me to reenter the real world. For the first time in a long while, my lovely wife Linda and I went out to dinner at a nice restaurant. Foolishly, I wasn't really that concerned. I successfully used a lot of the same strategies I talk about in this book to help me through dinner. The appetizers and the main course all went well and tasted delicious. I even had a beer. This was going to work, I thought to myself. Then it came time for dessert.

I picked up a dessert menu for the first time in many, many months. I looked it over, reading and rereading the descriptions. Then it hit me: **I would never have a real dessert ever again in my whole entire life.** Wow! I was floored.

My mind raced a mile a minute. I didn't know if I could do this. Like most people, I love dessert. The thought of going without dessert forever choked me up. At that moment I was sure I would fail. I could see myself dying a slow, horrible death.

A tight twisting feeling grew in the pit of my stomach. Tears started coming into my eyes, I had to choke them back. Dessert menu in hand, I almost cried like a baby in the middle of a restaurant.

I perfectly realize that in the scheme of things, my little problems don't matter. Most people have a much harder life than I'll ever have. Yet, this was my life and it mattered to me. These were my very real feelings of loss.

At that moment, all the main parts of this book, bits of which I had been thinking about for years, became clear to me. I then remembered Joyful Eating, a way of eating I had developed to help me deal with diabetes.

The idea behind Joyful Eating is that eating one bite of almost any food won't do me any harm. I can still have any food I want. Happiness, pleasure and satisfaction aren't in the quantity of the food eaten. One bite of truly excellent food is enough. I would be "normal" again. And Joyful Eating helps me lose weight too because I won't eat a full serving of dessert.

▌ There is Hope!

I had hope again. There was light at the end of the tunnel. Use every cliché in the book. Food wasn't a poison and my future had the pleasure and passion of eating still in it.

I then went on to research, develop, and perfect the strategies you see in this book. The same strategies that have worked for me will help almost anyone control their weight.

Certainly, life with diabetes hasn't been the same for me. Although, in many ways, by following the strategies, my life is better.

That's why this book offers a message of **hope.** It's not a false hope either. It's not a fad. It's real, practical, down-to-earth advice that works. **You can control your weight.** And we'll talk about exactly how in the next chapter.

Chapter 2

The 10 Designer Principles for Controlling Your Weight

O ut of control. That's how most people feel about their weight. Do you feel like weight just happens to you? Do you feel like you keep getting heavier and heavier and you don't know what to do about it? You don't have to feel that way any longer. Using the 10 Designer Principles you can learn to control your weight.

The Designer Diet is revolutionary because it adapts a powerful control technique that has been successfully used to solve some of the world's toughest problems. Following this process, you'll learn how to create a diet designed especially for you.

That's why the Designer Diet creates your **perfect** diet. At any time, your diet works perfectly. The instant you find your diet isn't working for you anymore, you change it so it starts working again. On the Designer Diet, you are always learning how to improve your diet. If your diet can be improved, you'll find a way to improve it. So your diet is always perfect for you.

Creating your perfect diet is powerful because it gives you your best chance of controlling your weight. Your typical one-size-fits all diet is hit or miss. It might work for you and it might not. Some parts of it might work better than others. We gather all different diets, all the different ideas and suggestions for losing weight, figure out which of those work for you, and then call that your diet.

That's what the Designer Diet helps you do. It helps you explore all the different ways you can eat less and exercise more and then helps you decide

23

which of those work best for you. So, part of the Designer Diet is searching for new ideas. Another part is testing to see if those ideas work for you. And by repeating this process you learn what works for you, and your diet constantly improves. **Constant improvement** is a big part of what it means to be in control of your weight.

Another part is to **understand your nature** as a human, your nature as an individual, and the nature of the world. All these forces impact on your weight. Your body is unique. Your life is unique. Your strengths are unique and your weaknesses are unique. You have your own way of being overweight that is different from everyone else in the world. It just makes sense that your diet plan should be as unique as you are. A big part of how the Designer Diet helps you control your weight is to teach you to understand your nature and how this information can be used to pick better and better weight controlling strategies. The better you understand your nature, the better you will control your weight.

Noticing changes in your life and then **responding effectively** to those changes is another overlooked aspect of controlling your weight. A simple one-size-fits-all approach to weight loss can't handle your complex life. Let's say a shock happens in your life. Perhaps you get sick or change jobs. How will you notice and what changes will you make to put yourself back in control of your weight? A diet based on just eating fewer carbs or more vegetables can't handle the constant change in your life. You need an approach to your weight that helps you overcome these life changes, not be victimized by them. The Designer Diet is that approach.

▌ Why do you need to create a perfect diet?

In the last hundred years, there has been a revolution in how people live their lives. Food used to be scarce, and mere survival required hard physical labor. Now cheap, tasty, high calorie food is everywhere and many people do very little exercise at all.

For the first time in history, **controlling your weight is completely and totally up to you.** You are among the first generation of people who can no longer rely on your environment to naturally control your weight. If your weight is going to be controlled it's you that is going to have to figure out how to control it. There's nobody else you can rely on to do it for you.

Isn't that a stunningly different way to look at weight problems in the world? It's not surprising so many people are having a hard time controlling their weight, because nobody has *had* to control their weight before! Why would anyone know how to do it?

Almost every human being has a bold new adventure ahead of them as they try to discover their own way of controlling their weight. The question that you and everyone else has to answer is **how,** exactly how will you control yours?

How to control your weight is what this book is all about. The essence of how to control your weight is described in these 10 Designer Principles:

1. Take responsibility.
2. Understand your three natures.
3. Identify the threats that sabotage your diet.
4. Discover your strategies for defeating the threats.
5. Follow the Designer Way for continuously improving your diet.
6. Nurture your Designer Mind.
7. Strive for improvement.
8. Whatever works.
9. Take the long view.
10. Ask for help.

We'll talk about each principle in this chapter and explore them all in the rest of the book. By following the ideas described in the principles, you will learn exactly how to control your weight, in your own way, for the rest of your life.

▌ Principle 1: Take responsibility.

Many people have problems with their weight because they expect someone else to tell them how they should control it. Unfortunately, that just won't work. We are all different and what works for one person may not work for you. You have to discover your perfect diet for yourself and keep on discovering it throughout your life.

That's why the responsibility for your weight is ultimately yours. Nobody else can tell you which strategies will help you. Nobody else can notice when changes in your life are making you gain weight. Nobody else can notice when there are opportunities to make your diet better. And nobody else can make the necessary changes in your life. Only you can do these things.

Yet responsibility is not the same as blame. You are not to blame for your weight. For many of us, weight problems are unavoidable. Our lives are very different than they were in the past and the same natures that historically have helped humans survive now make us overweight and threaten our health in the present. Remember the story of Hero and the Genie? There is nothing to be ashamed of. There is nothing wrong with you. In our current world, your body may simply be a perfect weight gaining machine. And that's not your fault. It's tragically unfair. But it's not your fault.

Many bad things happen to us in our lives. We do not ask for them to happen and seldom do we deserve them, yet it is still our responsibility to deal with them. Being prone to being overweight is just another unfair bad thing we must learn to deal with. The good news is you'll learn exactly how to control your weight in this book.

▌ Principle 2: Understand your three natures.

When you understand your three natures: your nature as a human, your nature as an individual, and the nature of how your environment influences you, then controlling your weight becomes common sense. That common sense helps you control your weight by building on your strengths and side-stepping your weaknesses. Everything in this book flows naturally from understanding your three natures.

You may not believe that now, but think of it this way: When your car goes too fast you put on the brake. Braking is just common sense because you know how to drive. In the same way, once you understand your three natures, controlling your weight becomes common sense because you'll know exactly why and how losing weight is so hard. It then becomes clear what you can do about it.

As a human being, you are a highly skilled survival machine. You can survive in any environment, outwit any threat, perform Herculean amounts of work, and outlast gnawing periods of hunger. Unfortunately, these super powers have a cost in our modern world. That cost is how easy it is for you to become overweight.

As an individual, you have a unique nature that can both help and hurt your weight. The problem is that there's almost no way for you to know your individual nature without experimenting on yourself. By experimenting you can find your unique way of being overweight and in the process answer questions like: Do you have a genetic predisposition to become overweight? Would you do better on a vegetarian, low carb, or low fat diet? Are you a person who naturally moves less? Nobody can tell you these things; you have to puzzle them out for yourself.

The Designer Diet helps you to understand your nature. In this process, you are connecting to a story that is as big as humanity. The knowledge you gain helps you find ways of amplifying your own strengths and minimizing your weaknesses. You'll finally start working with your nature and not constantly fighting against it. You aren't exploring your nature in order to highlight your failings, but to exploit your strengths.

This is hard work. It's hard to confront your weaknesses and work through your failures. In the end, you become a better person for it. A great person is someone who has triumphed over hardship and suffering. That's what makes life worthwhile. That's what character is made of. On the Designer Diet, you aren't just controlling your weight. You are also forging your character and you are working toward becoming a great person.

▌ Principle 3: Identify the threats that sabotage your diet.

Threats are the reasons you fall off your diet. You don't go quietly off your diet. The threats push you kicking and screaming, but push they do. Over 60 threats are presented in this book and you can find many more on our website. Some examples include not sleeping enough, having a genetic defect, living in the suburbs, hosting a particular virus or bacteria, eating from big plates, or simply having a body that doesn't like to move.

You don't even know most of the threats exist, because their effects are out of your awareness. Yet the threats are active every moment of your life, sabotaging your diet by tempting you to eat more and exercise less.

We'll cover six key power threats:

- **The Power of Starvation Threat.** Your body has an incredible ability to adapt to starvation by reducing your need for energy, making you hungry, and filling your mind with nothing but thoughts of food.
- **The Power of Genetics Threat.** Genetics has about the same effect on your weight as it does on your height.
- **The Power of Food Threat.** You fall off your diet not because you are so weak, but because food is so strong.
- **The Power of Rest Threat.** You don't have a drive to exercise; your instinct is to rest and conserve energy.
- **The Power of Environment Threat.** You probably won't become obese, even if your genetics make you prone to obesity, as long as your environment makes it necessary for you to work hard or food is scarce.

❖ **The Power of Slip-Ups Threat.** Small slip-ups over time equals obesity. You make well over 200 food and exercise decisions a day and research has shown as few as 50 extra calories a day leads to obesity. A few bad decisions a day is all you need to gain weight.

We are each affected differently by each threat. Each of us is overweight in our own way and is why you need to find your own way of losing weight that fits your nature and your life. You can read more about the threats by turning to Chapter 4, *The Threats—Why Your Diet Fails.*

Once you've figured out which threats are your worst enemies you are in a perfect position to defeat them.

▌ Principle 4: Discover your strategies for defeating the threats.

The good news is, once you learn about the threats, you can figure out your own ways to defeat them. These are called strategies. A strategy is anything you need to know or do to control your weight. Some examples include playing video games to lose weight, moving to a location that will help you exercise more, finding ways to take more steps, using smaller plates, pumping up the volume to eat more food for less calories, learning how to hide from food, and creating a more favorable environment in your neighborhood, home, school, and work.

Currently there are over a 150 strategies to help you lose weight. Many are covered in this book and the rest can be found on our website. Using simple strategies, you can realistically **lose a pound a week** by making only small changes to your life.

The strategies are organized into four major themes:

❖ **The Designer Way** is a revolutionary new process for controlling your weight on any diet that works, no matter how crazy your life becomes. We'll talk more about the Designer Way in Principle 5.

❖ **Joyful Eating** shows how to eat in moderation by extracting enough pleasure from food that you feel satisfied after only a few bites.

❖ **Weight-Proofing** is like baby proofing your home for your diet. Systematically remove diet slip-ups from your life by creating an encouraging environment in which you naturally achieve your goals without relying on willpower.

❖ **Lifeguarding** stops you from being a victim of your thoughts. Retrain your brain to stop the unwanted thoughts that make you start eating and stop exercising.

Joyful Eating

The Joyful Eating strategies teach you how to eat less by enjoying your food more. This is based on how your sense of taste works. You naturally stop tasting food after a few bites, so eating more than a few bites of any food is a waste of taste. Learn how to eat one glorious, delicious, perfectly eaten bite of any food you want and you can be satisfied with just a few bites.

The benefits of this simple practice are many and surprising. Cravings, restricted food choices, boredom, and eating too much are just some of the reasons for falling off a diet. Joyful Eating solves all these problems in one strategy. Joyful Eating makes it possible to eat any food you want in moderation. You won't have to restrict your diet to a small set of boring foods anymore, the pleasures of the entire world of food are there for you to explore.

Weight-Proofing

The Weight-Proofing strategies protect you from diet slip-ups by turning diet danger zones into Safe Zones. A slip-up is when you eat more or exercise less than you want because of the ever present threats that surround you. A Safe Zone is a protected area you create in which you naturally achieve your goals without relying on willpower every minute of the day. Using Weight-Proofing strategies, you systematically remove diet slip-ups from your life by creating ever widening circles of Safe Zones around you and your loved ones.

Weight-Proofing is about continually thinking how you can put yourself in the best position to succeed at four goals: eating to your diet, burning more calories, finding more joy, and preventing slip-ups. Weight-Proofing is like baby proofing your home. When baby proofing, you remove every possible way a baby might hurt themselves. When Weight-Proofing, you remove every possible way you might fall off your diet. In the Weight-Proofing chapters, you learn how to create Safe Zones for many important parts of your life: personal, home and family, exercise, portion control, car, shopping, work, school, and community.

Lifeguarding

The Lifeguarding strategies retrain your brain to stop the unwanted thoughts that lead to automatic eating and urges to stop exercising. You don't have to be a victim to your own random thoughts. You can learn to retrain you brain to stop unwanted thoughts, because of something called brain neuroplasticity. Neuroplasticity is the ability of your brain to change itself. Your brain is not hard-wired into its current behavior and can be retrained to reverse the years and years of bad habits that have been causing you to gain weight.

You can read more about the strategies by turning to Chapter 12, *The Strategies—How to Stop the Threats.*

All the strategies in the world won't help you unless you also learn how best to apply them in your life. That's what you learn in the next principle.

▌ Principle 5: Follow the Designer Way for continuously improving your diet.

The key idea behind this principle is: if you keep doing the right things you'll get the right results. The problem is figuring out the right things to do. Usually the right thing is said to be something simple like avoid fat, but these simple approaches rarely work.

The first reason diets don't work is because the chances are very high **you won't follow your diet.** You are not a computer mindlessly following instructions. The odds are you'll make enough mistakes on your diet that over time, you'll lose control of your weight.

Even following a diet perfectly is still not good enough. This leads us to the second reason diets don't work. Strictly following a diet won't work because **you constantly change,** your life constantly changes, and your approach to weight control needs to change along with those changes. If you don't adapt your diet strategies as you change, you'll naturally lose control of your weight. You can't do the same thing all the time and expect it to work when nothing around you stays the same.

Here we've finally found the deepest reason why your typical diet doesn't work. We talk about "controlling" your weight. Interestingly, how to control things is a field of study unto itself. It turns out there are different ways to control different types of things. These are called **process control** methods.

There are two general process control methods: **defined process control** and **empirical process control.** Your typical diet uses a defined process control approach, which doesn't work because it was meant to control simpler problems than your weight. *Your Designer Diet* introduces a new weight loss control method based on empirical process control ideas, which does work because it was designed to control very complex processes like your weight.

We are getting a little technical, but stick with me. It's worth it to know why *Your Designer Diet* will help you really control your weight when other approaches have failed you.

Let's start with understanding what a process is. According to Webster's Unabridged Dictionary, a process is "a systematic series of actions, changes, or functions bringing about a result." We are involved in processes all the time. There's a process for vacuuming your home. There's a process for controlling the heat in your house. When we want to achieve a result, there are a series of steps that need to be taken to make that result happen and whatever those steps are is called a process.

Controlling your weight is a process too. You take a series of steps with the goal of losing weight. The question is what is the best type of process for controlling your weight?

The defined process control method is used in your typical diet. It assumes the underlying thing to control (your weight) is completely understood, well-defined, repeatable, and predicable. They assume there is a well-defined set of inputs and the same results are generated every time from the inputs. Based on these assumptions, diets tell you exactly what you should do to lose weight and try to convince you their prescription will work the same for everyone, no matter what. Usually, defined process control methods are used for well understood processes like an assembly line where everything can really be thought out completely in advance.

But your life is not an assembly line and neither is your body. That's why diets based on this method just won't work. Very little is understood about the exact mechanisms of obesity, much less the unique ways in which you are overweight. And to make the problem worse, your life continually changes in ways no one can predict.

Right now, nobody on earth can tell you exactly what you will need to do to control your weight. Sure, they can give you generalities like eat less and exercise more, but what exactly should you as an individual do to eat less and exercise more right now? To know that, you have to know your genetics, everything that's happened in your life and the results from all the different strategies you've used to control your weight. Only then are you in a position to know how to control your weight.

This is exactly the type of problem where the empirical process control method shines. It is specifically designed to expect the unexpected and work with very complicated systems that change over time. This method has been used successfully by giant companies like Toyota to quickly and efficiently produce quality cars. And many of the world's most successful software companies use this approach to develop software.

What I've done is take the extremely successful and powerful empirical process control model and adapt it to controlling your weight. That's why this book is revolutionary. It's a completely new approach for weight control. I call this new process for controlling your weight the **Designer Way.**

A powerful way to think about being overweight is to understand that there are millions and millions of ways for you to become overweight. Threats are everywhere and they never let up. Yet, there are just a few ways for you to become lean and strong. The process captured in the Designer Way is how you sift through all the possible strategies to figure out which strategies are your ways of becoming lean and strong.

If all this just sounds like gibberish and you are bored to tears reading about it, don't worry. I just wanted you to be aware that there's some deep thinking going on in the approach used in this book and that the ideas have been used very successfully in other areas. There's no reason you can't be just as successful.

The Designer Way has a steady rhythm of three actions that happen once a week, once a day, and whenever the opportunity arises:

- **Start Spin.** A time for reflection. Every week, take time to check if you are meeting your goals, set new goals, and update your plan on how you want to meet your goals.
- **Daily Check.** A time for quick response. Every morning, perform a quick check to see if you unexpectedly gained weight. If you gain weight, quickly respond by adjusting your strategies.
- **Make a Move.** A time for immediate action. Always look for opportunities to prevent slip-ups, exercise more, eat to your diet and find more joy in your life. If you see an opportunity to implement a strategy, take it.

If you follow this deceptively simple process, you'll immediately notice when a new threat enters your life. Once you notice a threat, you'll immediately respond with a counter strategy. Ideally your counter strategy reduces your weight again. If it doesn't, then work out why not and use what you've learned to select another strategy to try. By reacting quickly to reverse any weight gain, you put yourself back in control of your weight.

The secret of the Designer Way is to make small changes in your weight control strategies in response to what is really happening in your life. The result is your diet continually improves and that is what finally empowers you to lose weight and keep it off.

This approach is stunningly effective. You can read more about the Designer Way by turning to *The Designer Way*, Chapter 13.

▌ Principle 6: Nurture your Designer Mind.

The Designer Diet is not just a list of goals and practices. It's a mindset. It's a way of looking at the world. Once you make this mindset part of who you are then your weight loss won't be a one time thing anymore. Keeping your weight off will be something you do naturally.

Why isn't the Designer Diet about goals? Because goals mean there's a finish line. There is no finish line. You are always trying to learn and improve your diet. There's no peak to climb where you can shout "Eureka, I am done!" The moment you think you are done the weight will fly back on and you'll be forever frustrated.

Why isn't the Designer Diet a fixed set of practices? Because the Designer Diet is a lifestyle, a mindset, a journey, not a destination. Once you understand that, you can ease up on yourself and relax. There is no list of things for you to do or not to do that will work for all time and every situation. You don't have to run around looking for the solution. There is no one perfect solution for weight loss. You can't be fixed because you are not broken.

That's the Designer Mind. Don't worry about goals or practices. Be steady. Don't get too low when you gain a pound. Don't get too high when you lose a pound. Just keep trying to do the right thing and over time your weight will work itself out.

It doesn't matter if you don't lose weight every day. It doesn't matter if you don't lose weight every week. It doesn't even matter if you gain a little weight. All that's normal and to be expected and can be handled. What matters is you keep on trying to do the right thing.

What else can you do? Give up? No, you can't give up. Can you eat less than what you should be eating? No, your body will think you are starving and do everything it can to make you gain weight. Can you exercise more than is reasonable for you? No, you'll just end up quitting or getting hurt.

There is no escape from your weight problems. No magic can turn you into a thin person. Weight problems are a natural and normal part of modern life. That means there's no reason to feel ashamed about your weight struggles. It's part of what it means to be human.

So, follow the Designer Way. Keep learning and getting better at your diet. That's what it means to have complete responsibility for your weight in the 21st century.

▌ Principle 7: Strive for improvement.

Never feel satisfied with where you are. You can always do better. The moment you start feeling you've learned all there is to learn or you've done everything you can do is the exact moment you'll start gaining weight again.

At some point you are almost certain to think you've got your weight problems solved. You'll abandon the Designer Way and go back to your old habits. Well, you don't have your weight problems solved, as your scale will soon tell you. So don't get down on yourself when a little weight comes back on. Just pick up where you left off and keep going.

Feel proud and happy with your progress. But remember, progress isn't a sign it's time to stop, it's a sign there's more progress to be made in your future.

▌ Principle 8: Whatever works.

Whatever works and be as extreme as you need to be is a good one line summary of the Designer Diet. What will work for you? Nobody can tell you. Nobody, not your doctor, not your partner, not your best friend, and certainly not the media. Nobody can know how you feel inside or how your body will respond to different strategies. **Believe in your own experience to figure out what works for you.**

To know what works you'll have to experiment with different strategies using the Designer Way as a guide. Don't feel bad if a strategy doesn't work, but keep trying and be creative. Try something and see what happens. Something will work.

When you do find a strategy that works, be as extreme as you need to be to make it work even better. Don't feel embarrassed. If you need to hide food from yourself at a table so you won't be tempted to eat, then that's just what you'll have to do. Remember: whatever works and be as extreme as you need to be.

The Designer Diet doesn't waste any time on the philosophy or the politics of weight loss. It doesn't try to tell you what foods you should eat or stay away from. It doesn't spend time trying to make you feel bad or guilt you into anything. No, the Designer Diet is about helping you understand why losing weight is so hard and then using that knowledge to explore all the possible ways of losing weight that work for you and your life.

On the Designer Diet, you don't accept anything on anyone else's authority. You test everything against your own experience and take nothing on faith.

It's completely practical. You try different things and if a strategy works for you then that's all that matters. What matters is what helps you control your weight, nothing else is important. Ultimately you must make up your own mind about what works for you.

▍ Principle 9: Take the long view.

Nothing is more frustrating than your weight. It magically fluctuates up and down for seemingly no reason at all. And it's so easy to let these little failures make you depressed or angry at yourself. We often let so much anger and disappointment build up in ourselves. Over time, constant failure often becomes a deep point of shame and that shame can easily cause an ever worsening downward spiral of dysfunctional behavior.

Let go of that anger, shame, and disappointment. How do you let go? By having perspective. Step back and remember the great challenges you face with your weight. You are a highly efficient weight gaining survival machine. Your hunger is real, natural and expected. Controlling your weight was never meant to be easy. And it isn't.

You will have weight problems. That's the way of it. That is your nature as a human, your nature as a person, and the nature of the world you live in. You are the way you are so you'll have the best chance of surviving in a dangerous, unpredictable world. That's why there is no need to feel shame or embarrassment. There is no reason to torment yourself. Weight control is simply a problem most modern humans must now learn to deal with.

You can control your weight if you keep doing the right things and don't quit. Nurture your Designer Mind and follow the Designer Way and you will put yourself back in control of your weight. By immediately noticing any weight gain, finding the cause, and then figuring out counter strategies, you will get your weight back down again. You can always control your weight. This is the long view.

So forgive yourself! Forgiving yourself is not a sign of weakness; it's a sign of mature strength. Realize you do not deserve to be punished for the rest of your life for weight problems that arise directly from your nature. Once you understand this in your heart, you can finally be honest with yourself and accept yourself for the complex being you truly are. And it's this honesty and acceptance that will keep you in control of your weight for the rest of your life.

Please see Strategy 28, *Forgive Yourself—Prevent a Lapse from Becoming a Collapse* for more discussion on this topic.

▌ Principle 10: Ask for help.

All the principles, threats, strategies, and ideas in this book aren't enough to free you from your weight problems. Most of them arise from impulses beyond your conscious control. These impulses can't be completely destroyed because they are part of your nature. And if you give in to your impulses you will gain weight and increase your health risks.

What you learn in *Your Designer Diet* is another way. You learn to be alert to your weight problems. Being alert gives you a gap, a window in which you can change how you would normally respond to the forces throwing your weight out of control. That gap gives you the space you need to see possibilities in your life you might not have considered before.

By being alert, you can choose to respond differently. You can respond using strategies in this book, strategies you've created for yourself, or strategies you've learned from other helpers along the way.

You can't be alert to everything. A lot of weight gain happens from unnoticed life changes. Perhaps a change in jobs, a change in season, or a lingering cold is the root cause of a recent weight gain, but you are too close to a situation to see it. Or perhaps you notice a problem but you've run out of creative ideas of how to respond.

What do you do in these situations? Ask for help! Do your best, but sometimes your best isn't good enough. Every problem can be solved with enough dedicated and friendly people helping you. Someone will have an idea or suggestion that will help you get your weight back under control again.

Please see Strategy 33, *Create Your Support Group—Long Term Support Systems Work* for more discussion on this topic.

▌ The Essence of the Designer Principles

If you extract the essence from the Designer Principles, here's what they ask you to do:

> *Understand the threats and how they make it hard to lose weight. Learn the strategies and how you can use them to control your weight. You are seldom done with a strategy; most strategies are endless. Sometimes you will do better. Sometimes you will do worse. This is the ebb and flow of life. Don't worry about where you are at now, it's what you do next that matters most. Seek help and give help, both are good for the soul. Pay attention to your life. Think about changes you can make for the better. Notice*

what works for you and what doesn't. Forget what doesn't work. Embrace what works. Be as extreme as you need to be. Be gentle on yourself, what you are trying to do is not easy. Keep trying. That's the best any of us can do.

▌ A Real-Life Example: My Unexpected Weight Gain

How do all these principles work together to put you back in control of your weight? A fair question. Let's look at an example of how I handled some unexpected weight gain using the 10 Designer Principles.

One morning I was a bit shocked to notice I had gained weight. But through my Daily Feedback System, which we'll talk about more in the Designer Way chapter, the evidence was right in front of my disbelieving eyes. My clothes looked and felt tight. And when I looked at myself in the mirror there was definitely some extra flab around the middle.

I was more than a little confused. Why had I gained weight? I was pretty sure I wasn't eating any more or exercising any less than usual. What was going on?

I started thinking about what new threats may have entered my life. Nothing came to me at first, but then it hit me: the weather had turned cold and rainy a few days earlier. That was it. I wasn't getting out as much so I wasn't burning as many calories as usual. I just hadn't noticed until my Daily Feedback System gave me an early warning of a train load of weight gain heading for me in the future.

I had my early warning so what was I going to do about it? I started by making a few small strategy changes to bring my weight back down. The first was to reduce my afternoon snack so I was eating 100 fewer calories. One hundred calories is about a mile of walking and with the horrible weather it would be hard to walk that mile.

I waited a few days to see how that strategy change worked. Using my feedback system I determined that my weight hadn't dropped. And that's really excellent news! Not gaining weight is a huge win. Just think how much better off you would be if you could just not gain any more weight. But I wanted to lose the weight I gained, so I decided I needed to be more extreme.

Next, I spent 5 extra minutes a day on the elliptical cycle. After a few days my weight was going down again. My clothes fit a little better, but it was clear I wasn't losing enough.

I realized I had to move more, even though the weather was like a prison cell with ropes of rain for bars. My strategy was to find more steps whenever and wherever I could. I took the stairs more. I cleaned the house more. I got up and walked more. I played with the dogs more. I did everything I could to find more steps to take.

All these little strategy changes worked. My weight went back down. That is, until the next problem popped-up causing me to gain weight again!

By finding the weight gain immediately and doing something about it immediately, I kept my weight from ballooning out of control. That's a big change from how I'd handled weight problems in the past. Previously, I would only have noticed I gained weight after I put on 20 extra pounds. And at that point it was hard to do anything about it. Finding problems early makes them much easier to fix.

This is just a simple example, but it shows how all the principles, threats and strategies can work together. You can always keep your weight under control by adapting to your changing life.

The true power of this approach is that it allows you to make things better by finding problems early. Actively finding problems rather than being the victim of problems is a real switch in the typical power relationship we have with our weight. Usually we feel victimized by our weight. Following the 10 Designer Principles changes that.

You become the powerful problem solver in your life. First you find problems and then you quickly solve them. That's the continuous cycle of improvement that puts you back in control of your weight. You continually improve yourself by making small changes in response to what is happening in your life, seeing how it works out, and then making more changes.

You are **learning by doing,** which requires you to act. Don't worry that you don't know everything and are unsure about what to do. Go ahead and **take action.** Taking action moves you forward, helps you learn, and makes you better and better at staying on your diet. **Constant improvement** is how you reach and maintain your goals over a lifetime.

Finding, rather than ignoring, problems has another not so obvious yet critically important benefit: **you can ask for help.** As we talked about in the *Ask for help* principle, there is no problem that can't be solved with enough dedicated and friendly people helping you. In my case, once I detected the problem I could have immediately asked for help from my friends, support group, or from the *http:// YourDesignerDiet.com* forums. Someone surely would have suggested the changing weather as a possible cause for my weight gain. And once the cause was diagnosed, some other people would have surely suggested small improvements I could make to bring my weight back down. It's amazing how much people in a group can help when you give each other a chance.

In this example, my problem was that I didn't notice the world had changed around me. I didn't notice I was spending more time inside and that was all it took to start the weight gain train in motion. You are always changing, your life is always changing, and your weight is always changing. You stay in control of your weight by quickly adapting to these changes.

▌ You Can Do This

It's a relief to know there's something you can do to control your weight. Most diets want you to do something you know deep down you can't do over the long run. Can you really eat low-carb for the rest of your life? Can you really go to the gym every day? The chances are against it.

The Designer Diet is something you can do because you create your own path for yourself. There's no need for you to give up. You can learn to channel your energy and effort in the right direction. You can do this.

The Designer Diet is the only thing I've been able to do consistently. I can't always exercise more and eat less. I can't always eat or do the right things. But I can do the Designer Diet because it's quick, simple and it works. It allows me to be who I am within a safe structure. That's the beauty of the Designer Diet.

▌ What's Next?

The rest of the book talks about the threats and strategies you'll need to implement the 10 Designer Principles. In the next chapter, we'll talk about a few initial strategies that will help setup the rest of the book. Then we'll spend a lot of time talking about the threats. And after the threats we'll talk about all the different strategies you can use to defeat the threats.

So, let's get started!

Chapter 3

First Things First
Strategies 1–3

Here are a few beginning strategies we need to talk about before tackling the threats.

· ·

 ## Strategy 1. See Your Doctor Now–What You Don't Know May Kill You

Make an appointment with your doctor NOW for a general checkup and blood panel. It could save your life.

This isn't the sexiest strategy, but it could be the most important point in the whole book.

It's advice I didn't take and I certainly wish I had. Then I would have known about my diabetes years earlier and I could have easily prevented a lot of damage to my body.

I know most people reading this probably won't go see a doctor. I know in the past I wouldn't. Why should I? I felt fine. If I had a time travel machine here's what I would tell myself:

> Dear Earlier Todd,
>   I am Future Todd writing to you to give you some advice. Don't ignore it. We both know how you can be.

The stock market bubble is going to burst, sell your stock now. Just do it. Now on to a more important topic...

You know how thirsty you get? You know how you drink glass after glass of water at lunch? That's a sign of diabetes.

You know how your feet and legs tingle at night? It's not just weird, it's nerve damage and it's a sign of diabetes.

You know how you think your wounds take a long time to heal? Don't bother with the multivitamins; it's a sign of diabetes.

What you don't know now is that virtually everyone on Grandma's side of the family has diabetes. Surprise! You only thought you had to worry about cancer.

And there's a problem you are ignoring. Look down. See that? You are way overweight dude (yes, the word dude has filtered down to middle class white guys). I suspect we were obese. Obesity can trigger diabetes.

Do you see the theme by now? You have Type II diabetes and you've probably had it for some time. Relax. It's not a death sentence. We'll figure it out and do OK. But we could have done better if we had caught it earlier, or better yet, prevented it completely.

You feel fine you say? That's what I remember too. But look at all the obvious symptoms. How could we have possibly known about all the symptoms and still thought we were fine? It boggles my mind to this day.

Go see a doctor. Now! I know you don't like doctors or hospitals or any sign of weakness. Just go. They'll run a few simple tests and ask you a few simple questions and then you'll know. The earlier you know there's a problem the longer we'll live and the better we'll feel.

Good luck. Oh, and rely on Linda, she'll be there for you in a big way.

Signed,
Future Todd Who is Doing Better But Should Have Started Earlier.

You probably don't even know if you have a medical problem. You probably have convinced yourself you feel fine. You probably are fine. I hope so. But maybe not.

Really good health can kill you. People in good health don't go to the doctor. Many of these people drop dead from a stroke later in life because they thought they were in good health, but weren't. Silent but deadly problems like high blood pressure, diabetes, heart disease, metabolic syndrome and hypothyroid can all be found by a simple checkup.

Many medical problems can make weight loss more difficult, so knowing your health status can help with weight loss. And many problems are simply a lot easier to treat when they are caught early. Don't wait for symptoms. Get a checkup now. Please don't wait, diseases never do.

Strategy 2. You are the Hero in Your Own Weight Loss Story

There's a way of thinking about having weight problems where you are the hero on a difficult hero's journey and you come out victorious in the end.

As an overweight person, you might be tempted to believe the story other people tell about you explaining why you are overweight. It usually begins by talking about how weak you are, how lazy you are, how you lack discipline, how if you just ate less and exercised more you would be thin, and how if you were just a better person inside you would look better on the outside. The story usually ends with a shake of the head, a sigh, and one inevitable conclusion: you deserve anything evil that comes from being overweight because it's all your fault.

You've probably listened to this story a thousand times. You may want to shout that the story isn't true. You may want to say it's not that simple. You may want to say something but you don't know what to say because when you say something you get shouted down by people just yelling the story even louder.

And you may have even come to believe this horrible story about yourself and why you are the way you are. You may think there's no reason to try anymore because you can't change how the story ends. But that's not so.

What if there was another story you aren't being told that would help explain why you are the way you are and that in this story you aren't the bad guy? What if in this story you are the good guy? What if you are really just a misunderstood hero doing the best you can against terrible odds? That's the story told in this book.

When you read a story, the hero doesn't know what comes next. But you as the reader can usually guess what will happen because the author has given you clues. In a scary movie, you might even yell out for the hero not to go into the basement because you know that they don't know there's a monster waiting for them.

The hero must work out everything for themselves making use of help from people along the way. Even then the hero won't know all the threats and enemies and troubles they will face. Yet the hero presses on. Sometimes the hero must be incredibly brave. Sometimes the hero must figure out a difficult puzzle. Sometimes the hero makes horrible mistakes and pays a devastating price to learn what they must learn before they can move on.

Later, when we talk of the threats sabotaging your diet, you'll hear a very different story about your weight than the one you've heard before. In this story you learn how you face monsters of all different types and descriptions on your hero's journey. Most of these monsters are unknown to you, yet you've been fighting them your entire life. And because you didn't know about them, you may have believed the earlier stories telling you how being overweight is entirely your fault. You may have even given up for a little while and put your journey on hold.

But once you learn about all the threats trying to throw you off your diet, you'll be ready and able to pick up your hero's journey once again. You'll learn that you really are a hero. You'll learn you have been fighting against terrible odds and that you've been doing much better than you thought. You'll learn how wrong all those old stories are about you and there's a different and more powerful way of understanding why you are the way you are. And this understanding points you the way forward.

This is the hero's journey of discovering your own nature. You can't believe the stories anyone else tells you about who you are. You have to write your own story for yourself.

 ## Strategy 3. Visit Our Website for More Information and Support

Get the support you need at *http://YourDesignerDiet.com.*

As you are reading, if you want to talk about anything covered in the book, then please visit our website. It was created so we could discuss all the ideas raised in this book and figure out how to apply them better in our daily lives.

When you visit you'll find a community of people like yourself who are interested in learning about the threats, who want to learn how to use the strategies to lose weight and stay on their diet, and most excitingly, who want to create new strategies we can all use. We'll be adding new threats and strategies as we keep learning more.

What can you expect in the community? You can expect a friendly group of like-minded people who are interested in staying on their diets. I can list only so many strategies in this book. There are many more. Wouldn't it help to have a group of people to share ideas with? Groups of people working together can be an amazing source of inspiration, knowledge, and help. That's the idea behind the on-line community.

I hope to see you there.

Chapter 4

The Threats—Why Your Diet Fails

T he threats are the reasons why it is so difficult to control your weight. Many people think saying this is making excuses for people being overweight. Not true. The responsibility for your weight is always yours. But how can you control your weight without understanding why you are overweight? Figuring out why things happen is not the same as making an excuse. A pair of cousins, who helped revolutionize obesity research, provide the best example showing how knowing isn't just another excuse.

▌ The Cousins Who Could Never Eat Enough

There are many fascinating threats, but I think the most interesting involves a pair of cousins from Pakistan whose amazing story opened up an entirely new scientific understanding of how we become overweight.

At four months, the cousins became unnaturally hungry. Starved for food, they could never eat enough. The problem was so bad that even after liposuction and surgery, the 190 pound eight-year-old girl still could not walk. Her two-year-old cousin, weighing in at 65 pounds, was destined to the same fate.

When the parents locked the pantry, the ravenous cousins went so far as to eat frozen fish fingers and search garbage bins for more food. They were obsessed with finding and eating food.

Dozens of doctors found nothing wrong with the cousins. You can imagine what people thought about the kids. They were gluttons. They had no willpower. They were lazy. They were weak. The parents must be bad parents. It was all in their mind. All they needed to do was eat less and exercise more.

Then scientists made a startling new discovery: the cousins didn't produce a hormone called **leptin.** It turns out leptin is used to regulate hunger in your body. If your brain can't sense leptin, it thinks you need to eat so your brain makes you feel hungry to make you eat. This is what was happening all the time to the poor cousins. They felt a strong and constant hunger because they lacked one simple chemical. Isn't it amazing how a simple fault could create such a dramatic change in behavior?

Once injected with leptin the cousins' hunger became normal, as did their weight. It wasn't about willpower at all; **it was about how their bodies worked.**

Interestingly leptin was only discovered in 1994, after years of hard and complex work by dedicated scientists. Before 1994, we had no idea hunger was regulated by hormones like leptin.

Since the discovery of leptin, scientists have found many different hormones and systems used by the body to regulate hunger and weight.

Now it's true, most people don't have a genetic problem as severe as the cousins. What people do have is a lot of small issues that when added together make it hard to control their weight.

Please keep an open mind as to why people find it hard to lose weight. We still have a long way to go in our understanding of how our bodies work. One thing we do know, it's not just about willpower, as the cousins could have told you.

The big question: were the cousins making excuses for their hunger or was a lack of leptin the reason for their hunger? Clearly it was the reason and a reason is not an excuse.

Notice **how finding the reason for their hunger allowed a treatment to be developed** to help the cousins. They were not cured because they still had to get continued leptin injections, but they were helped immensely.

And that's the whole goal with the threats: understanding all the different ways you can become overweight helps you create your perfect diet.

▍There are Many Different Ways of Being Overweight

I'll say it until you get tired of hearing it, but we each have different bodies and live in different environments, so we are each overweight in our own way. That's why you need to figure out which strategies work for you and how extreme you need to be in following the strategies. We'll talk a lot more about this idea when we begin covering the strategies.

While we clearly aren't all overweight because of genetic problems with leptin production, there are still a lot of other factors that can contribute to being overweight. You could be leptin resistant, for example. While you may produce enough leptin, your body may simply not listen to it anymore, this is called **being resistant.**

As a Type II diabetic I produce some insulin, but I am insulin resistant, which means my cells simply don't listen to the insulin hormone anymore. If you are leptin resistant, the effect is much the same as not producing any leptin at all: you are really hungry. Your brain simply doesn't get the signal to stop eating, so you just keep on eating and eating. Researchers at the Oregon Health and Science University have found at least one mechanism causing leptin resistance, so leptin resistance is a real physical problem you could have. This is just another reason why obesity is a disease, not a character flaw.

Are you leptin resistant? Even a little? How would you know if you were? You wouldn't. You couldn't possibly know if you are leptin resistant.

You could be feeling really hungry every day of your entire life because you are leptin resistant and you wouldn't even know it. Your willpower could be so strong that you only ate one extra candy bar a day because of this hunger, but in time eating that little bitty extra candy bar every day is still all it would take to make you overweight.

And what do you get for your heroic yet unseen battle with your very real feelings of hunger? Ridicule. Discrimination. Hatred. People laugh at you behind your back, call you weak, and say you aren't a good person.

Having leptin resistance would make you **feel hungry.** All the time. Are you really not supposed to eat when you are hungry all the time? Is it realistic to expect people who are really hungry not to eat even a little more than they should?

The problem is your feelings of hunger are private. Nobody knows how hungry you feel inside so they judge you on the outside according to their own experience of hunger. That's like judging how much another person's twisted ankle must hurt. You simply don't know the hunger another person feels, just like you don't know much hunger the cousins felt.

Is a thin person to be applauded for being thin, when it's because they have less intense feelings of hunger? Is a heavy person who wages a titanic battle every day with their weight to be looked down on because they have become overweight, but far less overweight than they would be without putting up such a tremendous fight?

Few people are leptin resistant, but many people have characteristics that make them prone to being overweight. **What are some other ways of being overweight?**

You could have a low NEAT quotient, which means you naturally burn 300–800 fewer calories on average than other people. Or your senses can be wired to get a lot more pleasure out of fat and sugar, which makes you an easy target for addiction. Or you could be a non-taster, someone with a relatively poor sense of taste. Non-tasters have been found to be more overweight than others. Or food could empty out of your stomach slower, which contributes to weight gain. Or you could have fewer dopamine receptors in your brain, which is related to food addiction. Or you could have a virus. Or you could have more efficient calorie extracting bacteria in your stomach. Or you could produce too much of the hormone ghrelin, which makes you hungry. Or you could live in a situation where you don't get much exercise. Or maybe your mother was starved when you were in her womb, which reprogrammed your metabolism to turn food into fat more efficiently. Or maybe you have a mix of very small genetic changes that add up to making you hungry. Or maybe you have impaired executive function, which reduces your ability to inhibit inappropriate actions. Or maybe you have lost weight and your body is burning fewer calories and making you hungry so you'll gain the weight back. Or maybe you have food close to you all day so you eat more. Or maybe you always buy popcorn in the super-humongous size, which makes you eat more. Or maybe you always put big bowls of food out so you'll eat more. Or maybe you are bored so you'll eat more. Or maybe you are under stress so you'll eat more. Or maybe you often eat in a large group which makes you eat more.

Phew, I need to stop and take a breath!

But do you start to see now? There are many, many ways you can become overweight. That's why I call all these reasons **threats.** They are threats to push your weight out of control.

Most threats center on making you hungry so you'll eat more. Some might say it's just hunger, tough it out and simply don't eat. But would you ask someone who is really thirsty to never drink? Would you ask someone who had to go to the bathroom to just hold it forever? Would you ask someone who was tired to never sleep?

The answer is probably "no" to all of these questions because these are all drives. While we can put off drives for a while, we all expect to give into them eventually. Eating is a drive too. Later we'll talk about strategies to naturally control the eating drive.

A number of other threats center on not getting enough exercise. Some might say just exercise more. Interestingly enough, exercise is not a drive, so we don't exercise naturally. In our modern world, exercise is strictly voluntary and not enough of us are volunteers. Later we'll talk about strategies for exercising more.

▊ The Magic Overweight Diagnosis Machine

I have a dream that some day a group of brilliant scientists will develop a magic machine you can use to diagnose all the different ways you are overweight.

You'd walk into the machine and it would gently attach probes all over your body. Then it would start calculating.

The machine would take a look at your DNA and be able to catalog all the little and big genetic mutations that impact your weight. It could take a look at your metabolism and your hormones. It could look into your memories and take a look at your environment to see what you could change. It would look at everything.

After a long while it would spit out why you are prone to being overweight and give you treatments and suggestions on how to fix everything.

But we don't have a magic overweight diagnosis machine, not yet anyway. And we aren't even close to knowing all the reasons why we are prone to be overweight.

In this book I am trying to do the next best thing. You'll learn about many of the threats we know about now and you'll also learn how to formulate your own plan for staying on your diet. It's not as good as the magic machine, but it's a good start.

Before I started thinking about the reasons for falling off a diet as a group of related threats, it was difficult to create a complete plan for staying on my diet. You need a wider perspective on what's going on or all the threats will keep getting you. The idea of threats provides a good framework for understanding the problems and finding practical solutions.

▊ Mark the Threats that Affect You

As you are reading the threats, please mark which threats you think apply to you the most. Use a 0–5 scale. If a threat doesn't apply you then write down a 0 by the threat. If the threat is 100% you then mark it with a 5.

We'll use this information later to create your personal plan for controlling your weight.

▌ Strategies to the Rescue

You may feel overwhelmed by the number of threats, but please don't worry. Some of them won't impact you at all. Those that do can usually be countered with a few strategies. That's why we are learning about the threats. Once you know about the threats you can then turn around and defeat them. We'll dive directly into the strategies after spending the next several chapters talking about the threats.

There are a lot of threats. Don't feel like you need to read every word of every threat right now. Just browse and focus on the ones you are most interested in. You can always come back later and read more.

Chapter 5

The Power Threats
Threats 1–7

The power threats are the most important reasons why your diet fails. Most of the other threats we'll be talking about are in some way derived from these main threats.

Threat 1. The Perfect Storm Threat

The modern world has unintentionally created the "perfect storm" for obesity.

I found a brilliant quote nicely summing up today's worldwide battle with obesity. The quote is from *Modifying the Environment to Reverse Obesity* by James O. Hill, Holly R. Wyatt, and John C. Peters:

> *We have unintentionally created the "perfect storm" for obesity. We have constructed an environment that is a perfect complement for our biology—if the goal is to produce weight gain. Our biology has evolved to the point that we eat when food is available and rest when we do not have to be physically active. We have created an environment in which food is inexpensive, readily available, served in large portions, and heavily advertised. This environment has eliminated the need for physical activity in our jobs and our schools and provides us with engaging ways to spend our leisure time being sedentary. Sedentary activities are heavily promoted. Our food and physical activity policies support*

high energy intake and low physical activity. Our cultural values have allowed super-sizing to become popular. In essence, we have achieved the "good life" that our ancestors were constantly seeking. Obesity is an unintended and unanticipated consequence of attaining the good life.

This is the **super-threat** because it shows how all the biggest threats are so interrelated.

You probably won't become overweight if you aren't genetically predisposed to do so, even when large amounts of food are available. If you live in an environment where food is scarce, then you won't be overweight either, no matter what your genes say. And if you have to work hard all day, then it won't matter how much food is available or what your genes say, you probably won't become overweight.

Being overweight is caused by an often bewilderingly complex mix of issues. We'll explore the many ideas presented in this threat in separate, more focused threats.

....

Threat 2. The Power of Starvation Threat

Your body has an incredible ability to adapt to starvation by reducing your need for energy, making you hungry, and filling your mind with nothing but thoughts of food.

Most threats relate to our need to eat to survive in a world where starvation waits to pounce as soon as we experience a long drought, a painful injury, or we just run into a little bad luck.

Today most of us don't consider starvation a realistic possibility. We have the exact opposite problem—too much food—so we may not understand what starvation can do to our bodies and our minds.

In an article titled "The Double Puzzle of Diabetes" in *Nature,* Jared Diamond, a famous and influential biologist, shares a telling story about how going without food was a perfectly normal part of life in our past:

So accustomed are we in the First World to regular meals that we find it hard to imagine the fluctuating food availability that was formerly the norm and remains so in some parts of the world.

I often encountered such fluctuations during my fieldwork among New Guinea mountaineers still subsisting by farming and hunting. For example some years ago, in a memorable incident, I hired a dozen men to carry heavy equipment all day over a steep trail up to a mountain campsite.

We arrived just before sunset, expecting to meet another group of porters with food, and instead found that they had not arrived because of a misunderstanding. Faced with hungry, exhausted men and no food, I expected to be lynched. Instead, my carriers just laughed and said, "OK, it's no big deal, we'll sleep on empty stomachs tonight and wait till tomorrow to eat."

Conversely, on other occasions when pigs were slaughtered for a feast, the New Guineans would consume prodigious amounts of food. This anecdote illustrates an accommodation to the pendulum of feast and famine that was very necessary in times when that pendulum swung often but irregularly—a situation that was much more typical of our evolutionary history than the state of plenty to which we are accustomed.

Later, when we talk about how your body makes you hungry and makes you eat, even when you don't want it to, think back to this section and give your body some credit. How your body reacts to food in today's environment makes no sense at all, but it made perfect sense 25,000 years ago and has allowed us all to survive through the most brutal trials.

My information for this threat comes from a startling report of an experiment on the effects of starvation published in 1950 by Ancel Keys and his colleagues at the University of Minnesota.

In the first line of the report Keys says, "A full account of human experience with starvation would cover all of history and would penetrate every phase of human affairs." Keys also observed that the history of man is in large part a history of the quest for food. Given the important role of starvation in history, it's interesting nobody had yet done a scientific study on starvation. Keys changed all that.

The experiment involved studying 36 men who volunteered as an alternative to military service. The 36 young men were selected from a larger pool of 100 volunteers and had the highest levels of physical and psychological health. The men were also selected based on their commitment to the goals of the experiment.

The implication is that these were men who were going to try their best and were tough both mentally and physically. Your average person off the street wouldn't have reacted any better than the men selected. And in fact might have reacted far worse. If the men developed problems we can't say it was because they were highly flawed test subjects.

For six months the men ate an average of 1,570 calories per day. On average they lost approximately 25% of their starting weight. Pictures of the men at the start of the study show a lean and healthy group. None of them were overweight or even pudgy at the start of the study, so the weight loss was significant. At the end of the study they looked like walking skeletons.

The World Health Organization defines starvation (the point at which the body is dying) as 900 calories or less a day. Most commercial weight loss programs target between 945 and 1,200 calories a day. Today the average male eats about 2,700 calories per day.

When I first read that they'd eaten 1,570 calories a day I didn't think it was all that low. But I was very wrong. When you see what happens to these poor fellows, you'll wonder how anyone stays on a low calorie diet for long.

What happened to them? The men experienced powerful physical, psychological, and social changes.

- They became obsessed with food, thinking, talking, daydreaming, and reading about it constantly. They found it hard to concentrate on their day-to-day life because their minds were filled by thoughts of food and eating.
- A lot of their day revolved around planning how they would eat their food. They devised ways of prolonging their eating experience so they could get the most out of it. When it came time to eat they would often eat in silence, devoting their total attention to eating their food.
- A few had extreme mood swings. One man feared he was going crazy and was losing his inhibitions.
- A few men mutilated themselves. One chopped off three fingers.
- Their physical endurance dropped by half. Their percentage of body fat fell almost 70% and their percentage of muscle dropped by about 40%.
- They began hoarding things like coffee-pots, hot plates, and other kitchen utensils. They even collected non-food items like

old books, unneeded second-hand clothes and other junk. After making these purchases, even when they couldn't afford them, they would often be puzzled as to why they bought such worthless junk. One man even rooted through garbage cans looking for even more "treasures."

❖ Binge eating was a problem for some of the men.

❖ Forty percent of the men considered entering a cooking related job after the end of the experiment. They hadn't considered cooking before the study. Three eventually became chefs and one went into agriculture.

❖ The men's resting metabolic rates declined by 40%, their heart volume shrank by about 20%, their pulses slowed and their body temperatures dropped. They had complaints of feeling tired and hungry; having trouble concentrating, and of impaired judgment and comprehension. One man said it was as if his "body flame [was] burning as low as possible to conserve precious fuel and still maintain life process."

❖ They were cold all the time. To conserve energy, their temperature dropped from the normal 98.6 degrees to an average of 95.8 degrees.

❖ The average heart rate slowed to 35 beats per minute. When they started the experiment the average was 55 beats per minute.

❖ Their testes shrunk and they lost all interest in sex. People often think sex is the strongest drive, but it's dispensable when you are starving.

❖ They had physical signs of accelerated aging.

❖ The men became nervous, anxious, apathetic, withdrawn, and impatient. They became self-critical with distorted body images and even felt overweight, moody, emotional and depressed. They lost their ambition and feelings of adequacy. Their cultural and academic interests narrowed. They didn't care about how they looked anymore. They became loners and neglected important relationships. They lost their senses of humor, love and compassion.

❖ When the men started eating again and regaining weight, many began having signs of heart problems, congestive heart failure and high blood pressure.

❖ At the end of the experiment, the men were at nearly the same weight as at the start of the experiment, which was some of the first evidence showing humans may have a natural weight set-point. Losing weight didn't reset their set-point to a lower level. The weight they regained was mostly fat; they ended up with approximately 140% of their original body fat.

What can we take away from the amazing results of this unique experiment?

❖ The men weren't truly starving. In the experiment they called it **semi-starvation.** Can you imagine how consumed with food you would be if you were truly starving? Unfortunately, you don't have to imagine. In the Leningrad famine of 1941, we have a real life example of what happens when people starve. Hitler's Siege of Leningrad lasted 872 days. Non-manual workers ate an average of 473 calories a day. When the siege started, hungry people first ate the zoo animals. Next they turned to household pets. Then they ate wallpaper paste and boiled leather. When that was gone they ate corpses. And eventually even the living.

❖ Your body has an incredible ability to **adapt to starvation by reducing your need for energy and by making you hungry,** and filling your mind with nothing but thoughts of food. This is often called being in **starvation mode.** If you were just a dumb computer you would simply note you were starving and then die. But that's not what happens. Your body has ways of getting you to eat. These aren't extra special abilities it only uses sometimes, but capabilities your body uses every day to get you to eat. When the desire to eat pops up in your mind, where do you think it comes from? It's your brain telling you to eat so you won't starve. The longer you go without eating, the stronger the urge becomes. In some people these urges are strong all the time.

❖ If your body didn't have the ability to conserve energy and obsess you with thoughts of food, then **you would simply die when food became scarce** or when your attention was focused on other interesting events in your life. The starvation study shows how humans become more focused on food when starved and how other goals important to the survival of the species, like sex, become unimportant in comparison. Food is the most important thing in your life. Don't forget that. Don't blame yourself for it either.

❖   If you think you are going to stay on a **low calorie diet** for any length of time, then you are **fooling yourself.** Think about how the body reacts to any hint of starvation. Trying to lose weight by eating a lot less won't work, your body won't let you. You'll stop losing weight.

❖   The physical performance of the men deteriorated greatly, yet their mental performance did not. Although the men thought their minds performed worse, tests showed differently. Even when starving, your body maintains your ability to think because your mind is your best survival tool.

❖   Another interesting conclusion from the study is that **people varied a lot in how they handled starvation.** Some coped well and others didn't. This goes to show we are all different. What works for you may not work for someone else. **Your personal call of hunger may not be the same as anyone else's.** Try to remember that when judging your own difficulties of losing weight and staying on a diet.

❖   One of the most interesting implications of the experiment is that **your body doesn't care about your willpower.** It will defend a set-point weight with all the tools at its disposal. Your body doesn't seem to adjust to a new lower weight. It wants to gain the weight back.

Todd Tucker wrote an excellent book on this study called *The Great Starvation Experiment.* In summing, Tucker says:

> *When he [Keys] looked at the big picture drawn by the thousands of tests, graphs, and X-rays they had created, Keys concluded that the human body was supremely well equipped to deal with starvation. Eons of erratic food supplies and natural disasters had built into the body an array of mechanisms for conserving energy until the floodwaters receded, the crops were restored, or the drought ended. In later years Keys would say it was the most significant finding of the study.* **The human body was very, very tough** *(emphasis added).*

....

⚠ Threat 3. The Power of Genetics Threat

Genetics has about the same effect on your weight as it does on your height.

We are going to take this threat slow and easy because many people object to the idea their weight may be strongly influenced by their genetics.

We now accept genetics as an explanation in many areas of life. I've heard a lot of people say they are worried about heart disease because it runs in their family. I've also heard a lot of people say they aren't worried about cancer because it doesn't run in their family.

But when you say someone is overweight because obesity runs in their family, many people look at you like you are crazy. People are quick to judge someone who is overweight as lazy with no self control. It wasn't long ago when being sick meant you were possessed by evil spirits. Likewise, there's still a lot of misunderstanding around the topic of obesity and genetics.

▌ There isn't an Eat a Donut Gene

Genes generally don't work by directly causing a specific behavior. The effect of genes is much more subtle than that. So, it's true that genes don't make you eat in the sense that there is no gene that says "stop when you pass a donut shop and order three maple bars." No, there's no gene like that.

What do genes do? Technically speaking, genes make regulatory factors, signaling molecules, receptors, and enzymes that interact with your brain and influence you to have tendencies for a particular behavior.

That explanation of what genes do is a bit obscure because genetics is a complex topic, so let's go back to the cousins as an example.

The cousins had a genetic defect that kept their bodies from making leptin. Without leptin, the brains of the cousins thought they were starving and made them very hungry. The result of being hungry is people will create and carry out a plan to find and eat food.

A cruel person could still say the genes didn't directly force food down the cousins' throats, but that's not how genes work. Genes influence. And as we saw in *The Power of Starvation Threat,* when you are hungry enough, you will eat anything and you'll do what it takes to get the food you need.

▌ Your Hunger Drive is Like Your Drive to Procreate, but Stronger

Most people will say that they want to procreate because it's instinct. It seems clear to them that they want children because it's a drive, not because of some rational thought like "I am going to ensure my genes survive by having children." It's not like that at all.

People seem to accept the drive to procreate with no problem. When you say we have a drive that means it's genetic. We want to procreate because it's in our genes. Sex has been made pleasurable precisely so we'll have children.

Why is it so hard for people to apply the same sort of logic to eating? You eat because you have a strong drive to eat and that drive is implemented in your genes. The strength of the drive depends on a lot of factors, many of which we will be talking about in various threats to come.

Some people have higher sex drives than others and the difference has been found to be genetic. Though some people remain celibate through their entire life, it's difficult because over time the drive to procreate is often stronger than the mental control needed to stay celibate.

Let's imagine that, for some reason, someone is born with a very low sex drive. How hard would celibacy be for them? Let's imagine another person who was born with a very high sex drive. Wouldn't we expect celibacy to be much harder for this person? Would you be surprised to find out the person with the higher sex drive slipped-up more often than the person with the lower sex drive?

You would be right to say your sex drive is under mental control, but is your sex drive under perfect mental control? Maybe for some people, but over time it certainly isn't for all people.

Now let's imagine we put a person with a high sex drive, who is trying to stay celibate, into an environment where they are continually around people they find extremely attractive and who are willing partners. Wouldn't you expect people to slip-up more in this situation? Some people will still stay celibate, but we would expect fewer people to succeed.

Why would we expect fewer people to stay celibate over time when surrounded by temptation? Because the drive to procreate is pretty strong. That's why many people serious about celibacy minimize temptation by living in a monastery-like environment. Unfortunately, you can't create an environment without food. You must eat to survive and food is all around you.

▌ Drives Like Hunger Succeed Because They Operate Over Long Time Periods

One reason biological drives like breathing, sex, thirst and hunger are so successful is because **drives operate over time.** A drive works 24 hours a day, every day of your life.

You may be consciously motivated not to eat and you can stop yourself from eating for a while. But the drive will be operating over days, weeks, and years. When you finally give in and eat, you'll likely think it was a loss of will-power when it was really the expression of the basic biological drive to eat.

The same discussion we've had about the drive to procreate also applies to the drive to eat. Only the drive to eat is stronger because without the energy provided by food you can't do anything else.

Complicating weight loss is that you can't stop eating or you'll die. Having to eat continually opens you up to the possibility of overeating. And overeating is so easy when you have a strong drive to eat and you are in an environment filled with tempting food. Many of the strategies try to create a more favorable environment where it is easier not to overeat.

▌ The Human Obesity Gene Map

I was surprised to learn that researchers maintain a website *(http:// obesitygene.pbrc.edu)* documenting the Human Obesity Gene Map. The map identifies over 300 genes and regions of human chromosomes linked to obesity in humans. More than 70 specific gene variants are thought to cause a person to become obese. The obesity map keeps growing as researchers make discoveries using new and more powerful technologies.

There are generally three different ways genes impact on weight: by affecting appetite, overall metabolism, and how fat is stored in the body.

The most common effect of your genetic inheritance is to directly impact on how hungry you are, how full you feel, and how much food you eat. Most people still think genetics either cause a metabolic problem or somehow cause more calories to be stored as fat, but that's not so, **the biggest genetic effect is on your appetite.** Human obesity is more a problem of how genes influence your brain than it is a metabolic disease.

There seem to be a large number of genes affecting obesity, but most of them have relatively small effects. You may have many small genetic contributions to your weight rather than having one major defect, like the two cousins with their leptin gene defect. This is one reason why obesity is so hard to treat: even if you figure out how to treat one problem that still leaves all the other problems in place.

Why are there so many genes controlling eating behavior and weight regulation? It gets back to survival again. **Eating and weight are so crucial to survival that they need to be regulated by multiple and redundant mechanisms.** If one pathway fails then another must be ready and willing to take over.

▌ What is the Genetic Heritability of Obesity? As Much as 80%

Studies in twins, adoptees and families show as much as 80% of the variance in your weight can be attributed to genetic factors. What does this mean exactly? The whole idea of heritability is very confusing.

Heritability doesn't mean some gene(s) is 80% responsible for obesity. What heritability means is that 80% of the variance, the difference in weight between people, is explained by genes. The actual weight for people is explained by a lot more than genetics. The environment is a key if not the most important factor in explaining your weight.

▌ Americans are No Longer the Tallest People in the World

A fascinating example of the interaction between genes and environment is **how quickly height has changed** in the world. At one time Americans were the tallest people in the world. After World War II, the Dutch were on average four inches shorter than the average American. But Americans stopped growing in height in 1955 and the rest of the world is catching up.

The Dutch are now three inches taller than the average American and have become the tallest people in the world. Why the sudden change? Could their genetics have changed so quickly? Not likely.

What has changed is their environment. The Dutch are now eating better and have better health care, which has increased their average height. Yet height is still a function of genetics too. You won't grow to be seven feet tall no matter how good your diet is if it isn't in your genes. **Genes and environment work together.**

▌ What Accounts for the Height of the Mystery Plant?

As another example of gene-environment interaction, let's consider a species of plant called the Mystery plant. The **Mystery plant** is a fake plant name for this example, so please don't go searching your plant dictionary for it.

Looking in the handy dandy genetic handbook, we read that the heritability of plant height for the Mystery plant is 80%.

For our example, picture a clump of three Mystery plants growing in the desert, next to a rock at the base of a small hill. One plant is 2 feet tall, the second plant 2 feet 2 inches tall, and the third plant is 3 feet tall.

What is the biggest factor determining the height of the plants? Is it genetics? Or is it the environment?

Think about this a bit. A desert lacks what? Water. Even if a plant has the best genetics in the world it can only get so tall without enough water. The amount of water available to the plants in the desert is probably the biggest factor in determining how tall the plants are.

If you found yourself a big wide brimmed hat and a gigantic watering can and watered only one of the plants every day, that plant would probably be taller than the other two plants. So, the biggest factor in determining height is the environment, not genetics.

Now, let's assume nobody has watered the plants and all the plants are getting close to the same amount of water. What explains the difference in height between the plants? The plants aren't the exact same height. Something must explain the difference variance between the heights of the three plants.

Recall that the heritability of height for the Mystery plant is 80%. That means 80% of the difference between the plant heights is due to genetics and 20% of the variability is due to the environment.

We have our crack team of scientists analyze the three plants and they noticed the tallest plant has a genetic mutation that makes it process water more efficiently than the other plants, so that's why it is so much taller.

Now, what would happen if those same Mystery plants were planted in my garden where they would get all the water they need? In this new scenario, the first plant is now 5 feet tall (it was 2 feet tall), the second plant is now 4 feet 10 inches tall (it was 2 feet 2 inches tall), and the third plant is now 4 feet tall (it was 3 feet tall). It's a complete reversal. The tallest plants are now the shortest and the shortest plants are now the tallest. What happened? What explains the differences in plant height this time?

All the plants are taller because there is so much water available. But why is the third plant when grown in my garden now the shortest plant where it was the tallest plant in the desert?

Every mutation has a cost. The genetic mutation that helped the third plant grow taller in the desert now hurts it because it is unnecessarily spending energy on efficiently processing water instead of spending the energy on growing. With so much water available, the efficient water mutation now hurts instead of helps. The other plants don't have this mutation so they can spend all their energy on growing.

What's interesting is how the same mutation can help in one environment and hurt in another. Even more interesting is how genetics still wasn't the biggest explanatory factor for the height of the plants. It was their environment that provided a better explanation. So if you wanted taller plants you would change their environment, not their genetics.

▌ How does inheritance influence weight?

We've looked at the big inheritance number where as much as 80% of the variance in weight can be attributed to genetic factors, but what does that mean for how your body works and how you live your everyday life?

To answer that question, John M. de Castro of the Department of Psychology, University of Texas, has done some really amazing research on the many startling ways inheritance influences how much you eat.

Your food intake is controlled by a wide range of physiological, genetic, psychological, social and cultural influences. Each individual responds to each of these influences differently. How differently you respond to each influence depends, at least in part, on your genetics.

Here's a list of some of the different ways heredity influences eating:

- How much you eat.
- The size of your meals.
- How often you eat.
- The amount of food you tend to have in your stomach before and after a meal. Some people tend to eat their meals with their stomach relatively empty, while others with it relatively full. This matters because if you eat when your stomach is relatively full, you eat smaller meals.
- How hungry you need to be before you start a meal.
- How much you will eat when hungry.
- How hungry you will feel after you eat.
- How many people you eat with. The more people you eat with, the more you will eat.
- What time of the day you eat. Meals eaten later in the day are associated with higher weight.
- How much you like the taste of a meal.
- How much you will eat when you like the taste of a meal.
- How much you like the taste of fat and sugar.

All these pieces fit together to influence how much you will eat. Each of us is overweight in our own way because each of us will have different internal settings for all these factors.

More Frequent Genetic Variations are Being Discovered All the Time

The genetic defect afflicting the two cousins is extremely rare, but new technologies are finding more and more weight-related genetic variations.

In April of 2006 scientists using a new gene-mapping tool found that 1 in 10 people carry a common genetic variation that may make it very hard for people to keep their weight down. This one genetic variation impacts one in 10 people. That's a lot of people. You could have this genetic variation and not even know it.

University of Florida researchers found nearly 6% of morbidly obese children and adults have a genetic defect that keeps them feeling like their stomach is running on empty, no matter how much they have eaten. Only 6% of the morbidly obese were found to have this gene, but 6% is still a lot of people. Research reports like this are coming out all the time now.

In another report, researchers shared their discovery of genes that control where fat is stored on your body. If fat is more likely to be stored around your stomach, then you are more likely to become insulin resistant, which can lead to diabetes and obesity. This isn't even a genetic defect. These are simply genes controlling how fat is distributed on your body.

Scientists from the Peninsula Medical School, Exeter, and the University of Oxford found people with two copies of a particular gene have a 70% higher risk of being obese than those with no copies. Over 16% of people were found to have both copies of this gene. Are you one of these people? If so, your chances of being overweight just skyrocketed.

Some genetic influences are because of a defect: something is broken. But most of the genetic influences are genetic variations and it's just how you are.

The Dynamic Duo of Genes and Environment in Depression

We've seen how genes and the environment can interact to affect your weight. Another interesting example of the subtle interplay of genes and environment can be found in clinical depression. The connection between genes and the environment is hard to make, so I am including this example to help you build up a better understanding of the interaction between genes and the environment, not because it relates directly to weight.

Researchers found that a variation in a single gene combined with major life stress more than doubles a person's chance of becoming clinically depressed. Some examples of stressful events are losing a job or the death of a loved one.

Not all people become seriously depressed after experiencing serious stress events. Why not? One difference between the group that became depressed and the group that didn't could be found in their serotonin transporter genes. Serotonin is a chemical messenger in the brain, but don't worry too much about what it is, how it affects you is more important.

The gene for the serotonin transporter comes in a short and a long form. Each person carries a copy of the gene from each of their parents, so you have two copies of the gene.

Forty-three percent of those who had two copies of the short form developed depression while only 17% of those with two long copies became depressed. And those with two long copies seem to be protected from stress as they had the same rates of depression regardless of how many major life stress events they experienced.

What does all this mean? There are several important take-home messages in this example.

The first take-home message is that it's not just your genes *or* the environment. It's your **genes *and* the environment.** If you didn't have the genes that made you susceptible to stressful events then your chances of becoming clinically depressed are a lot less. And if you lived a life without a lot of stressful events, or if you somehow could react more calmly to stressful events, then it wouldn't matter if you had the genes. It takes both genes *and* the environment to bring about your reactions to events.

The second take-home message is that **genes and the environment are still not destiny.** Having both the genes and the stressful events only *increased your chances* of becoming clinically depressed. Not everyone became clinically depressed. Why not? Good question. Hopefully scientists will be able to answer that some day.

. . . .

Threat 4. The Power of Food Threat

You fall off your diet not because you are so weak, but because food is so strong.

Eating is so important for your survival that you have **two separate yet overlapping systems to control hunger:** the **life** and **love** systems. The **life system** is feeling hungry so you'll eat enough to replace the energy you use in daily life. The **love system** is feeling hungry because of the reward—you eat because you **want** food.

Individual differences in either of these systems can make it hard for you to stay on a diet because they give food the power to make you eat. Your willpower is strong. Your diet is strong. But if you are prone to obesity, food is strong enough that, over time, becoming overweight is almost certain without dramatic changes in how you stay on your diet.

▌ Why Is Food So Strong? Survival.

Why is food such an overwhelming force for those prone to obesity? **Survival.** And how does your body get you to eat? It makes you hungry. Hunger is the big stick your body has to control your weight. Remember in *The Power of Starvation Threat* how the men in the experiment became obsessed with food? That's simply a more extreme version of our normal urge to eat. And as we learned in *The Power of Genetics Threat*, a large number of genes interact to control obesity and we all have different genes, so we all have our own unique way of being overweight.

Almost all the genetic syndromes that clearly and obviously cause obesity work by making people hungry. Remember the story about the cousins who could not produce leptin? They were voraciously hungry nearly all the time. Those prone to obesity may simply have a greater basic drive to eat, depending on their own genetic makeup.

▌ Why can you taste food at all?

A few simple-sounding questions helped connect the dots between food, eating, and weight: Why do you have a sense of taste at all? And why do you crave ice cream but you don't crave cardboard?

So you can survive! Survival is the obvious reason behind why you eat, but it's easy to forget.

Your brain doesn't keep a big mental dictionary of the foods you should eat. You aren't born with a picture of an apple in your mind and a drive to eat apples. How would you survive in a world without apples if this is how your body really worked? How would you learn about new foods when you entered a new environment?

Instead, your body has developed a more general and far more clever way of making you eat the foods you need to survive. It gave you the ability to taste fat, sugar, protein and salt because they are all flavors in the foods you need to eat to survive.

What happens when you taste these flavors? Do you feel pleasure? I certainly do. Why should you feel any pleasure at all from tasting food? If you were a computer, you wouldn't feel pleasure, but you're not a computer.

Pleasure is how your body tells you that what you're doing is good and that you should do more of it. Pleasure is your reward for doing what your brain thinks will help you survive. Rewards are the way Mother Nature ensures you will perform the behaviors indespensible to your survival.

You seek out food because you can taste it. Tasting food gives you pleasure. Pleasure is your reward for eating food. And as a result of this innocent series of steps, you naturally eat a wide enough variety of foods that give you all the calories and nutrients you need to survive. **Pleasure seduces you into good behavior and Mother Nature always thinks that eating is good behavior.**

It's a pretty good system. Here's how this system helped our anscestors survive.

To our ancestors, food with a sweet taste meant fruit because fruit would have been almost the only sweet flavor available to them. Why is eating fruit important? Because fruit is chock-full of vitamins and energy, both of which we need to survive. We love salt because we need salt for our cells to work properly. We love protein because protein is the most important building material for muscles and other critical body functions. We taste sour and bitter flavors to warn us off bad foods. We love fat because fat has the highest number of calories and we need vast amounts of energy to survive. A 26 calorie chocolate kiss, for example, provides enough energy to lift a large SUV over six feet in the air!

The end result is, you're attracted to these flavors. Food marketers and manufacturers know this. Do the ingredients of fat, sugar, and salt sound familiar? They should, because some combination of fat, sugar, and salt is in all **junk food.**

You love junk food precisely because it mimics the tastes your body is driven to love. But junk food is worthless as a food. It packs on pounds while providing next to zero nutrition. What a cruel trick to play on Mother Nature.

▌ How Long Can You Hold Your Breath? Our Basic Drives are Strong

Jeffrey Friedman, a medical doctor and a famous researcher, illustrates the power of our basic drives with a wager. He says he will give someone $10 million if they can hold their breath for about one hour. Though everyone is extremely motivated to collect the reward, you know you can't because your body will force you to breathe. Intuitively you know you can't win the wager because you know your basic drive to breathe will win out over time and you will breathe. Can some people stop breathing until they pass out? I am sure there are such people, but there are very few who have the willpower necessary to overcome the drive to breathe.

What if the drive to eat is similar?

▌ Drive to Eat About as Strong as the Drive to Drink When Thirsty

Friedman estimates the drive to eat isn't quite as powerful as the drive to breathe, but he says the drive to eat after losing weight is about as strong as the drive to drink when you are thirsty. When I read that I was astonished. I just didn't think of hunger and the drive to eat as being that strong. When you are thirsty, how long can you resist a tall glass of water? Not long. Yet on a diet, that's the force you must be able to continually counter with your willpower. **How possible do you think that is?**

Is it reasonable to expect people to withstand such a strong drive to eat? As we'll talk about in Threat 7, *The Power of Slip-ups Threat,* people really do an amazing job using their willpower to stay on a diet. The problem is you don't need to slip-up very often to gain weight. And given the constant compulsion to eat **it is unreasonable to expect people to rarely slip-up.**

▌ The Two Ways of Making Us Eat

Eating is so important for our survival that we have **two separate yet overlapping systems to control hunger.** I was quite surprised to learn we had two different mechanisms for making us eat. To the extent I had thought about it all, I had simply thought we ate to make up the energy we burned while going about our daily activities. But there's a lot more to hunger and eating than simple energy balance.

▌ Out with the Old Standard Model of Eating

My original idea of why we eat is what Michael Lowe, a professor of psychology at Drexel University, and Allen Levine, a professor of food science and nutrition at the University of Minnesota, call the **standard** model of hunger.

The standard model of hunger says there are two types of hunger: **physical** and **psychological.**

Physical hunger results from the need to replace the energy used in daily life by eating food. Physical hunger is part of what is called our **homeostatic** system, the natural system we have for maintaining weight. An important tool used in weight maintenance is the control of hunger.

Hunger exists to make you eat. Eating supplies energy and nutrition. Hunger is balanced by signals to the brain when you are full, so your brain will stop you from eating. A number of threats involve malfunctions in the homeostatic system. In the standard model, physical hunger is thought to be the only "real" form of hunger because it is motivated directly by your energy needs.

Researchers have learned quite a bit about the homeostatic system in recent years and there's a mad dash to learn even more by those developing drugs to solve the obesity problem. The homeostatic system involves many important mechanisms, some of which we'll see later in this book: insulin, leptin, neuropeptide Y, ghrelin, peptide YY, serotonin pathways, and many more.

Psychological hunger, in the standard model, isn't thought to be real, because we aren't eating when we are "truly" hungry. Instead, we are thought to be eating because we are sad or happy or for other non-physical reasons. Psychological hunger is eating based on emotion. The easy implication is that you should be able to control your emotions which will then control your eating. This is why you are thought to be weak if you can't control your eating. The hunger isn't real so you should be able to stop it. If you can't stop your emotional eating then it must be because of some weakness from within you. If you were just stronger and had more willpower then you wouldn't get fat. I am sure you have heard this many times.

Most of us still think of the standard model as the way hunger works. But what if the standard model is wrong? What if your body had another way of making you eat? If that were true, would you still be weak and lack willpower for eating?

▌ In with the Life and Love Model

Does psychological hunger really exist? The theory of psychological hunger may not be needed if a new hunger model proposed by Lowe and Levine, called the **homeostatic-hedonic model,** turns out to be true. Yes, homeostatic-hedonic is quite a catchy title, but they are scientists after all.

The homeostatic part is the same as physical hunger in the standard model. It's eating because of **need.** This is what I call the **"life"** reason for eating. We eat to replace the energy we use to live. The hedonic part means eating for reward. We eat because **want** food. This is what I call the **"love"** reason for eating.

Why might we want food? One explanation some people will jump to right away is that we want food because we are pigs who can't control ourselves. Let's examine that a bit.

If I place a piece of cardboard in front of you, will you want to eat it? No. Why not? Because it's not food. What you want is good tasting food. What defines good tasting food? That's a surprisingly difficult question to answer. A good place to start is by asking what can you taste? Your taste buds can sense fat, sugar, and salt. That's the kind of food you want. You want food made from fat, sugar, and salt. Why? Because that's the kind of food you need to survive.

The food you want makes absolutely perfect sense from a survival point of view. You need to eat when food is available and your body needs a way to make you eat even if your immediate need-based food requirements have been satisfied. Any other approach would make you very vulnerable to famine.

▌ The Better Food Tastes the More You Want to Eat

You may think it obvious, but it is well documented that people eat more the better food tastes. It's not as obvious a statement as you might think. If hunger is only tied to your need to refill energy supplies, then the taste of food shouldn't impact how much you eat. But the taste of a food at the start of a meal does predict how much you will eat. The better the taste the more you will eat. This is the "love" reason for eating.

What does this mean for those of us in the modern world where large portions of good tasting food are in near infinite supply?

This is our first link in the chain describing the Power of Food.

▌ The Better Food Tastes the More You Eat, Even When You Are Full

When you are full, common sense would tell you that your body should stop you from eating more. After all, you are full. You have all the energy you need for now, what's the point in eating more?

Surprisingly, research shows that's not how eating works. In fact, it's just the opposite. Good tasting food makes **you eat more, especially when you are already full!** Good tasting, high energy food simply overwhelms the "I'm full" signal in your brain with a stronger "it's time to eat" signal. You keep eating even if you previously felt full.

This makes perfect sense from a survival point of view. You have to eat when calories and nutrition are available; you can't wait until later because later may never come.

What does this mean for those of us in the modern world where good tasting high energy food is in near infinite supply?

Add the second link in the Power of Food chain.

▌ Seeing, Smelling and Even Talking About Food Makes You Hungry

Several studies have found the mere sight and smell of a food can make you hungry. Even talking about food can make you hungry! After all this talk of food, are you starting to feel a little hungry?

How do we explain getting hungry simply by seeing, smelling, or talking about food? Is it for homeostatic reasons? Nope, you aren't hungry because you need more energy. The trigger is the presence of food you like.

The standard model of hunger would probably say you were experiencing psychological hunger, a hunger driven by emotional eating. But it's not psychological, it's physical and it's in your brain.

Gene-Jack Wang, a physician at the Brookhaven National Laboratory, led a study using PET brain scanning techniques that discovered that the mere display or smell of one of your favorite foods causes the parts of your brain associated with the desire for food to light up like a Christmas tree. The study found new evidence that brain circuits involved in drug addiction are also activated by the desire for food.

"These results could explain the deleterious effects of constant exposure to food stimuli, such as advertising, candy machines, food channels, and food displays in stores," says Wang. "The high sensitivity of this brain region to food stimuli, coupled with the huge number and variety of these stimuli in the environment, likely contributes to the epidemic of obesity in this country."

The significance of this study is that the volunteers did not eat the food. Their hunger didn't come from the pleasure derived from the eating of food. Mere exposure to food **motivates your brain to eat** in the same way addicts experience when craving drugs. Isn't that interesting? Craving is your brain telling you something is important and you should pay attention.

From a survival point of view, becoming hungry when you are exposed to food you like makes perfect sense. You need to eat when food is available. The problem is in our modern world food is always available and the foods we like are usually high in fat and sugar.

Is your willpower strong enough to continually resist the hunger every time you see or smell food you like?

Some people tell me they don't get hungry every time they see their favorite food so they don't believe the results of these studies. It doesn't have to be every time to have an impact on your diet. How about just sometimes? When I go into the bakery section of the store and I see and smell fresh donuts I am immediately hungry for them. Not every time, but enough of the time that if indulged on those times I would gain weight.

And what if everyone is not like you? What if some people have a much stronger attraction to certain foods than you have? Would you cut them some slack then? We'll see in later sections how people can vary quite dramatically in their reaction to food.

Add another link in the Power of Food chain.

▌ Overweight People Like Fatty Foods More

Many studies have shown the heavier a person is, the more they like fatty foods.

One study found that when compared to leaner people, heavier people who were fed high-fat foods ate more and reported greater feelings of pleasantness, satisfaction and tastiness from the high-fat foods.

Twin studies confirm that fatter twins also have higher preferences for fatty foods.

Now combine liking fatty foods with the finding that you'll eat more of a food you like, even when you are full. What could be a worse scenario for becoming overweight?

Well, unfortunately, there is a worse scenario. Obese women have been shown to have a much greater preference for **sweet high-fat foods** than do lean women. Think chocolate. I bet many women you know passionately love chocolate. A preference for both sweet and fatty foods is the worst case scenario for becoming obese.

I think these findings are fascinating. I always assumed people loved foods pretty much equally. Again, I hadn't given the issue much thought, but then I don't think many of us do. We all eat. We all have a sense of taste. So why wouldn't we all pretty much like the same foods equally?

It turns out **we don't like all foods equally.** As we'll cover throughout this book, we are all different and we all have individual quirks that set us apart from each other.

The conclusion is that a big reason some people become obese is because their body prefers fatty food. If your body preferred lettuce, for example, what would be your chances of becoming obese?

The downside of liking fatty foods is that fatty foods have the most calories. One tablespoon of butter, for example, has about 100 calories. Fat calories add up fast. If you eat a lot of fatty foods, there is almost no way you can exercise enough to burn off the excess calories.

When it comes to the choice of which foods you eat, more often than not, isn't it likely you will choose to eat the foods you like? Even if your willpower is excellent, the preference for fatty and sweet foods operates on you every moment of every day of your entire life.

Is it reasonable to expect in our modern environment, offering endless access to sweet and fatty foods, that your willpower is perfect enough to prevent obesity?

Add another link in the Power of Food chain.

▌ Your Biology Helps Determine Which Foods You Like Best

You may be thinking obese people like fatty and sweet foods for psychological reasons. You may be thinking that if these people were just right in the head they wouldn't like fatty and sweet foods anymore. As attractive a theory as this may be to some, the preference for fatty and sweet foods has deep roots in your biology. The next several sections will show this.

▌ Overweight People Get More Pleasure from Eating

If for some reason a person got more pleasure from eating than you did, would you expect them to naturally eat more? I would think so, yes.

In a fascinating research finding, scientists found overweight people get more pleasure from eating than do lean people.

Researcher Gene-Jack Wang at Brookhaven National Laboratory used a PET scan machine to compare the brain activity of obese and normal weight volunteers who had fasted to make themselves hungry.

Results from the study suggest that overweight and obese people may overeat because the parts of their brains that are stimulated by sensations in the mouth, lips and tongue are more active than in those at a healthy weight.

"This enhanced activity in brain regions involved with sensory processing of food could make obese people more sensitive to the rewarding properties of food, and could be one of the reasons they overeat," Wang said.

The brains of overweight people are set up to get more pleasure from food and eating. Obese people are very sensitive to the pleasurable sensations of food! And as we have seen, more pleasure means you'll eat more and eating more leads to obesity.

This study found real physical reasons why overweight people like and consume the foods they do. It's hard wired. Each person responds differently to the rewarding aspects of food.

Is it reasonable to expect people who get more pleasure from food to be able to counter the consequences for the rest of their life?

Research by Duke University psychologist Susan Schiffman has also shown that overweight people have heightened requirements for foods that are fatty, flavorful and highly textured. These exaggerated needs doom most diets because, she says, "When you cut back calories, you frequently cut out the fat. You also cut out a lot of the taste, smell and texture." The trick is to add these qualities back into the food or you'll find it hard to keep the weight off.

A lot of people may overeat because they get a big reward out of food. Some people play the lottery. Other people can get a big payoff simply by eating.

Add another link in the Power of Food chain.

▌ Food Demands Your Attention

The ultimate power of food comes from recent research showing that for certain people, food is addictive. The addictiveness of food is a very controversial idea. Some don't want food to be addictive because they think it gives others an excuse to eat whatever they want. Once food becomes addictive the thought is people can't help it anymore and they are absolved of responsibility.

The addictiveness of food does not absolve anyone of responsibility, just like being more prone to nicotine, alcohol, or cocaine addiction doesn't absolve those addicts of responsibility. **We are all responsible for our actions.** It's just for some of us being predisposed to an addiction makes that responsibility much harder to live up to.

We have all been dealt a different hand. Character is how you deal with the hand you've been dealt.

But in the case of food, how can you deal with an addiction you don't even know you can have? Most people still buy into the psychological theory of hunger, so most people won't think they are addicted, they will think they are just weak.

In another study lead by Gene-Jack Wang, they found dopamine, a brain chemical associated with addiction to cocaine, alcohol, and other drugs, may also play an important role in obesity.

Dopamine is now thought by researchers like Dr. Nora Volkow, director of the National Institute on Drug Abuse, to **tell us what we need to pay attention to in order to survive.** New information is bombarding us all the time, what information should we think is important? Dopamine is released when something surprising and important happens.

What is important could be an unexpected reward like a cheeseburger or a painful accident like placing your hand on a hot burner. With the help of dopamine, we are able to pay attention to the information we need to survive, act on the information, and remember the information later.

Given all that the dopamine system does, it's impossible to think of surviving without it. But rarely is anything all good and dopamine's downside can be found in drugs and addiction.

A drug like cocaine **pumps five to ten times the normal amount of dopamine** into your system. What do you think that does to you? It makes the drug the most important thing to pay attention to in your life. The drug effectively hijacks the system your body uses to regulate attention by turning all your attention back to the drug. If you have noticed addicts have a hard time thinking of anything but their drug, it's because that's exactly what is happening.

Addicts have been found to have fewer dopamine receptors in their brain. Receptors are the parts of your brain that sense the dopamine in your system. An analogy is a radio that tunes into a particular radio station. With fewer receptors, the dopamine signal is weak. If you heard a weak signal on your radio you would try to tune to a station with a stronger signal. But there's no way to change the "dopamine" station. What you have to do is make the dopamine signal stronger by upping the power.

How does an addict boost their signal? They take more and more of the drug. An addict needs to take more of the drug to feel anything at all.

Even scarier, because your brain is paying most of its attention to the drug your prefrontal cortex stops functioning normally. Your prefrontal cortex is the part of your brain responsible for judgment and stopping you from doing things you shouldn't do. It's in charge of doing the harder thing. With an impaired prefrontal cortex, your judgment is worse and you are more likely to engage in risky behaviors.

What we then have is a combination of extreme motivation for a drug and a reduction of the ability to stop taking it. That's one reason addiction is so difficult to defeat.

▌ What has all this got to do with obesity?

People are born with different numbers of dopamine receptors. Obese people were found to have fewer dopamine receptors than people at a normal weight. In fact, the more obese a person was, the fewer dopamine receptors they had.

Oh boy. All the drug addiction problems we talked about with a drug like cocaine apply to food as well, but with one important difference: **food isn't nearly as strong a drug as cocaine.**

There's evidence, however, that a high calorie meal made up of fat and sugar can approach the strength of a drug in the release of dopamine. Hmm, a high calorie food made out of fat and sugar, does that sound like fast food and junk food to you? So the addiction may not be as powerful, but it seems powerful enough to lead to obesity.

Why does having a lower number of dopamine receptors lead to addiction? At first I thought having a higher number of receptors would lead to addiction. My reasoning was if you had a higher number of receptors then you would get more pleasure from food so you would want it all the more.

I was wrong. Having a lot of receptors means you are **very sensitive,** so a little goes a long way. Too much and you don't like it.

I think of it like loud music and someone who is hard of hearing. If you are hard of hearing, you have to turn up the volume really loud so you can hear the music. If your hearing is excellent, then loud music hurts your ears and you will immediately plug your ears with anything handy to escape the loud sounds crashing into you.

Eating food while having more dopamine receptors is like listening to loud music with excellent hearing. You won't be able to handle the over-stimulation of eating more and more food if you have a lot of dopamine receptors, so you will stop eating sooner. This is how thinner people react—they stop eating, the stimulation becomes too much.

But if you have fewer dopamine receptors, then you want to keep enjoying the pleasure of food, so you keep on eating. This is how people prone to obesity react to the rewarding properties of food, they keep on eating.

If you have fewer dopamine receptors, you are not eating to get high; **you are eating to feel normal.** You need to keep on eating to keep feeling pleasure so you can feel good, so you can feel well, so can feel like a normal person.

The fewer receptors you have, the more you will have to eat to feel something. That's probably why the heaviest people had the fewest receptors. The heavier people need to eat more to trigger their dopamine system. Why food? Heavier people have been found to have bodies that extract more pleasure out of food than thinner people so food is a very convenient and practical drug.

Interestingly, mice bred without dopamine receptors quickly starve themselves to death. Goldilocks wanted her porridge just right, not too hot or too cold. That's how we need our dopamine receptors too, not too many or too few. The number of receptors you have is determined by the genetic lottery that was held when you were born. The results of this lottery heavily influence your fate.

But like almost all the topics we'll talk about in this book, it's not all a lottery. You are still the biggest influence in your own destiny, even if it doesn't feel that way sometimes.

Exercise, of course, has been found to increase the number of dopamine receptors. Why is the answer always more exercise? But, exercise is just one of the things you can do to change the lottery results. The strategies in this book give a lot of other things you can do too.

▌ More Evidence for Food Addiction

In yet another study, Gene-Jack Wang and his team found obese people may be as addicted to the drug of food as junkies are to other drugs. The study monitored the brains of test subjects who had a device implanted in their stomachs, allowing researchers to trick their brains into feeling full.

They found that the brain circuits motivating obese people to overeat are the same that cause addicted people to crave drugs. These circuits are also linked to eating to soothe negative emotions.

The implications of the study are that even if you lose weight you will still feel food cravings that you can't suppress. This adds up to a high chance of relapse—that means regaining your weight.

Believe it. Food has all the power it needs to get you to eat.

▌ Changing How We View Obesity

For the longest time, society thought drug addicts were simply morally weak people who couldn't deal with life. Now many people think of addiction as a medical problem. There has been a similar change of heart on depression. Depression was also once thought to be a weakness of character. Now depression is often diagnosed as a problem of brain chemistry and may be treatable using drugs.

There is still research needed to establish the relationship between food and addiction, but it's clear to me that over time we will change our view of obesity to be more like how we now think of depression and drug addiction. What motivates us to eat is clearly much more complicated and powerful than the outdated psychological model of hunger that is now the default view of obesity.

Add another link in the Power of Food chain.

▌ Why do people become addicted to food and not other drugs?

People who have a hard time thinking of food as an addictive substance often ask this question. Here are two possible answers:

1.   People attracted to food also become addicted to other drugs. A big problem for many people who have lost weight is that they move on to become addicted to other drugs. It's not an either/or situation.

2.   A more interesting answer is to remember that people prone to obesity often feel more pleasure from food than people not prone to obesity. Their brains are particularly sensitive to food. So, for them food is a very attractive drug. They really don't need to find another drug. And when you consider that food is legal, relatively cheap, endlessly varied, socially acceptable, and in great supply, why would you need another drug?

▌ The Power of Food Chain Is Strong

In this threat I have added a lot of links to the Power of Food chain. Link by link I've tried to show how food itself has the natural power to make us hungry and eat. You don't need to make up psychological reasons for why you eat. Tasty high-fat and high-sugar foods are all the reason you need to eat because that's the kind of food that helped humans survive in the past.

Now add that many people, for genetic reasons, are more prone to obesity because they are physically more vulnerable to wanting good tasting food.

Now add to that the 24 hour a day availability of and exposure to high calorie good tasting food.

The real question that comes to mind is: **how is anyone not overweight?**

The common treatment for drug addiction is to stay completely away from the drug you are addicted to. Drugs are so strong a single exposure can cause a relapse. Food addiction is so hard because you can't stay away from food. You must eat to survive.

Given the extreme Power of Food isn't losing weight and staying on a diet hopeless? It's not easy, but it's far from hopeless. You can't just break one link in the chain and solve all your problems. All the links must be attacked simultaneously.

By understanding the true power of food, you become capable of devising strategies to beat its power. Many of the strategies that follow are directly targeted at defeating the Power of Food.

....

Threat 5. The Power of Rest Threat

You don't have a drive to exercise, yet you have a drive to be NEAT.

Your body doesn't tell you when to exercise. You are built to rest and conserve energy when there's no work to do. Twenty-five thousand years ago, people continually worked hard and burned a lot of calories. Hunter-gatherers covered 6 to 12 miles a day on foot in a hunt for vegetables, fruits and small, lean game. None of these foods would lead to obesity, especially with such high levels of exercise.

In our past, **exercise drove how much we ate.** We exercised a lot so we could eat a lot. It was nearly impossible to get enough fat and sugar in our diet, so there was little risk of becoming obese.

Today, many people can survive without exercising at all. And your body won't care. Your body is happy to be a couch potato. And when given a chance, most people won't exercise.

A couple of studies help show our lack of interest in exercise. Seven out of 10 American adults don't exercise regularly. And when people were given free access to high-quality exercise facilities, they did not significantly increase their use of them. It was thought cost might be a barrier to exercise. It wasn't.

My favorite study showed that when people had to walk 5 extra minutes to get to their exercise facility, it reduced the amount people exercised by over 50%. I always imagine people going to their hour-long aerobics class and driving off if they can't get the parking spot closest to the entrance!

▌ Maybe You Don't Love Exercise as Much as the Next Person

Some people seem to love to exercise. They'll get up early in the morning and knock out a 7 mile run and then hit the gym for a few sets in the weight room. Other people look at the gung-ho exerciser like they are crazy. You might think these are two different kinds of people. And you might be right.

A study based on data collected from a large group of twins living in 7 different countries found the heritability of the amount people exercised ranged from 48% to 71%. This means individual genetic differences help explain a lot about why some people love to exercise and others hate it. The study also found that men tended to exercise more than women. People gradually exercised less as they got older, and only half the study participants were active regularly.

I wish there was a magic spell to turn me into a lover of exercise. Then I might naturally exercise more. But like me, most people aren't that excited about exercise. And I bet there are a lot of people, maybe even you, who are even less excited about exercising than I am.

Unfortunately you can't rely on magic. And **you can't let the fact that life isn't going your way become an excuse.** Instead, you have to figure out ways of using your other strengths to get enough exercise, even when exercise may not be on your personal top ten list. A great many strategies in this book are targeted at helping you naturally get more exercise.

▌ How NEAT are You?

Exercise isn't your only form of activity. There's another form of activity you don't have conscious control over, called NEAT (non-exercise activity thermogenesis), which may be one of the key reasons some people are obese and others are lean.

NEAT is all the everyday activities you do that aren't formal exercise. Think of tapping your toe, fidgeting, wiggling your ears, pacing, cleaning your house, playing the piano, even playing a video game. You know those people who never seem to sit still? Are those people usually lean or obese? Here comes the science.

How many calories could all this NEAT activity add up to? James Levine, MD, is the Mayo Clinic endocrinologist who led a study on NEAT that found obese people sit, on average, 150 minutes more each day than those people who are "naturally" lean. This means, if you are **obese you burn 350 fewer calories a day** than lean people. That's 35 pounds a year! Thirty-five pounds is easily the difference between being obese and being lean. That's stunning to even think about.

Dr. Levine thinks the differences in NEAT between obese and lean people is biological, not a matter of conscious choice. A person's NEAT level may be fixed. Obese people seem to have a biological need to sit more. Even after losing weight, obese people sat as much as they did before, so the lack of activity wasn't due to their weight. And when the naturally lean people gained weight they still managed to stand, walk and fidget more.

Many people have thought their obesity was because they had a low metabolism, though research has shown very few people really have a low metabolism. In fact, obese people have higher metabolisms to support their increased size. The difference in weight gain between two people eating the same amount of food may turn out to be their NEAT level.

Naturally obese people simply may not have a biological drive to fidget. Without that drive, obese people are missing an enormous source of calorie burn.

The trick for people with a low NEAT is to figure out ways to purposefully increase their NEAT level. Many of the strategies aim to increase your NEAT level.

. . . .

⚠ Threat 6. The Power of Environment Threat

You probably won't become obese, even if your genetics make you prone to obesity, as long as your environment makes it necessary for you to work hard, or food is scarce.

I am often challenged to explain why obesity has increased so much in the last 50 years. Our genetics couldn't have changed that fast and people in the past weren't as overweight, so doesn't that mean people today are lazy and weak willed? Don't we just need more willpower?

Sort of. People are naturally inactive, as we talked about in *The Power of Rest Threat*. Survival requires that we conserve energy. And for people prone to obesity, tasty food is particularly hard to resist, as we talked about in *The Power of Genetics Threat* and *The Power of Food Threat*.

The thing is the **people of yesterday were just like us.** They had the same love of food and the same love of leisure as we do. It just didn't matter, because the environment they lived in **forced** them to exercise and made tasty high calorie foods unavailable to most people.

Given a chance, our ancestors would behave exactly as we do today. We are them and they are us.

A good example historically is how **rich people have been overweight.** Rich people in the past lived like most everyone can live today. They didn't have to do hard physical work to survive and they could afford large quantities of the best food. When given a chance, they became overweight by moving less and eating more. So, has the character of people changed, or is it more likely that more people are now able to live the life they naturally prefer?

What has changed dramatically in the last 50 years is the environment. Modern technology has given us the world we most desire. Food is cheap, available everywhere, served in monster portions, and comes filled with large quantities of wonderful tasting fat and sugar. You can't escape food. Food is everywhere you look.

At the same time, we have engineered physical activity out of almost every aspect of our lives. Most jobs today require little activity. We spend our leisure time watching TV, movies, and playing video games. We drive everywhere. We buy labor-saving devices and, if we can, hire other people to do the hard work. It all adds up to a lot less work than even a person two or three generations ago would have done to survive.

Today, if we wish to eat less, we have to **make ourselves eat less.** In the past the environment didn't provide enough food for most of us to become overweight. And today, if we wish to exercise, we have to **make ourselves exercise more.** In the past the environment demanded we exercise in order to survive. Now the responsibility for your weight is completely yours.

Four of the Power Threats *(Power of Genetics, Power of Food, Power of Rest,* and *Power of Environment)* conspire together. If one threat weakens you, then your chance of being overweight increases, which is why obesity is such a difficult problem to combat and understand. You'll likely stay lean if you aren't genetically predisposed to be obese no matter how tempting the environment. Even if your genetics makes you prone to obesity, you probably won't become obese as long as your environment makes it necessary for you to work hard or keeps food in short supply.

But what happens when we turn lose people who are prone to obesity into a world where little activity is required and great tasting food is available for next to nothing everywhere you look? **You get exactly the world we see today.** Isn't expecting any other outcome a bit unrealistic?

Can we make ourselves exercise more and eat less? Much of the time, we can. But can we consciously make ourselves exercise more and eat less, 24 hours a day for the rest of the lives?

Most of us can't. If you have to rely on willpower 24 hours a day for the rest of your life, then your chances of staying on your diet are very small. You just have to look at the very high failure rates (up to 95%) for diets to see the likely results.

What you need is an approach that doesn't rely on continual conscious control for success. That's why this book introduces the strategy of Weight-Proofing. You are in a good position to control your weight once you can create an environment in which you don't have to rely on a constant supply of willpower.

. . . .

Threat 7. The Power of Slip-Ups Threat

Small slip-ups over time equal obesity

It's too difficult for most people to constantly remind themselves to pass on all the attractive foods in their environment. Wait, you say, if someone is truly motivated enough, they can do it. Probably not. It only takes a few slip-ups to gain weight. Some people may be able not to slip-up, but most people, over time, aren't able to consciously minimize their slip-ups enough to lose weight.

By a *slip-up* I mean any time you eat more than you planned or exercise less than you wanted. Maybe you have an extra big helping at dinner. Maybe you have an extra drink. Maybe your dessert was larger than you expected. Maybe you skipped an exercise session. Add up all the little slip-ups and over time you can gain a lot of weight really fast.

Research has shown that as few as 50 extra calories a day over 10 years can lead to obesity. **Small slip-ups over time equal obesity.** I know this doesn't seem possible. After all, 50 calories is nothing, isn't it? Let's run the numbers. Fifty extra calories a day means you gain about 5 pounds a year. Over 10 years that's about 50 pounds. You are considered obese if you are about 30 pounds over your ideal weight. That's the power of slipping-up. How can that be?

▌ Small Slip-ups Add Up to Big Weight Gain Numbers

Let's use another example where a slip-up costs about 200 calories. A slip-up could easily cost a lot less or a lot more, but let's say each slip-up is 200 calories on average. Even a much lower number leads us to the same overall result so the actual number isn't that important.

Dr. Brian Wansink of Cornell University estimates **you make well over 200 food decisions a day.** These decisions can be subtle like which plate to use, or obvious, like which foods to eat. You could make more or fewer decisions. Again, the actual number isn't that important. The important thing is the small number of slip-ups you get to make before sliding into obesity.

Let's say you make just one slip-up out of 200 eating decisions. That's like getting a score of 199/200 on a test. That's excellent, almost impossible, better than I ever did in school. You would get an A. Unfortunately this isn't school. This is the exacting world of calorie balance and on that test you get an F.

How can just making one little slip-up a day matter so much? It works on the same principle as your savings account. You know how people keep pestering you to put a little away each month so you'll have enough money when you retire? They want you to put a little away each month because it all adds up. It all adds up for calories too.

▌ The Cost of Those Extra Calories

Here's what your weight gain will be if you make one slip-up a day, at different calorie imbalances. Remember, one pound of fat is created by eating about 3,500 extra calories.

- ❖ Eating an extra **10 calories** a day means you gain an extra pound a year. One Lifesaver® has 10 calories.
- ❖ Eating an extra **100 calories** a day means you gain 10 extra pounds a year. One 12 ounce can of soda has 152 calories. One bottle of beer has 139 calories. One cup of orange juice has 110 calories.
- ❖ Eating an extra **200 calories** a day means you gain 20 extra pounds a year. One small order of McDonald's french fries has 209 calories. One 16 ounce can of soda has 202 calories. A typical candy bar has over 230 calories. A donut has about 250 calories.
- ❖ Eating an extra **500 calories** a day means you gain 50 extra pounds a year. One slice of pepperoni pizza is over 500 calories. One cup of ice cream is almost 500 calories. A bagel with cream cheese has over 500 calories. A realistic bowl of cereal and whole milk can be over 500 calories.

You may be saying to yourself, "Wow, that can't be right!" Unfortunately, it is. It's easy to see now why making even one slip-up a day leads to huge weight gains in a really short amount of time. And if you only make a few slip-ups a week, you'll still quickly gain a lot of weight. Even if you fall off your diet for just a little while, you can still ratchet up your weight.

▌ What Does It Take to Prevent Obesity?

It's estimated that 90% of obesity could be prevented if people consumed 200 fewer calories a day, burned 200 more calories a day in exercise, or through some combination of the above. A mere 200 calories a day separates the overweight from the obese. The bad news is it doesn't take many extra calories to tip us into obesity. The good news is it doesn't take many fewer calories to prevent obesity either.

▌ Your Willpower Is Really Pretty Good

One very positive note you can take away from the discussion of eating slip-ups is that your willpower is really pretty good. You succeed far more than you fail, you just don't have to fail very often for it to make a big difference in your weight.

Willpower is not enough to control your weight because after just a few slip-ups the weight starts piling on. The chances of most people making zero slip-ups are pretty small. That's why preventing slip-ups is the major focus of many of the strategies we'll talk about later.

To Learn More

❖ *Mindless Eating* by Brian Wansink. After I was nearly done writing this book, Dr. Wansink published his own very interesting book on his research. Please take a look if you would like to learn more about the hidden reasons we eat.

Chapter 6

Threats from the Power of Genetics
Threats 8–24

This chapter is a collection of threats rooted in the ideas we talked about in *The Power of Genetics Threat.* Few threats are just about genetics, but I felt these threats made the most sense when thought about from a genetic point of view. There are so many ways genetics makes staying on a diet hard. Yet knowing all these reasons helps you figure out strategies for countering their influence.

⚠ **Threat 8. The Double Whammy Threat**

Obese people remain hungry longer and don't feel full as quickly as other people.

The Double Whammy Threat was expressed by Endocrinologist Stephen Bloom of Hammersmith Hospital of London:

> *Compared with other people, the obese remain hungry longer and don't feel full as quickly. No wonder these poor people can't lose weight.*

Parts of your body communicate with your brain through your bloodstream using chemical messages called **hormones.** Sometimes these messages don't work as well as they should.

That's what is happening in *The Double Whammy Threat.* Your body may be misreading or ignoring messages that tell your brain when you are hungry or full. Bloom's study found these messages do not work as well as they should in obese people.

The **first part** of the whammy is that the **"I'm full"** message to your brain doesn't work as well in obese people. A hormone called PYY is released in your stomach as you eat. PYY is a message telling your brain "I'm full."

PYY has been found to increase less after a meal in obese people. This means the "I'm full" message isn't being sent at full strength. Your brain doesn't get the "I'm full" message, so you think you are still hungry even though you have eaten.

The **second part** of the whammy is that obese people are less satisfied and more hungry than normally weighted people after eating. Because of this, **obese people may eat more because they don't feel as full as normally weighted people.**

The culprit this time is a hormone called **ghrelin.** When your stomach is empty, ghrelin is released as a message to your brain telling your brain **"It's time to eat."**

A shot of ghrelin gives a person a ferocious hunger. Ghrelin levels should increase when you haven't eaten and fall off after eating.

In normally weighted people, less ghrelin is sent after eating a meal. So, a normally weighted person will feel full after eating.

Not so for obese people. The stomach of an obese person will keep sending the "It's time to eat" message to their brain. So, the feeling of fullness after a meal for obese people was much less than for normally weighted people.

Scientists used to think it was a silly idea that your stomach sends messages to your brain, but Mother Nature is clever. She wants you to eat so she has created multiple overlapping systems, like PYY and ghrelin, to get you to eat that both independently control hunger using different strategies. Unfortunately, either mechanism can go bad, or both.

How much PYY and ghrelin does your stomach send? You have no idea. Everyone will send different amounts. This is another reason why everyone is overweight in their own way.

Think about what this means for a second.

By your stomach sending wrong messages to your brain you don't feel as full as you should. What do you do if you don't feel full? You keep on eating. If you think a person is a pig, it just might be that their brain isn't getting the right message.

This is a key point: **your brain makes you feel hungry.** Your brain is looking at dozens and dozens of messages about how hungry you are, it then merges all the messages, and then your brain makes you feel as hungry as it thinks you should feel. You could feel hungry because of too much ghrelin or not enough PYY or for a lot of other reasons. But no matter what the cause, you won't know why. Keep in mind that some of **the reasons you might feel hungry could be wrong.**

....

Threat 9. The Two Brain Threat—The Ant and the Grasshopper

You have two brains for decision making: one emotional for making short term decisions *(eat junk food now)* and one logical for making long term decisions *(don't eat junk food at all).*

Let's say one fine day you come home and follow a familiar and delicious smell into the kitchen. On the table you see a dozen freshly baked cookies just sitting there begging to be eaten. Your hand is half way to the cookies before you stop yourself and think, "I've already had enough calories today so I can't have the cookies." Then you say, "what the heck" and chomp down a few cookies.

Has anything like that ever happened to you? Doesn't it feel like parts of your brain are fighting each other? Doesn't it feel like you are being torn between two different decisions?

Well, you are! Brain imaging studies of people making decisions clearly show there are two different parts of your brain competing to see which makes the ultimate decision.

Who is doing the battling? When it comes to decision making, you have **two brain systems:** one **emotional system** for making short term decisions based on immediately available rewards and one **logical system** for making long term decisions based on long term rewards. Different brain systems have developed to handle different types of problems.

Your emotional brain is all about getting the short term reward. It doesn't deal well with imagining the future consequences of current actions; that's the job of your logical brain. The more immediate the reward, the more likely it is your emotional brain will win out against the logical part of your brain.

Borrowing from Aesop's classic *The Ant and the Grasshopper* fable, your emotional brain is the grasshopper, always thinking about the now. Your logical brain is the ant, always planning for tomorrow.

The sight, touch, and smell of food kicks in your emotional brain and makes it very likely you'll give in and eat. Your brain is putting a higher value on getting precious calories now and less value on more abstract rewards like better health when you are 70.

Later you may regret eating the cookies as your logical brain gets a chance to chip in, but the chances are you will still eat. It's like your brain is saying "food now or health later? Duh, I'll take the food now. You never know when our next meal will come from. We may not even live to 70."

Is your brain wrong? Should you eat the cookie or not? For our ancestors, the choice was clear: eat when food is available. We aren't our ancestors, but we still have their brain. Your decision will likely be to eat the cookie, because for most people the long term reward (health, etc.) of not eating the cookie is less than the short term reward (pleasure) of eating it.

Logically, you may have decided junk food is bad for your health so you don't want to eat it. But when face-to-face with junk food, and especially when you are hungry, your emotional brain will win enough of the time that you will slip-up. And slip-ups lead to falling off your diet. Even one bad decision a day is enough to tip the balance toward becoming overweight.

The big questions are: **How can you make the long term perspective more rewarding? How can you give your emotional brain as little opportunity to operate as possible?** We'll consider both of these questions in later strategies.

▌ The Single Mind Illusion

Just to be clear, this "two brain" idea is not a metaphor; it's actually how your brain physically works. And the idea of "competition" between the parts is not a metaphor either. The two parts of your brain are actually competing to make decisions.

Your ancient limbic system, which includes your dopamine system, is involved in decisions regarding immediately available rewards, and your more modern prefrontal cortex gets involved for decisions about longer term rewards.

Your thinking appears seamless to your conscious mind when really, behind the scenes, many different parts of your brain coordinate their actions to bring you your thoughts.

It's like ordering dinner at a restaurant. Behind the scenes, all the chefs in the kitchen work together as a team, talking, coordinating, gathering ingredients, mixing them together, and then cooking them properly. If they do their job right, all parts of your meal are done at the same time and the waitperson brings you your plate with everything on it. When you get your dish, you don't see all the hard work that went in to make it. You just get to enjoy a fine meal.

That's how your brain works too, you just don't notice because the chefs are so good at their job. It is even more amazing when you consider your brain has 100 billion chefs (neurons).

Through your conscious mind, your brain creates the illusion that all thinking is the same, but on the inside, thinking happens in different areas of your brain and you'll make different decisions based on where and how your thinking happens.

You have this "short term/long term" split in thinking we've been talking about. There's also a "you/other" split in thinking. You'll make different decisions when thinking about yourself than when you are making decision involving other people. There's also a "like/dislike" split in thinking. You'll form different conclusions from the same information for someone you like when compared to someone you dislike.

All this makes sense from a survival perspective. It's not necessarily bad, but it is difficult to deal with because you don't consciously know it's happening. So you have to structure your life to reduce the chance of making decisions you would rather not make. This is what the Weight-Proofing strategies are all about.

. . . .

Threat 10. The Weight Defense Threat

Your body tries hard to make you gain back every pound you lose.

Your body doesn't mind if you gain weight, but it really doesn't want you to lose weight. This is a built-in imbalance of your weight regulation system. Weight gain happens effortlessly because it means you will have fat for the time when no food is available. Yet any weight loss is fought fiercely.

Your body is quite clever and helps you regain your weight by making you hungry and by reducing your energy expenditure by 15%. This is a potent combination of effects. You are hungry so you'll eat more when food is available and your body uses less energy so more of the calories you eat can be stored to fat.

This effect is often called the **set-point** because it's like your body is trying to return to some predetermined weight.

▌ Making You Hungry

If you don't eat for 4 or 5 hours, your body starts to think you are starving and kicks off a bunch of processes to protect your body from starvation. This is called the **starvation response.**

Your body first notices the amount of leptin has decreased, which signals it to start protecting its stores of energy. You will start feeling hungrier so you will eat to provide more energy. Your body will also start decreasing the amount of energy it uses so you don't use up the energy you do have. This is the why eating a low calorie diet doesn't work. Your body, quite understandably, wants to protect you from starvation, so when you starve yourself, it will take action to save you. Your hunger will get worse and worse until you have no choice but to eat.

Your body thinks overeating enhances survival while under eating, like when you diet, puts you on the extinction train. In a different environment you would joyously thank your physiology for helping you survive. But in today's abundant food environment, the drive to gain back weight just makes your job of losing weight and maintaining weight loss that much harder. Not impossible, just harder.

▌ Reducing Your Energy Expenditure by 15%

Compare the amount of energy someone expends after losing weight to a person of the same weight who didn't lose weight. Amazingly, you'll find that the person who lost weight burns about 15% fewer calories.

What does this do for you? You'll regain weight because it's unlikely you'll be able to reduce how much you eat by 15%. Tricky, isn't it?

How does this happen? The majority of the change is from burning fewer calories during physical activity. A small amount of the change is from burning fewer calories when at rest.

Scientists are still trying to figure out how this works, although after weight loss people often complain of feeling cold, hungry, and just not normal in general.

This means that if you take two otherwise identical people and one has lost weight, the person who lost weight will have to eat 15% fewer calories or burn 15% more calories to maintain the same weight. It's not fair, but that's the reality of it.

Once you drop your weight by about 10% or more, you kick in the 15% energy reduction. Even if you keep the weight off for a long time, this effect will not go away. It's thought, however, that exercise helps prevent weight regain not just by burning calories, but by making other changes that counteract whatever your body is doing to reduce your energy expenditure.

You should be getting the feeling by now that losing weight is much more complex than you may have thought.

· ·

⚠ Threat 11. The Bored Taste Buds Threat

You get bored of a taste after a couple of bites, which causes you to eat a wider variety of foods.

When you take your first bite of a beautiful, tasty food, the flavor explodes in your mouth and you may think to yourself, "Ah, you know, this eating ability we have is pretty good."

You take the second bite expecting the same zing of flavor, but you don't get it. That bite doesn't taste as good as the first.

And then you take the third bite and the same reduction in flavor happens. The more of a food you eat the less flavor you taste and the less pleasure you experience from eating. At the end of a large dish, it's likely you taste almost nothing at all.

This effect is called **sensory-specific satiety.** Bite by bite, as you eat a food, your brain is dialing down your response to that food. Why would your brain do such a dastardly thing?

You become bored by the taste of a food so you'll switch to another food. You see, the sensory-specific satiety effect works on the foods you have been eating recently. Switching to a new food brings back the full pleasantness, taste, smell, and pleasure of the new food. Switching to a new food also **resets your hunger level** so you feel hungry again, even though you may have eaten a lot already.

You can demonstrate this effect with a quick test using chewing gum. Chew a piece of gum until you stop noticing the flavor. Take the gum out of your mouth and put it somewhere safe. You'll need it again. Where do you think the flavor went? Did the gum run out flavor? It didn't go anywhere. The flavor is still there. Your brain turned the flavor off so you will switch to a new food. To prove this, wait about five minutes and start chewing the gum again. The flavor will magically reappear.

Why would your brain want you to switch foods so often? The wider the variety of foods you eat the better chance you have of meeting your nutritional and caloric needs.

Think back to what we said about why you taste particular flavors. Your brain can't tell you what specific foods to eat because you have to eat from what's available. Neither can your brain tell you what combination of foods to eat, so it tries to get you to eat as many different flavors as it can, on the bet that this will maximize your chances of getting all the nutrients you need.

As a result, humans have an incredibly varied diet. We eat a wider variety of foods than any other animal.

Now think what happens at a buffet! You have access to lots of different kinds of foods, many of them highly caloric. Poof! Your diet goes down the drain. This is an unconscious process you don't even realize is going on.

....

Threat 12. The Value Threat

Finding a good food value means buying bigger portions which leads to eating more.

For a great many people, finding good value and convenience are the most important factors in selecting what they eat. Nutrition may only be a small part of their decision making process.

Finding a good value is so important consumers will choose a restaurant based on the portion sizes it serves. This rings true, doesn't it? The more food you get for your money the better the deal. And the better the deal the more likely you are to buy.

Food manufactures know how to tap into this love of the deal. Using nutrition information from several major fast-food chains, researchers Rachel Close and Dr. Dale Schoeller at the University of Wisconsin-Madison estimated that super-sizing a soda and fries costs consumers only 67 cents, on average. And for the small price of 67 cents you buy about 400 extra calories. That's a good deal!

Offering a lot of food for a little money is called **value pricing.** For example, in 2002 McDonald's offered a "value meal" of a Big Mac, medium fries and a medium Coca-Cola™ for only $2.99. This meal provides 1,250 calories. For a little more money, if the fries and Coke were super-sized, the meal would have a total of 1,640 calories. This single meal would then amount to 73% of the average Recommended Daily Allowance (RDA) for calories.

Restaurants can afford to offer large portions because the cost of the actual food is a relatively small part of a meal. Labor and overhead are a large part of the total cost and increase very little with portion size. So, increasing portion size is a cheap and hugely effective strategy for restaurants.

It's not only fast food restaurants that use value pricing. We see value pricing in all areas of the food industry now. Why? Because it works! People are attracted to a deal.

To see why, think about how most people on a budget would vote on the following choice. You can go to a fast food restaurant and get an unhealthy, huge, great tasting meal for very little money. Or you can go to a more upscale restaurant and buy a healthy, smallish, good tasting, and expensive meal.

With their dollars, most people have voted for fast food restaurants. What are some of the consequences of this choice?

✦   You eat more because the portion sizes are huge.

✦   You eat more very fattening food because it is made primarily
     from fat and sugar.

Fast food restaurants dominate the landscape for good reasons. For next to nothing, at a fast food restaurant you can buy a hot, fresh, tasty meal that is served almost immediately. Unfortunately, your meal will also likely be high in fat, sugar and calories.

Why are fat and sugar such popular ingredients? Customers love the taste of fat and sugar. For restaurants, those ingredients are dirt cheap. This compelling combination of taste and economics has made fast food available throughout the land.

▌ Not So Good a Deal After All

When is a good deal really a bad deal? When it costs you more in the end.

Close and Schoeller found that for every 100 calories a person eats beyond their daily needs, the price in terms of food, medical care and gasoline rises anywhere from 48 cents to nearly $2. The more you weigh the higher the cost. Over the long run these food deals end up being no deal at all.

We learned in *The Two Brain Threat* how short term rewards often win over the promise of long term rewards. Finding good food value is a powerful short term reward. Perhaps learning about the high long term cost of cheap food can boost the long term reward part of your decision making process enough to overcome the weight of the short term reward.

Is getting a good deal bad? Not at all. But you need to remember it comes with a cost.

Threat 13. The Stress Threat

You eat fat and sugar under stress because they physically make you feel better.

Imagine you are sitting quietly, reading this book after finishing a nice meal. You look up and notice a lion stalking you. Do you: A) Think, how odd, a lion is about to eat me, but rather than react I'll digest my meal, or B) Forget about all non-essential activities; mobilize every last bit of energy to run!

Hopefully you chose B. But how does your body switch from resting and relaxing to running so quickly? Because stress activates your fight-or-flight response.

When your brain first notices a lion stalking you, it tells your adrenal glands to pump out the stress hormone **cortisol.** Cortisol signals your fat cells to quickly release energy. Your muscles use this energy to boost the "fight-or-flight" response. After you've either outrun the lion, or vanquished it with your trusty spear, your cortisol stays elevated a little while to tell your body to refill its fat stores. Then your cortisol level returns to normal. Your body gets you to refill fat stores by making you crave high-energy comfort foods loaded with fat and sugar.

The whole lion-related stress event was over quickly because you either escaped the lion or became its dinner. But in the modern world, stress never seems to end. We may not face lions anymore, but we do fight a continual stream of worries about mortgages, jobs, traffic, kids, bills, and well, I am sure you have your own list of ferocious worries you could add.

If the stress doesn't end, then levels of cortisol stay high, which both does damage and tells your body to keep on storing fat. A lot of women will store this fat in their belly, which puts them at greater risk of heart disease and stroke.

Persistently high cortisol levels, like you would experience under chronic stress, keep telling your body you need to eat to refuel your energy stores. It also spikes the hormone insulin, which controls blood sugar levels and affects your feelings of hunger and fullness.

Stress makes you want to eat and continual stress makes you want to eat continually. So overeating when chronically stressed is biologically driven, you eat when stressed for a reason.

What do you want to eat? Good healthy food? Of course not! You **want to eat high energy food** to replenish your energy stores and fat and sugar are the high energy foods of choice. If you are under constant stress, you'll have a constant desire to eat high-fat and high-carbohydrate food. The likely result is, you will eat extra calories and gain weight.

But providing high quality energy isn't the only effect eating fat and sugar has on your body. Eating fat and sugar when you are stressed may be the way your body copes with the sometimes overwhelming stress of modern life.

Physiologist Mary Dallman at the University of California, San Francisco, says fat and sugar calm the brain, lowering levels of stress hormones. "That's why we call them comfort foods," she says. **Eating comfort food switches off stress by calming down brain systems linked to anxiety.** It's like a little mini-tranquilizer.

If the temptation to eat junk food wasn't already enough, stress hormones may turn on your brain's reward centers so in times of stress **comfort foods will taste better, making you eat more of them.** Clearly your body wants you to eat high-energy foods in response to stress. You don't have to make up reasons why you like comfort foods, there are good physical reasons for this under stress.

One study in rats showed a hormone called CRF, which humans also release under stress, **tripled their desire for sugar.** University of Michigan psychology professor Kent Berridge, who worked on the study, says:

> *People who feel bad during stress cope in part by overeating or pursuing other incentives. It turns out that a stress chemical also activates the same brain mechanism that goes wrong in drug addiction to make us excessively want pleasurable things. This could* **trap individuals into chasing incentives they could normally resist,** *pulled in by tempting cues or images that become more powerfully wanted.*

In other words, you might normally be able resists that delicious double scoop of your favorite ice cream cone, but when you're under stress, just seeing a glossy color picture of a cone might make it irresistible.

While stress affects us all, women may have a harder time with it. A study conducted by researchers at Rush University Medical Center in Chicago and the University of Pittsburgh has found that **stress can lead to weight gain in women.** "Under stress, people conserve more fat, and we think that is perhaps what's going on here," says the study's lead author, Dr. Tene T. Lewis. Women who reported more negative life events (such as the death of a relative, loss of a job or divorce) at the beginning of the study were more likely to gain weight.

Try not to let this bother you, but your stress over weight loss may cause a **cycle of weight gain.** The cycle goes something like this: losing weight is literally stressful; the stress hormones then make you crave fat and sugar so you'll feel better; eating more fat and sugar cause you to gain weight; you try harder to lose weight. And the cycle starts all over again.

Isn't it amazing how our ancient survival instincts for dealing with lions can go so wrong in our modern environment? Fortunately, there are other ways of dealing with stress. We'll talk about some options in later strategies.

....

Threat 14. The Sleep Threat

People who get only five hours of sleep are 50% more likely to be obese.

You may find this threat hard to believe, but the less you sleep the more you weigh. The numbers go like this:

- ❖ People who slept four hours or less per night were 73% more likely to be obese than those who slept between seven and nine hours each night.
- ❖ People who slept 5 hours per night were 50% more likely to be obese than those who slept between seven and nine hours each night.
- ❖ People who slept 6 hours per night were 23% more likely to be obese than those who slept between seven and nine hours each night.
- ❖ Children who sleep less than 10 hours per day are 2.5 times more likely to be overweight.

The results are a bit counterintuitive. If you sleep less you should be burning more calories. On the other hand, if you sleep less you have more opportunity to eat.

What researches have found though is people who are sleep-deprived have decreased levels of leptin and increased levels of ghrelin released. Remember, leptin tells you brain not to eat and ghrelin tells your brain it's time to eat. With the changes in leptin and ghrelin, you become hungry, eat, and store the excess calories away as fat.

Just getting a good night's sleep may not be enough. A study at the Yale School of Medicine found a link between insomnia and stress. Stress can stimulate you so much that it triggers sleeplessness and, as we've seen, leads to overeating.

Tamas Horvath, the lead author of the study said, "...people with weight and sleep problems could benefit from cutting back on stressful aspects of their lives, rather than trying to specifically medicate either insomnia or obesity." Is there any end to the bad things stress does to us?

An interesting observation is that the obesity trend and the sleeplessness trend might be related. Weight has risen as the modern world has gotten more stressful and people sleep less. It's just a thought.

....

⚠ Threat 15. The Menopause Threat

Women gain on average 5 pounds during menopause; about 20% of women gain 10 pounds or more.

For most women, menopause sets in between the ages of 45 and 50, when a woman stops producing eggs and her monthly period stops. Without a job to do anymore, less of the reproductive hormones estrogen and progesterone are produced.

Menopause is a threat because the Healthy Women's Study found women gained on average **5 pounds** during menopause. About 20% of women gained **10 pounds** or more.

In general, women either gain weight or find maintaining their weight more difficult during menopause. The end result is the number of overweight middle-aged women jumps 12% when compared to women in their 20s and 30s. It doesn't matter if you were thin to start. Women of all sizes are likely to gain weight during menopause.

The reason for this has always been in question. Is it because of lifestyle changes or the radical hormonal changes women experience during menopause? It's probably a bit of both.

Research at the Oregon Health and Science University found evidence that falling hormone levels increase hunger, which leads to rapid weight gain. Lower estrogen may not only affect hunger, but also your metabolism and activity levels.

Other studies have found postmenopausal women to be less active than pre-menopausal women. If you are less active, you are burning fewer calories and will gain weight, especially if menopause makes you hungrier at the same time. The good news is that increasing physical activity can prevent a lot of the weight gain.

This is another area where you are overweight in your own way. Some women gain little during menopause and for some reason other women gain a lot of weight.

Another consequence of reduced estrogen levels is the weight women gain tends to accumulate around their belly rather than around their hips and thighs. Belly fat is associated with higher heart disease risks.

All the strategies in this book will help you mange your weight through menopause. But, one option for treating menopause we won't talk about is Hormone Replacement Therapy. Menopause is a complex subject and you really need to talk to your doctor about treatment options.

 ## Threat 16. The Andropause Threat

Andropause is often called the male version of menopause.

Men go through their own change because of reduced testosterone production. As you age, you lose muscle and that causes you to gain weight. One of the reasons men lose muscle mass is that they produce less testosterone as they grow older. If you notice a "pot belly," "beer belly," or a "spare tire," low testosterone might be part of the cause. Low testosterone is associated with weight gain around the belly.

It's not known how many men have andropause, but testosterone levels are estimated to decline by 1% per year after the age of 50. In some men the decline is much faster. Nearly 50% of men over the age of 80 have lower than normal testosterone levels.

You may have andropause if have less energy, a decreased sense of well-being, a decreased sex drive, weaker erection strength, decreases in strength and muscle mass, changes in height (due to osteoporosis), and increased body fat.

These same symptoms are shared by a lot of medical conditions so, as always, you need to see your doctor to know for sure.

 ## Threat 17. The Growing Old Threat

After 30 you will gain about one pound per year unless you take steps to stop it.

When you are under 30 years old you, can look marvelous without a lot of effort. You are at your peak. After 30 you start having to put in some work to keep it all from going down hill.

The reason is, after 30 you start losing muscle. After 30 an inactive person will lose between ½ and 1 pound of muscle every year. And after 50 the rate of muscle loss becomes much higher. Your strength will decline 15% from 50 to 60 and 30% a decade after the age of 60. Don't stress, you can do something about it.

Why does this matter? It matters for a lot of other reasons, but let's just talk about weight in this book.

About 75% of the calories are burned by your metabolism, not by physical activity. We'll talk about what your metabolism means in more detail later, but in short, your metabolism is all the calories you burn to maintain your body. That includes keeping you warm, digesting food, fighting a cold, thinking, and so on.

Your muscles burn a big chunk of the calories burned by your metabolism. So, when you lose muscle, you burn fewer calories, which makes you gain weight. How many calories will you fail to burn because of muscle loss? A lot.

One pound of fat burns about 4 calories a day. One pound of muscle burns a whopping 50 calories a day. Starting at age 30, if you sit on your butt for 10 years, you'll slow your metabolism down by over 400 calories a day!

That's why, if you do nothing, **you gain about a pound a year** just from aging not so gracefully. Many people turn 40 and wham! They find themselves overweight, even if they have never been overweight before.

Now let's say you go on a diet and lose weight. Congratulations! Not so fast. If you lose weight by just reducing the number of calories you eat, then 25–50% of your weight loss is really muscle loss. Not good.

After losing the weight, your metabolism is actually lower than it was when you started because you have less muscle. This means you need to eat even less than you think, or the weight will pile back on. Perform this cycle—gain weight, lose weight, gain weight, lose weight—a couple of times and you won't have much muscle left at all.

If the problem is muscle loss, then there's an obvious solution: lift weights. Lifting weights keeps the muscle on and can make a dramatic difference in your life. Adding resistance training to your exercise routine will help you lose 44% more fat than if you don't.

The fun thing about adding muscle is that muscle burns calories 24 hours a day. It's like a magic weight loss genie granting your weight loss wishes.

As you grow older, you need to make a special effort to change your strategies to counter the impact of growing older. Hey, growing older is just one more threat to your diet. You can beat it, especially if you use a dumb bell!

Threat 18. The Race Threat
Some races are at a higher risk of obesity than others.

African women, Native Americans, South Asians, Pacific Islanders and Aboriginal Australians are all at a higher risk of obesity than Europeans.

Black women, for example, for reasons we still don't completely understand, become obese more than twice as fast as white women. Hispanic women become obese at a rate about midway between black and white women. "We found Hispanic men became obese 2.5 times faster than U.S. men of European ancestry," said Dr. Kathleen M. McTigue, a Robert Wood Johnson clinical scholar at the UNC School of Medicine. "We saw no difference in the rate of obesity development between black and non-Hispanic white men until after age 28, when black men in this country became obese 2.2 times more rapidly than white men."

You want some more startling statistics? Sixty-six percent of African-American women are overweight and 37% are technically obese. The statistics for Mexican-American women are similar. Forty-nine percent of Caucasian women are considered overweight and 24% are obese. It's hard not to notice the rates are high for everyone, but the rates for non-Caucasians are significantly higher.

What is the difference among races?

As you might expect, the explanations aren't simple and as with everything concerning race, they can be controversial.

As you read this section, there will be a lot of references to particular races and genders because those are the subjects of the studies. That doesn't mean other races don't have the same problem to one degree or another, it just means I don't know about the research or that it hasn't been done yet.

▌ Black Women are Naturally Hungrier

Black women were found to have significantly higher levels of the hunger hormone ghrelin after eating than white women.

We've talked about the ghrelin hormone in other threats. Ghrelin is the message your stomach sends to your brain saying, "It's time to eat." It makes you hungry. And if you are hungrier you'll naturally eat more.

So ghrelin and other hormones may differ by race. Hopefully more research will help clear things up.

▌ Black Women Have More Cortisol

Black women were found to have higher levels of cortisol than white women. If you remember from the discussion of cortisol in *The Stress Threat,* cortisol is associated with weight gain.

▌ Discrimination Leads to Stress

Experiencing poor treatment because of your race or gender increases stress levels. And as we've seen, stress is associated with obesity.

▌ More Likely to be Inactive

More than 25% of women are not active at all. African Americans and Hispanics are more likely than whites to be physically inactive. If you aren't burning calories through physical activity, then you'll find it really hard to maintain your weight.

▌ Insulin Resistance Related Obesity

Insulin resistance (IR) is linked to heart disease, diabetes, high blood pressure, **and obesity.** IR is important because it seems that a lot of people have it.

Researcher Philippe Froguel from the Pasture Institute in Lille, France, and colleagues from the Imperial College London, have found a hereditary gene mutation that causes IR. What's amazing is this faulty gene is present in up to 20% of Caucasians and 50% of black people.

Other studies have found 47% of black women of normal weight to have insulin resistance, compared to less than 20% of the Hispanic or Caucasian women. Usually, obesity has been thought to contribute to IR; now it's found even black women of normal weight have high rates of IR.

And researchers at Cedars-Sinai Medical Center, in collaboration with investigators at UCLA, have found a gene that is linked to insulin resistance in Mexican-Americans.

So, a lot of people have IR. **What is IR and why does it matter?**

When you eat, your body releases the hormone insulin to tell your cells to soak up the sugar (glucose) in your blood you get from eating. Insulin resistance is when your cells don't listen to the insulin message and the sugar stays in your blood stream.

There's has been a lot of debate whether IR causes obesity or is the result of obesity. Philippe Froguel thinks their study shows that IR might be a cause of obesity, not just be a consequence of obesity.

The idea is that all the extra glucose in your blood stream is soaked up by the fat-storing adipose tissue, which becomes layers of fat, leading to obesity.

IR also impairs the release of insulin, which leads to increased risk of Type II diabetes. The researchers didn't find any evidence of behavioral changes, but as insulin plays an important role in controlling appetite, there might be some impact.

Froguel says the mutated gene may have an effect on the brain, causing people not to feel as full. He says the effect won't cause people to always feel hungry, but be more subtle.

But as usual with genes, there are environmental factors that cause the genes to kick in earlier than they might otherwise. Froguel found that younger generations were getting IR much earlier than the older generations, most likely from a lack of exercise and eating sugary foods.

▌ Individual Differences in Weight Loss and Weight Gain

Even if we all ate exactly the same food, in exactly the same environment, and exercised exactly the same amount, we would all respond differently. Even identical twins respond differently to all these factors.

For example, researchers from East Carolina University found African-American women burned 30% less fat during low-intensity exercise, like walking, than do Caucasians. This might help explain why African-American women have been found to have a slower rate of weight loss than Caucasians.

But it goes deeper than just saying African-American women are different from Caucasian women. **We are all different.**

Research has shown that not everyone responds to exercise the same way. You can put in the work, but you may not get as much out of it as the person walking on the treadmill right next to you. Some people are more likely to store energy as fat, while others are more likely to convert it into lean tissue. Some people lose weight more easily than others. Sometime the differences can be dramatic.

We are all overweight in our way. You'll have to do some experimentation to figure out what works best for you and how you need to overcome the challenges your body has created for you.

▌ The Thrifty Gene

The "thrifty gene" is the idea that there's a set of genes that allow people to utilize food more efficiently, and rapidly gain weight when food is available. If you had these genes you would be much more likely to survive the next famine. But these genes would also make you an ideal candidate for obesity when put in an environment where lots of food is available.

This may be why we now see high rates of obesity and diabetes in Pacific Islanders, Native Americans, Aboriginal Australians, and other native populations. The people who survived famines were the people who had the thrifty gene, so all their descendants are more likely to have it too. The thrifty gene probably isn't one gene, but is many different genes.

One explanation for racial difference in obesity rates is that groups who historically suffered the most starvation are the most prone to become obese in our modern environment. People whose ancestors moved away from the hunter-gatherer lifestyle and adopted agriculture have had longer to adapt to the dietary changes brought on by agriculture. So, people descended from Western societies would be at less risk from obesity in our modern environment.

And the reason we might see more diabetes and obesity in America versus Europe, even for similarly weighted people, is that the people who immigrated to America were the poorer people, more likely to have the thrifty gene. The people who stayed in Europe were richer and thus had better access to food, so it's less likely they had the thrifty gene. This is just a theory, nobody knows for sure.

This is a hard hitting threat. It may seem almost inevitable you'll gain weight. But this threat is just another problem you can solve. You can still create your perfect weight loss plan.

· ·

Threat 19. The Womb Threat

Your appetite may have been programmed in your mother's womb.

Your mother's diet while you were in her womb can permanently change your appetite levels and where fat is deposited on your body, all the way into adulthood.

Who would have thought that either increased or decreased levels of nutrition before birth could lead to an increased risk of obesity? Until recently, not many people would have thought it possible, but it looks to be true. If your mom ate too much or too little, you may be "programmed" to have a higher chance of obesity, diabetes, high blood pressure and heart disease.

And you are not affected just by your mother's diet. You may also be affected by your grandmother's diet! This research was on rats; time will tell if it applies to humans too. The research showed the grandchildren of rats fed an inadequate diet during pregnancy were more likely to become obese and insulin resistant. Amazing.

It's not just diet. Smoking can "program" you for obesity too. If **your mother smoked** you have a higher chance of being obese. By age 33, the children of smokers had about a 40% higher chance of being obese than the children of non-smokers.

Early evidence for *The Womb Threat* came from tragic circumstances.

During the winter of 1944–1945, Dutch citizens experienced a period of starvation called the Dutch Hunger Winter. The German administration put an embargo on all food transports to the western Netherlands. It was a harsh winter and adults found it difficult to find more than 1,000 calories of food a day. Approximately 30,000 people starved to death before the famine ended in 1945.

Some good did come out of this horrible situation. The Dutch kept excellent medical records, which allowed for a very interesting study on how the mothers' nutritional levels affected the health of their children.

What they found was fascinating. Mothers exposed to famine in the first two trimesters had children who were heavier over their lifetime than the children of mothers who didn't face famine or who faced famine in the third trimester. Not only were they heavier, they had a lot of other health problems too.

The idea is that the fetus adapts to a limited supply of nutrients, which permanently alters its physiology and metabolism, which could increase the risk of disease and obesity in later life.

How can this happen? A fetus and its mother share the same environment. It's easy to see how if the mother isn't getting enough calories then the fetus can't get enough calories. But there's more to it. The mother's hormones can reach the fetus too. And the mother's hormones can change the development of the fetus.

That's why these effects can be passed generation to generation without involving genetic changes. Stress is a good example of this chain of events. If the mother is under stress, the fetus may be programmed to be more sensitive to stress. Once born, the child will grow up to be a more stressed adult. And the cycle can start all over again. No genetic changes are involved at all.

As surprising as it sounds, obesity can start in the womb.

Threat 20. The Hypothyroid Threat

Hypothyroidism contributes modestly to obesity by slowing your metabolic rate.

Your thyroid gland is a small butterfly-shaped structure located in the front of your neck. Its job is to make a substance called **thyroid hormone,** which helps to regulate your body's metabolism.

Your thyroid gland doesn't always work perfectly. Sometimes it can make either too much thyroid hormone, which is called hyperthyroidism, or too little, which is called hypothyroidism. We'll only be talking about hypothyroidism in this threat, since it is the problem associated with weight gain.

Hypothyroidism means that your thyroid gland can't make enough thyroid hormone to keep the body running normally. As many as 10% of women and 3% of men have hypothyroidism.

What does the thyroid hormone do for you?

Low thyroid hormone levels slow your body's processes down. You may notice that you feel colder, you tire more easily, your skin is getting drier, you're becoming forgetful and depressed, you may be constipated, and you may gain weight.

With a slower metabolism, your body doesn't burn as many calories, which means you'll gain weight and find it harder to lose weight. The double whammy is that you feel tired, which means you'll probably exercise less than you otherwise would.

The only way to know for sure whether you have hypothyroidism is with blood tests. Please see a doctor if this sounds like you.

⚠ **Threat 21. The Nontaster Threat**

Supertasters are thinner than nontasters.

Taste buds are little structures on your tongue that send information to your brain about the taste of food as you eat. Everyone has a different number of taste buds, though the average is about 10,000.

Interestingly, the number of your taste buds has a profound effect on which foods you think will taste good and which foods you think will taste bad. And which foods you prefer strongly influences how heavy you become.

People are divided into taster types based on the number of taste buds they have on their tongue. The types are: nontaster, medium taster, and supertaster. About 25% of people are supertasters, 50% are medium tasters and 25% are nontasters.

Nontasters have very few taste buds. Supertasters have 10 times the number of taste buds as nontasters and have taste experiences at three to five times the level of the other taster types.

With their vast number of taste buds, supertasters are more sensitive to bitter, sweet and fat flavors. How does this help you stay thin? If you are sensitive to a taste, then you'll stop eating it sooner because you'll become over stimulated by the flavor. A supertaster may find sweets too sweet and stop eating. A supertaster may eat less of fatty foods like cream because it's too greasy for them. It's not hard to imagine how this helps keep your weight down.

A nontaster on the other hand will love fatty foods and sweets like cotton candy. They can eat anything and everything. It's not hard to imagine how this helps you gain weight.

You can see how your taster type makes a difference in real life by a study testing to see if the different taster types could distinguish between a salad dressing with 40% fat and one with 10% fat. From a calorie point of view that's a big difference.

They found medium tasters and supertasters could tell the difference between the two salad dressings, but the nontasters could not. More importantly, for weight loss purposes, the nontasters liked the higher fat dressing more. The medium tasters and supertasters liked either dressing.

Imagine what this means over a lifetime of eating. If you like either dressing, you can pick the lower fat dressing without losing any satisfaction from your meal. To experience the same amount of satisfaction, the nontaster picks the higher calorie dressing. Over a lifetime, all those simple decisions add up to a huge number of additional calories for the nontaster.

Surprisingly, your taste bud count is traceable to a single gene. A simple genetic difference in the number of taste buds you have can impact your weight. Amazing, isn't it?

To Learn More

❖   There is a test on our website to determine which kind of taster you are.

Threat 22. The Fast Stomach Threat

How quickly food empties out of your stomach is related to overeating.

There is evidence showing that overeating can be related to how quickly food empties out of your stomach. Obese people have been found to have faster emptying stomachs. The thought is the faster food leaves your stomach the less of a chance your body has to know it should be full. This means you will be hungrier, eat more, and eat your next meal sooner.

Without complicated tests, you won't know if you have a fast stomach, so it's just another way we are all overweight in our own way.

Another interesting possible threat is that in many studies obese people have been found to have **larger stomachs.** A larger stomach means you will eat more before feeling full. The evidence on stomach size and obesity is mixed or I would have made it its own threat, but there was a strong enough case for it that it should be mentioned.

It's fascinating to think how such simple reasons like having a fast or big stomach could explain at least some of why you are overweight.

 Threat 23. The Gumption Threat

Your ability to resist temptation is reduced each time you use it.

It takes continual concentrated effort to resist temptation. You can't just resist temptation once and be done with it. You have to resist temptation each and every time for the resistance to be effective. And with food temptation all around, we have a lot of temptation to resist.

Most of us probably assume willpower to be in infinite supply and we can always resist temptation. But what if that's not true? What if willpower came from a well holding only a limited supply? What if using a bit of willpower, in the form of self control, left just that much less willpower in the well for you to use to resist the next temptation?

That's what Professor of Psychology, Roy Baumeister, has found in his research. Your ability to resist temptation is weakened each time you use it. Baumeister speculates that we have a sort of mental energy, like physical energy, that drains away when we use it.

In one test, a group of students were asked to resist eating chocolate chip cookies and eat a radish instead. Another group was given permission to eat the cookies and didn't have to resist any temptation. The group that had to resist temptation gave up faster on a difficult puzzle when compared to students who were given permission to eat the cookies. It's as if resisting the cookies used up bits of the students' gumption so they were less able to put forth the effort necessary to solve the puzzle.

Let's say you have spent all day resisting the continual attack of advertisements on the radio, TV, and magazines. Then you resist all the smells and sights of food assaulting you at work, at school, in stores, and in all the shops that you pass while driving. How much mental energy do you think you have left as the day goes by? Is it any wonder you eventually give in to your cravings?

Many of the strategies, especially the Weight-Proofing strategies, help keep your will power well full of mental energy by removing temptation from your life.

....

Threat 24. The Food-Free Threat

You can gain weight without overeating.

We've always been told we gain weight because we eat too much. Timothy Kieffer, a University of British Columbia researcher, has found that's not always true. He found how an "imbalance in the action of the leptin hormone" can cause obesity and major disturbances in blood sugar levels—**even when eating normal food levels.** It is thought the problem causes an over-production of insulin, which leads to putting on more fat. This process is independent of overeating.

I'd love to tell you more about this threat, but it's a new area of research. Hopefully we'll learn more later.

This threat is a good example of how we are each overweight in our own way. We don't know how many people have this problem. Even if it's only a few, they could be tearing themselves up over their weight problems when it's really just how they are built.

Chapter 7

Threats from the Power of Food
Threats 25–32

This chapter is a collection of threats rooted in the ideas we talked about in *The Power of Food Threat*. Food has an undeniable power to tempt you off your diet. In this chapter you'll learn all about the vast number of ways you are influenced by food.

⚠ **Threat 25. The Eat When Food Is Available Threat**

In the modern world you are rarely hungry, yet you can almost always be seduced into eating.

You naturally eat when food is available. Since food is almost always available for us, it's not surprising people prone to obesity are overweight.

Why would you be built to eat when food becomes available? **Survival.** In humanity's past, food supplies were scarce and unpredictable, so humans needed to eat all the food they could when food became available. Any excess calories are stored as precious fat reserves for use later. Not eating would be foolish and potentially deadly.

Why would you have this incredible ability to store nearly unlimited amounts of fat if you didn't also have the ability to overeat? If you couldn't eat more when you were full, there would be very little chance of you eating enough to store excess calories as fat.

Many studies show that you will eat when food becomes available, even if you think you are full, even after a big meal. And when a food tastes good, you will naturally keep on eating, even when full.

Another piece of evidence can be found in how often you eat. Do you ever go long without eating? Probably not. Do you think you only eat when you are really hungry or when you really need energy? It's unlikely. You probably eat on a fairly regular schedule even when you don't need the energy and there's no reason for you to be hungry. So you already know you can eat a lot of food when you don't need to.

Even stranger, you will eat even when you are overweight and don't need any additional weight. And stranger still, you will eat when you desperately don't want to eat more. How can this be?

Passing up available food doesn't make sense from a survival perspective. For most of human history, humans did not have a way to store food. There was no refrigerator or grocery store.

Your natural food storage mechanism is to eat and store the excess as fat. Later, when food is scarce, the fat is used for energy and survival. As there was rarely too much food, obesity wasn't a problem. Preventing you from becoming too fat was never a capability the human body had to develop.

When I put it this way, can you imagine your body not having a way to make you eat when food becomes available? It makes no sense to think otherwise.

The end result is you eat when food is available and because food is always available you can eat all the time. This is one role the environment plays in obesity. If the environment didn't have an endless supply of food, then you couldn't eat it and you couldn't become overweight.

. . . .

Threat 26. The Boredom Threat

A reason people often give for going off their diet is that they are bored.

When you are at home and bored, do you drop by the refrigerator to check if there is anything good to eat?

I know I do. Intuitively, most of us would say boredom is a big part of why we eat, but there have been surprisingly few studies showing a relationship between boredom and weight. Perhaps researchers think it is just obvious.

One study did find that when people were bored they ate more. And another study found the reason most people gave for going off their diet was boredom.

What could boredom have to do with eating? In one bizarre study, researchers found overweight people may have a **different sense of time when bored.** They found that, when bored, overweight people experience a slower passage of time, which leads them to eat sooner because they think it's time to eat again.

What else about boredom could lead you to eat? I think it's because of what we talked about in *The Power of Food Threat:* **food has power.** Food in your house is like a giant neon sign saying "come eat me," especially when you don't have other thoughts to crowd out the thoughts of eating.

Your brain isn't stupid. Your brain knows where the food is and is drawn to it because it wants a reward. Your brain wants to feel satisfied and food makes people feel satisfied, especially those people with fewer dopamine receptors and a biology that makes food more pleasurable.

If you are one of us, then food isn't just a small little neon sign, it's more like the spotlight at a red carpet premiere of a Hollywood blockbuster movie. When you are bored, the spotlight zooms in on the refrigerator and you walk the red carpet, open the door to the fridge, and you do what comes naturally...eat.

You are drawn to the fridge because food activates a common mechanism in your brain for getting your brain what it wants. What your brain wants isn't exactly sugar or fat or salt or sex, what it really wants is another shot of dopamine. Dopamine is how your brain knows what is important and how it knows what it should learn to help you survive.

Food is just one of the ways your brain can get dopamine, it has other ways. You can get dopamine from interaction with friends, art, music, shopping, and of course, drugs.

But have you noticed how the feeling of satisfaction you get from food and other activities doesn't last? You get a quick hit of a sense of well-being and then it goes away. If the pleasure didn't fade quickly, you would probably die because you wouldn't want to do anything other than what brought you the amazing sense of well-being.

From a survival perspective, you can't stay too interested in any one pursuit for too long. You have to keep chasing satisfaction. Satisfaction doesn't stick around and you can't save it in a bank for later.

What happens when the sources of satisfaction in your life become fewer and fewer? You lock on tighter to the sources of satisfaction you have left. This is why you can become addicted to anything supplying a hit of dopamine. Drugs like cocaine work through dopamine, but dopamine is released by a lot of things, not just drugs.

If you had a lot going on in your life that interested you, the spotlight couldn't shine on just one source of satisfaction. It would have to flit from one source of satisfaction to another. But if your only satisfaction is food, then the spotlight will shine so bright and hot on food you won't be able to ignore it.

Food can become your whole world without anything being broken in your body at all. All you need is a small enough world where food is your best source of satisfaction.

....

Threat 27. The Finish Your Plate Threat

You eat what is put in front of you. The more food available, the more you eat.

The sad simple fact is you try to eat as much food as is put in front of you. It's not just the voice of mom in your head telling you to clean your plate. From a survival point of view this makes perfect sense, from a diet point of view it's a disaster.

A study by Dr. Brian Wansink at Cornell University found portion sizes are as big a factor in how much you eat as is taste. For example, moviegoers ate 50% more popcorn from a big bucket than when they ate from a smaller bucket. They ate more even when the popcorn was stale and horrible tasting!

Just using a bigger bucket encouraged people to eat more popcorn. And the key is the people didn't even realize they were eating more. In fact, they thought they would eat the same amount no matter what size container they ate from. People have no idea they unconsciously eat more from large containers and over a whole lifetime this can have a big impact on weight.

Other studies show people don't even notice when they are given 50% or even 100% more food. This conclusion is backed up by study after study. It doesn't matter how hungry you are: **you eat more food when you are served more food.**

Imagine it's 25,000 years ago and you bagged a deer. You couldn't store the deer for later, so you had to eat as much as you could. If your body stopped you from eating when food was available, that would be the real problem.

▌ You Eat More from Bigger Packages

Dr. Barbara Rolls, a nutritionist at Pennsylvania State University, found in her research that you'll eat a lot more calories when package sizes are increased.

In a snack study, participants were given a snack of potato chips in an unlabeled opaque package on different days in five different sizes ranging from 1 to 6 ounces.

Do you think people will eat more from the larger package of potato chips? If you said yes, why would that be? If you are hungry, shouldn't you just eat until you stop feeling hungry? If how much you eat depends on the package size, wouldn't that imply hunger has a lot less with how much you eat than you might think?

It turns out package size does matter. A lot.

Men ate 311 more calories and women ate 184 more calories from the largest bag of chips than they did from the smallest package.

In a similar study using sandwiches instead of potato chips, it was found men ate an extra 355 calories and women ate an extra 159 calories when they ate the largest sandwich compared to the smallest sandwich.

Perhaps it's not just hunger that determines how much you eat. Perhaps there are many more subtle and deeper mechanisms at work.

▌ Your Stomach Doesn't Count Calories

Amazing research by Dr. Wansink has shown **people use their eyes to count calories,** not their stomach. Your stomach doesn't count calories for you. You need accurate **visual cues** to prevent unintentional overeating. And because food disappears while you are eating, keeping track of how much you have already eaten can be tricky.

One fascinating study found that people would eat 73% more soup when eating from a self-refilling soup bowl. In this clever study, people ate soup, but the soup level didn't go down in the bowl. The bowl kept refilling! As the people ate they couldn't tell how much soup they had eaten, so they just kept on eating and eating.

Without the visual evidence of the quantity of food you are eating, you will eat a tremendous amount more than you would otherwise. Your stomach won't tell you to stop eating until after you have overeaten.

▌ Eating What You See is Called Unit Bias

Andrew Geier, of the University of Pennsylvania, performed a number of experiments that all confirmed the same basic idea: **you eat what you view as a unit, independent of the actual size or number of servings.**

"Whatever size a banana is, that's what you eat, a small banana or a big banana," says Geier. And "whatever is served on your plate, it just seems locked in our heads: that's a meal.

"In terms of food, unit bias applies to what people think is the appropriate amount to consume, and it shows why smaller portion sizes can be just as satisfying," said Geier. "A 12-ounce can of soda and a 24-ounce bottle are both seen as single units. But be careful, the 24-ounce bottle, though viewed as one unit, is actually more than two and a half servings of soda."

In one experiment they put a large bowl with a pound of M&Ms® in the lobby of an upscale apartment building. Below the bowl hung the sign: "Eat Your Fill…please use the spoon to serve yourself." Sometimes the bowl had a small serving spoon and other times it had a much larger serving spoon.

And just like we've seen with Dr. Rolls's and Dr. Wansink's research, people consistently took a lot more M&Ms when using the larger spoon.

The unit bias doesn't always work. If people are served what is considered less than the normal serving size, they will go back for more.

Are you more satisfied with more food?

Not really. Rolls performed an experiment in a restaurant where on one day they served a standard size portion of pasta and on the next day they served a larger portion with 50% more pasta. They kept the entire meal identical, including the price.

What was the result? People ate nearly all the larger portion and they ate more of the side dishes as well. All-in-all people ate 172 more calories when eating the larger meal than when eating the small portion. You'll gain 17 extra pounds a year if you eat the larger portion size every day, for just one meal!

Survey responses show that the diners thought both the small and larger portions were appropriate. So they didn't feel cheated by either meal.

That's OK, you might say, but in these studies people ate more food yet they didn't report feeling more satisfied. People didn't even notice when they were served more food.

Surprisingly, you will feel just as satisfied with smaller amounts of food.

The conclusion: **eating more doesn't make you happier.**

Threat 28. The Snack Threat

The more snacks you eat, the more total calories you eat, up to 830 calories more per day.

Obese men who ate one snack a day consumed 330 more calories than obese men who didn't eat any snacks. Eating two snacks a day added an additional 448 calories per day. And eating three snacks per day added an additional **830 calories** per day.

A similar increase of calories was found for women, though the number of calories added was lower.

The lesson is: **snacks don't replace food from later meals,** but are additional food you eat in a day. If you have a snack you'll still eat a full meal later too.

Deciding to eat a snack is deciding to eat more total calories for the day. It's certainly your choice to make, but people often think a snack won't add calories because they think they'll just eat less later. Unfortunately that's not true.

And what do you eat when you snack? Carrots? Nope, you eat sweet, fatty foods. The amount of chips, crackers, popcorn and pretzels consumed has nearly tripled from the mid-1970s.

Threat 29. The Craving Threat

Almost everyone has cravings. Cravings continually tempt you to fall off your diet.

Most of us crave foods at one time or another. Almost 100% of young women and nearly 70% of young men said they have experienced cravings during the past year. Cravings can easily make you snack and go off your diet, which can in turn cause you to quit your diet completely.

You might think cravings are just silly thoughts stuck in your head. But they are much more than that.

University of Pennsylvania researchers used functional magnetic resonance imaging (fMRI) to show that food cravings activate brain areas related to emotion, memory and reward—areas also activated during drug craving studies. The study lead Marcia Levin Pelchat, PhD says, "This is consistent with the idea that cravings of all kinds, whether for food, drugs, or designer shoes, have common mechanisms."

Dr. Pelchat goes on to say, "During a craving we have a sensory memory or template for the food that will satisfy the craving. The food we eat has to match that template for the craving to be satisfied. It's as if our brain is saying 'It has to be chocolate ice cream, lemon pie just won't do.' ...Cravings are also like habits. We often reach for a craved food without thinking of it."

By trying to totally avoid certain foods, people tend to over-consume them in the end when the craving becomes too great to resist.

....

Threat 30. The Calorie Bomb Threat

You will eat far more calories than you realize when eating high fat and high sugar foods.

Telling people to "eat less" isn't the whole story on weight loss because it's not just large portion sizes that make you overweight. How many calories are in the food you eat matters just as much. It's possible to eat less while eating more calories. And it's also possible to eat more while eating fewer calories.

How many calories a particular amount of food has is called its *energy density*. Water, for example, has the lowest energy density because it has 0 calories for any weight of water. Fat has the highest energy density because it has the most calories.

Why does energy density matter? Dr. Barbara Rolls has found in her research that, over the course of a day or two, you will tend to eat about the same volume of food, regardless of its energy density or the number of calories in it.

This is probably related to the fact that your stomach needs a certain volume and weight of food before it will send the "I'm full" signal to your brain. You'll most likely eat until your stomach has enough food in it to send this signal.

Volume simply means the amount of space the food takes. What Rolls is saying is pretty interesting: you'll consistently try to eat the same volume of food. So picture how big a salad you need to make you full. Now picture how many candy bars you would need to eat to fill the same volume as the salad. Which has more calories, the salad or the candy bars?

This is the key point of the threat. You will have to eat a lot more high energy density foods to reach a satisfying volume of food. And what are the high density foods? Junk foods. Foods chock-full of fat and sugar.

If you eat foods with a lot of calories in a little package, then you will eat far more calories than you realize. But if you limit yourself to smaller portions of high-calorie foods, you will end up feeling deprived and hungry and the chances are you'll fall off your diet. It's a no win situation.

The calorie bomb is when you **eat large portions of junk foods.** You'll eat more to reach the necessary volume of food. The total number of calories you eat skyrockets.

In one study, students ate over 1,600 calories in a single meal at a food court. That's about 62% of the recommended daily intake. There was no way they realized how many calories they were eating. Combining large portions of high energy density foods is a sure diet killer.

In another study, women were served a casserole in three different sizes and two different energy density levels. You can easily lower the energy density of a casserole, for example by replacing cheese with more vegetables. This will keep the volume of the dish the same, but it will have fewer calories.

Amazingly, the **women were just as full from the smaller** low density casserole as they were from the larger high density casserole. Now get this, the large high density dish had 620 calories and the small low density dish had 398 calories. So you can save 220 calories by eating the smaller lower density meal and you will feel just as full!

Another variation on this theme is that by eating a large salad as the first course of a meal, you can eat significantly fewer calories in total. Eating a salad fills you up so you'll eat fewer calories from later courses. You may have heard this advice before. This works because you feel full by eating larger portions of a lower energy density food—the salad. You need to eat a certain volume of food and the salad helps you reach that volume for fewer calories. Eating the same volume in steak or pasta would be a lot more calories.

In another study, Dr. Rolls found that increasing the amounts of **fruits and vegetables in meals** could **reduce your total daily calorie intake by more than 400 calories a day.** And you won't feel hungry. That's amazing stuff.

And the advantages just keep on coming. Researchers have also found that eating vegetables and fruits make you stay fuller longer. You can keep hunger away by simply adding a few more veggies to your meals.

In another interesting finding by Dr. Rolls, men eating a low energy dense diet ate 425 less calories and women eating a low energy dense diet ate 275 fewer calories when compared to people eating a higher calorie density diet. People on the low energy density diet ate significantly more food too.

Dr. Rolls found people with normal weight had diets with lower energy densities than did the obese people. And the people who ate more fruit and vegetables had the lowest energy density diets and the lowest obesity rates.

Now, why might some people eat higher density diets than others? We talked about why some people are attracted to junk food in *The Power of Food Threat* and *The Stress Threat*. But many others simply haven't heard of this amazing research.

You don't need to eat small portions to lose weight. You can eat satisfying portions of lower energy density foods. You don't have to starve yourself. You can change your diet, eat more, lose weight, and still feel full. What at deal! Knowing how your body works can teach you a lot about how you can have the best of all worlds.

···

 # Threat 31. The Devil's Bargain Threat
Food tastes better than being thin feels.

Many of us try to lose weight because we think we should, rather than because we really want to. We hear that being obese is bad for our heart. We would like to look better. But when it comes down to it: **food tastes better than being thin feels.** So we accept the devil's bargain: **experience the pleasure of food now and worry about health later.**

Why would anyone accept the devil's bargain? Is it really a bad deal?

Food is the number one pleasure in many people's lives. Tasty food is cheap. We can eat what we want when we want. Food is always available. There is a huge variety of tempting food for us to choose from. Food is less complicated than pleasure from love or sex. Food links us socially at work and with family. Even our body conspires to make food our primary source of fun by being able to convert food directly into pleasure. Food is a legal indulgence. **Food is the perfect drug.**

Except for one thing: we know obesity leads to all kinds of health problems. The result of our rising weights is that for the first time in generations children may die sooner than their parents.

As with any deal, it's up to you to decide if it is worth the cost. As an adult you can make the choice for yourself, but as a parent you are also making the choice for your child. **Is obesity a good deal for your child?** That's a much trickier question for you to answer.

Threat 32. The Pink Elephant Threat

People who limit the types of foods they can eat end up eating significantly more than those who don't.

Quick, try not to think of a pink elephant. What do you think of? A pink elephant of course. That's what it's like going on a diet. Simply planning to go on a diet can trigger overeating. Research has found that people who limit the types of foods they can eat end up eating significantly more food than those people who don't.

As soon as you are told you can't eat something, you want it all the more. When people are told they can't have a food it often increases their preference for it. It doesn't matter if it's you or someone else telling you that you can't have a food. This seems a little odd, but people don't like being told what to do, even when they are doing the telling.

Restrict yourself from a food and you start thinking about it. You start craving it. And the cravings eventually become strong enough you fall of your diet. You might find yourself throwing your hands up and saying to yourself "I'll eventually break my diet anyway, so I should just enjoy myself and pig out."

To make the situation worse, when people go on a diet they usually plan their meals around a small selection of boring foods. This triggers cravings. A monotonous diet has been shown to lead to large increases in the number of food cravings. And once you experience cravings the same cycle we talked about previously happens and you fall of your diet.

The craving for food is no joke. These are the same cravings people have for drugs and they are extremely powerful causes of relapse in drug addicts. When you crave food and fall off your diet it's like a drug addict relapsing and going back to drug use.

Chapter 8

Chapter 8

Threats from the Power of Rest
Threats 33–35

This chapter is a collection of threats rooted in the ideas we talked about in *The Power of Rest Threat*. Staying on a diet would be so much easier if we had the same drive to exercise as we do to eat. But we don't, and these threats show some of the diet destroying implications of staying at rest.

⚠ Threat 33. The Lost Exercise Threat

You probably won't consciously exercise over an hour each day, so you need a plan that doesn't depend on unrealistically high levels of exercise.

Why not just control your weight with exercise? That's how our ancestors controlled did it the past, why can't we do it now? Well, we can. And if that works for you then great. Whatever works.

Unfortunately, it may not be realistic for most people to use exercise alone to control their weight. Why do I say that? Because of the high amount of exercise necessary to maintain weight without using other measures. Let's take a look at why.

In our past we exercised much more. In order to survive, it was nearly impossible to eat enough to become obese. This was still true 100 years ago and was mostly true as little as 50 years ago. Today we can survive while doing almost nothing, which means **how much we eat becomes the key driver for obesity.**

The best estimates are that people 25,000 years ago, a period of time called the late Paleolithic, on average burned about 1,240 calories a day in physical activity. Your average American is thought to burn up an average of 555 calories a day.

More modern non-industrial people burned about the same number of calories as did those in the late Paleolithic. For example, lumberjacks could burn up to an amazing 10,000 calories a day. Growing up in Oregon, I lived next to lumberjacks and they worked hard and had the muscles to prove it. Fortunately, through the miracle of modern technology, most of our lives are much easier.

So each day we burn about 700 calories less than our ancient ancestors. I thought the difference would have been greater. I thought our ancestors would have burned far more calories than we do, but they didn't really.

One reason for the relatively small difference in calories burned is the surprising fact that exercise doesn't burn as many calories as you might think. Walking a mile burns about 100 calories. The difference between us moderns and our ancestors is that they walked 6 or 7 miles more than we do each day.

But our ancestors did a lot more than walk. They were the **ultimate cross-trainers.** They didn't just lift weights or run marathons, they did a bit of everything: walk gathering food, walk while hunting, walk when visiting neighboring camps, run after prey, carry children, carry game, carry roots and nuts home, carry water, carry firewood, make shelters, gather plants, make tools and clothes, prepare food, shell nuts, clean, butcher animals, dig for roots and tubers, train in survival skills, participate in ceremonies, gossip, groom, and play.

So, what did you do today? Not much? Me either.

It turns out people who are successful at losing weight and maintaining their weight loss have a lot in common with our more active ancestors: **they exercise.**

There's a registry of people who have lost significant amounts of weight and have kept it off for long periods of time, it's called the National Weight Control Registry.

Successful weight maintainers in the National Weight Control Registry burn an average of 2,817 calories per week on exercise. Exercise means any physical activity, not just time spent in a gym. It could be housework, taking the stairs, or in short, any physical activity.

This translates to an average of about 60 minutes of exercise a day, which is more than most recommendations for exercise. There's an interesting argument over how much exercise is enough. Different organizations make different recommendations.

It's commonly recommended to exercise 30 minutes at a moderate intensity five or more times a week. A moderate intensity is walking or jogging at 4–5 miles an hour, which is actually pretty fast. In the military you are supposed to maintain a speed of 3 miles per hour while carrying heavy gear.

For weight loss and weight maintenance purposes, 30 minutes a day may not be enough, though it is still an excellent target for overall health benefits. This is another one of those "you are overweight in your own way" issues. Some people can get by with almost no exercise, others will find 30 minutes a day enough, and for others 30 minutes a day isn't close to enough.

That's why some organizations recommend for weight loss and weight maintenance you need to burn a minimum of 2,500 calories a week from exercise. That works out to about 7 hours of brisk walking per week or about **60–90 minutes per day** of moderate intensity physical activity.

The recommendation for 60 minutes of daily exercise is in line with what the successful weight maintainers in the National Weight Control Registry do, so I'm inclined to think it is a more realistic target than 30 minutes of exercise a day.

At first blush, 60 minutes a day doesn't seem like a lot of exercise. You might think to yourself "Oh, I can do that." But when you actually go to do the exercise it's quite a bit.

It's too much exercise for me and I suspect it's too much for a lot of other people too. Again, if you will exercise that much, then more power to you. Exercise has so many benefits it's an undeniably great strategy for those who can pursue it.

Realistically, most people won't consciously choose to **exercise over an hour every day.** Given most people hardly exercise at all I don't feel this is a very bold statement.

If only people would exercise then everything would be great. We could spend all our time on if-onlys if we wanted to. I hate if-onlys. We can if-only ourselves out of any problem, yet nothing will ever be solved. If-only people weren't so lazy. If-only people wouldn't do this or if-only people wouldn't do that.

Playing the if-only game doesn't work and it's a frustrating waste of time. Any solution must be based on what people can and will actually do in the real world.

Don't get me wrong, exercise is an important part of this book. It's hard to lose and maintain your weight without exercise, but large daily blocks of exercise are not a winning diet strategy for many people.

It turns out you don't have to set aside time for a formal exercise session for it to be counted as exercise. For instance, walking from your car to the store counts as physical activity. Many strategies will make good use of little bits of natural exercise like walking to the store. It all adds up.

··

Threat 34. The Convenience Threat

Convenience shapes the world, which means you exercise less and make more fattening food choices. You burn between 100 and 200 calories fewer per day because of modern conveniences.

Something is more convenient if it takes less time or less effort than it did before. Why do we love convenience so much? Perhaps it has something to do with *The Power of Rest Threat:* We naturally do as little as possible to save energy.

▌ Time Pressures Drive the Convenience Trend

Americans lead busy, stressful lives. There never seems to be enough time so people look for every convenience. Many people might want to exercise more and eat better, but they don't think they can find the time.

If you are a parent shuttling your kids around and you have 10 minutes for lunch, where will you eat? A fast food restaurant. If you have spent 10 hours at work and two hours commuting where will you pick up the family dinner? A fast food restaurant. The pressures to eat poorly are enormous because the easiest course of action is always to do what is the most convenient. If what is convenient also happens to taste the best, serve giant portions, and is inexpensive, how hard must people work to go against the convenience driven fast food lifestyle?

Whatever the reason, greater convenience is a hot selling point in every area of life. That's why **convenience literally shapes the world you live in.** The world you experience has been created to be ever more convenient and this force shows no sign of slowing.

▌ More Convenience Means Less Exercise

Physical activity has been engineered out of our lives because of our love of convenience. We want it now and we want it easy. Businesses know we like convenience and work hard to make life as convenient for us as they possibly can.

Think about how much our lives have changed as a result of innovations like dish washers, cars, remote controls, lawnmowers, drive-through services, electronic games, elevators and snow blowers. Communities and businesses are designed to be drive-through so we can save time. Everything can be delivered, bought pre-assembled, pre-packaged and pre-made.

How many fewer calories do you think we burn each day because of these conveniences? It's estimated that when added together the changes due to mechanization in our non-work lives, **we burn between 100 and 200 calories fewer per day.** That's enough calories to account for much of the rise in obesity.

If you aren't burning calories from work, then you'll need to burn calories from some sort of regular physical activity. Usually we think of regular physical activity as either exercise or play. But people aren't exercising or playing very much.

Less than one-third of adults exercise moderately at least 30 minutes several days a week and about 40% of adults do not participate in any leisure time activity. Unless the environment demands we work, most of us won't work on our own.

All is not lost. You can include more activity naturally without relying on a formal exercise program. In later strategies, we'll talk about this interesting approach.

▌ More Fattening Food Decisions

The love of convenience also impacts on the food choices available to you and those you make.

The "fast" comes first in "fast food restaurant" for a reason. In our busy world, we are always looking to save time, and eating quicker meals is a major convenience.

The problem is fast foods are less healthy. They have more fat and sugar because the ingredients are cheap and people like the flavor. In *The Restaurant Threat* we'll learn eating fast foods is associated with weight gain and account for half of all meals eaten away from home.

Food is available virtually everywhere, and this is an amazing convenience. In an urban/suburban environment tasty, cheap, high calorie food can usually be had in fewer than 5 minutes. But you don't have to wait that long, because there's probably food near you in a gas station, drug store, vending machine or just about any place you turn.

By seeking convenience we are almost automatically deciding to eat a less healthy, more fattening diet. You can say it doesn't have to be that way; people can make different choices. But these are the choices people are making. This book attempts to deal with how people really behave and how they really are, not how we want them to be under ideal conditions. Convenience is an enormous factor in modern life, to expect people not be drawn to convenience is not very realistic.

Is convenience bad? Not at all. But we need to remember it comes with a cost.

 ## Threat 35. The TV Threat

The single biggest impact a parent can have on their kid's weight is to get them to watch less TV.

Some parents spend less time at work than their kids spend in front of the TV, playing video games, being on the Internet, and listening on their MP3 players. The Kaiser Family Foundation found that the average child spends 6.5 hours a day consuming all types of media. Imaginative play is becoming a lost art.

Media consumption isn't the only consumption going on. Kids are chowing down food to the tune of 600 calories while watching TV. This has been found to be a major cause of obesity. It's not so much watching TV that's the problem, it's eating while doing it.

You can see the effects of TV watching in weight statistics. Teenage girls who watched television for 1–3 hours per day were 40% more likely to be overweight than girls who watched less than an hour a day. Girls watching 4 hours of TV a day were 50% more likely to be overweight. Similar results were found for boys.

What has been said about TV seems to apply to electronic games too. Kids who play electronic game get less physical activity and are more likely to become obese.

A report by the Institute of Medicine found "strong evidence that television advertising influences the food and beverage preferences of children aged 2–11 years." The report said that most of the food and beverage products promoted to children are high in calories, sugar, salt and fat and low in nutrients and many are promoted with popular cartoon characters.

So, TV encourages your kids to make poor food choices, to play passively, and to eat while watching TV. After all this, is TV bad? Not at all. But watching too much TV is bad.

Chapter 9

Threats from the Power of Environment
Threats 36–50

This chapter is a collection of threats rooted in the ideas we talked about in *The Power of Environment Threat.* The environment has many surprising influences on weight. It is more than where you live. It's all the factors in your home, work and community that impact on how much you exercise and how and what you eat.

⚠ Threat 36. The Portion Distortion Threat

Larger portions of food are being served. Larger portions have more calories. When combined with *The Finish Your Plate Threat,* large portions make you gain a lot of weight.

A 7-Eleven Double Gulp holds 64-ounces of soda and comes in at a whopping **800 calories.** Most people are shocked when they hear that. Eight hundred calories is almost half the calories an average woman should eat in one day. That's also 10 times the number of calories in the original Coca-Cola when it was introduced.

For some reason, people don't think about larger portion sizes as having more calories. A drink is just a drink and a burger is just a burger. How big a food item is and its calorie count doesn't spring to mind. It's as if food performs a certain role in our mind and as long as it satisfies that role we are satisfied.

When thirsty we get a drink without consciously thinking about portions or calories, we just want a drink. Then we evaluate the drink based on value, convenience and taste, not nutrition, or calories, or portion size. We want the most for the money so we get the biggest item we can afford.

We are attracted to good deals offering the best value. That's why value meals from fast food restaurants have been so stunningly successful. And that makes perfect sense. Who doesn't want more for their money, especially on a good tasting food that's immediately available?

But combine large portions with *The Finish Your Plate Threat*, which shows how people eat more from larger servings, and you have a recipe for obesity.

Americans are eating at least 200 more calories a day than we were in the 1970s. Some studies show we are eating up to 500 calories more a day. Over the same period, obesity has increased in adults and children, while portion sizes have jumped. Many people think larger portion sizes and increases in obesity are strongly linked.

Portion control has been shown by research to be the number one strategy needed to lose and maintain weight. If your portions are correctly sized, it's almost impossible to gain weight. Yet over the years, portions sizes have gone up as cost has decreased, so finding proper portions has become difficult.

The very idea of a proper portion size has changed over time as **we have come to expect big portions as the norm.** Who wants a tiny 8-ounce cup of soda when we can get a 48-ounce cup of soda for the same price? The 48-ounce cup as become normal now.

The original McDonald's meal had 590 calories. Now it has 1,550 calories. A serving of McDonald's french fries had 200 calories in 1960, 320 calories in the late 1970s, 450 calories in the mid-1990s, and 610 calories at present.

A typical hamburger in 1957 contained a little more than one ounce of cooked meat. Today a typical hamburger has six ounces of cooked meat.

Bagels and muffins that used to be 2 to 3 ounces are now typically 4 to 7 ounces. A jumbo muffin has between 400 and 700 calories. Bagels have doubled in size and have the equivalent of six slices of bread, or over 400 calories.

Candy bars and potato chips used to be packaged in 1-ounce servings are now marketed in 2- to 3-ounce single-serving packages. A 2.1-ounce Butterfinger has 270 calories and the 5.0-ounce version has 680 calories. At one time I would automatically buy the bigger one without thinking about calories, because it seemed like a better deal. And so do most people.

Restaurant meals are growing too. Many meals now contain enough food for two people.

Are increases in portion sizes wrong or bad? Not once you realize what's happening and adjust. But if you are like the 25% of people who clean their plates no matter how much food is on it, then it's disaster. As food portions increase, so will your weight.

If you can learn correct portion sizes, as you will in the *Perfect Portions Strategy*, then increased portion sizes are a great value. You get more food for less money. The only problem is when you eat more food than you should.

· ·

Threat 37. The Proximity Threat
You eat more when food is closer.

People will only walk so far—even for food. One study found people ate 9 chocolates from a clear bowl placed on their desk. Move the bowl 6 feet away and they ate only 4.

That's a difference of 125 calories simply from moving a bowl a little father away! If you eat 125 extra calories just a few times a week, that's an extra 4 pounds gained each year.

Other studies have found that employees will eat more if their desks are stocked with food, or when a package of food is open, or if the food is nearby. Being hungry doesn't matter. What matters is the food.

Merely having food closer encourages you to eat more. It seems that the **harder** you make something to eat, the less likely people are to eat it.

· ·

Threat 38. The See Food Threat
You eat more when you can see food to eat.

One study found that people ate many more chocolates served from a clear bowl when compared to when the same chocolates were served in a cloudy or opaque bowl.

Merely having food more visible encourages you to eat more.

· ·

Threat 39. The Variety Threat
You eat more when a greater variety of food is available.

A surprising study found the more variety of colors you see, the more you eat. Why should you unconsciously eat more just because of color? Brian Wansink, a professor of marketing and nutritional science at the University of Illinois, co-authored some interesting experiments showing how increased variety increases eating.

Let's say you put six colored flavors of jellybeans in separate bowls and keep track of how much people eat. Now mix all the jellybeans together in one bowl. Will people eat more or less? People ate 69% more when the colors were mixed together.

Another interesting experiment showed movie goers given M&Ms in 10 colors ate 43% more than those offered the same number of M&Ms in seven colors.

"People eat with their eyes, and their eyes trick their stomachs," Wansink said. "If we think there's more variety in a candy dish or on a buffet table, we will eat more. The more colors we see, the more we eat."

Other studies have found that providing more sources of food can make you eat more. You will eat simply because the food is there, not because of nutritional reasons. Food availability has a lot to do with how much you eat.

· ·

Threat 40. The Dish Threat
The bigger your dishes the more you eat.

▌ Big Plates, Big Meals

Most people fill their plate with food and we've already seen in other threats how you eat everything on your plate. So the size of your plate has a lot do with how much you eat.

The typical American dinner plate has an 11-inch diameter. If you lay a ruler through the center of a plate, the diameter would be the length from one side of the plate to the other side. European dinner plates typically have a 9-inch diameter. And many restaurant dinner plates now have a 13-inch diameter.

You might think a 2 inch difference in diameter can't make a big difference in how much you eat. Well, through the magic of math (the area of circle is πr^2) it turns out to make a really big difference.

An 11-inch plate has 50% more surface area than a 9-inch plate. And a 13-inch plate has twice the surface area of a 9-inch plate. That's a huge difference!

When using an 11-inch plate you can fit about 50% more food than on a 9-inch one. And a 13-inch plate can hold an astonishing two times as much food compared to a 9-inch plate.

This difference is completely unintuitive as is the effect it can have on how much you eat. But the size of your plate can cause you to eat a lot more than you expect.

▌ You Drink More from Short Wide Glasses

People naturally pour up to 32% more of a drink into shorter and wider containers. That's a lot of extra calories from just the shape of a glass.

▌ Big Bowls, Big Servings

In a study called *Ice Cream Illusions* from Cornell University and Eastern Illinois University, researchers think they have found a tendency for humans to judge object sizes based on comparisons with neighboring items.

This means that in real life **you will serve yourself more food when using big containers.**

This study found that people served themselves 31% more ice cream when they were given a 34-ounce bowl instead of a 17-ounce bowl. A 34-ounce bowl is the same size as a typical salad bowl. In my power eating days I always used a salad bowl for ice cream. If you try hard enough, you can fit a lot of ice cream in a salad bowl. ☺

▌ Big Spoons, Big Servings

The *Ice Cream Illusions* study also found that you will serve yourself 14.5% more when using a 3-ounce spoon instead of a 2-ounce spoon. To get a feel for the sizes, because nobody knows how big spoons are in ounces, a 3-ounce spoon is 6 tablespoons and a 2-ounce spoon is 4 tablespoons (¼ cup).

When people are given both a big bowl and a big spoon, they served themselves an astounding 56.8% more ice cream, **without being aware they were serving themselves more.**

Who were the people in this study? A group of nutrition experts! You can imagine, if nutrition experts are so bad at estimating serving sizes, then the rest of us must be even worse.

▌ You Eat What You Serve

In *The Finish Your Plate Threat* we saw how people tend to eat everything put in front of them. *The Ice Cream Illusions* researchers found the same thing. They found people ate 92% of the food they served themselves.

This threat seems subtle. We don't often pay attention to what dishes and utensils we use to serve our food, but as we've seen it makes an enormous difference. People really just aren't very good at estimating how much food they are eating or serving.

....

Threat 41. The Low Income Threat

People on a lower income are more overweight.

For a long time, obesity has been considered a problem of the poor. But the times they are a-changin'. Dr. Jennifer Robinson of the University of Iowa lead a study that found obesity is growing three times faster among Americans who make more than $60,000 a year than it is among their low-income friends.

Now everyone can be overweight, regardless of class, creed, or color!

Why do we see such growth? Dr. Robinson gave longer commutes, longer work hours, and the popularity of dining out at restaurants as possible reasons.

Traditionally, it has been thought that higher income people had lower obesity rates because they had better access to education, health care, and affordable fresh vegetables. Now we find obesity is an equal opportunity threat.

But lower income people are still more likely to be obese. In 2002, 32.5% of people earning under $25,000 were obese. In 2002, 26.8% of people earning above $60,000 were obese. Not that big a difference. But the rates of extreme obesity—being 90 to 100 pounds or more overweight—have skyrocketed among lower-income groups.

Why might lower income people have higher rates of obesity?

▌ Stress Levels Vary by Income

We've already talked about how stress can lead to weight gain. An interesting question is who is under the most stress?

A Carnegie Mellon University study found the lower the levels of income and education, the higher the levels of cortisol and other stress related hormones. This association is independent of race, age, sex or BMI.

Being under chronic stress is really bad for your weight, and if you are in the lower income bracket, it looks like your stress could be chronically high.

▮ More Likely to be Inactive

Lower income people have been found to be less physically active than wealthier individuals. Clearly, if you are less active it's more likely you'll gain weight.

▮ Lack of Time

Lower income people have to work long hours to make ends meet. They often lack the time to prepare healthy meals. This kicks in *The Convenience Threat* where fast food is convenient, and more likely to be eaten.

▮ Food is an Affordable Indulgence

If your family has very little money, food is one of the few indulgences you can afford. Guilty feeling parents, having little money for other treats and presents, can go to a fast food restaurant and make their kids and their family happy. And once there, *The Restaurant Threat* kicks in and you eat more from large portions of good tasting food, which leads to weight gain.

▮ Some Fix-it Strategies Not Easily Available

The usual advice if you are overweight is to eat healthier food and get more exercise. Both can be hard if you live in an inner city. We'll talk more about these issues in *The Unsafe Neighborhood Threat* and *The High Cost of a Healthy Diet Threat*.

This is a very controversial threat. A frequent reaction is that lower income people could eat healthier meals with a little more work. They could shop more efficiently, eat at home more, buy in bulk, buy at farmers' markets, buy frozen vegetables, skip expensive restaurant meals, and so on.

On the surface this line of logic is hard to argue with, so I won't try. This isn't what real life people do in a real life environment. You can play the if-only game if you want, but as we can see with the rising obesity rates in higher income people, it's not just a low income problem, it's just worse in the lower income brackets.

After a long day at work, maybe working two jobs, it's understandable that the choice of fast food is often made, for people of all income ranges. You can make an entire family happy; it's a cheap, fast, tasty, and filling meal. It may not be the healthiest option for a family, but it is understandable.

. . . .

Threat 42. The Unsafe Neighborhood Threat

People living in unsafe neighborhoods are 150% more likely to be overweight.

People, regardless of income level, are more likely to exercise when it's comfortable and convenient. If you live in an unsafe neighborhood, exercise is neither. In an unsafe neighborhood you are much less likely to go outside and get some exercise. It makes a lot more sense to stay safe indoors.

Even if you did go outside, a poor neighborhood is much less likely to have public facilities like parks and recreation centers. And even if you did have these facilities, would you use them if you didn't feel safe?

Why not join a health club? Because it's too expensive. You probably live in a dangerous neighborhood to begin with because money is tight. That doesn't leave much money for gym fees.

Why not buy a treadmill? Because it's too expensive and space in your apartment is tight, so there's not enough room.

The bottom line is, a fear of crime makes people less likely to leave their homes and if you don't leave your home you aren't going to get the exercise you need.

. . . .

Threat 43. The High Cost of a Healthy Diet Threat

A healthy diet costs more, which means people are less likely to eat healthy, especially when low-cost alternatives like fast food are available.

A healthy diet is often said to consist of lean meats, fish, fresh vegetables and fruits. But these foods cost a lot more than pre-packaged foods, rice, beans, potatoes, pasta and other low cost favorites.

A bunch of grapes costs more than a bag of cookies, for example. The reason is cookies, like a lot of junk foods, are made out of fat, flour, and sugar which are very cheap ingredients.

Nutritionists recommend that each person should eat between 4–5 servings of fruits and vegetables a day. Let's take as an example adding one peach per day for a family of four.

Peaches are about $2.50 per pound where I live, with about 3 peaches in a pound. A family of 4 would need 28 peaches a week, costing over $23 a week. It's definitely expensive.

One estimate had shopping for a healthier diet increasing a grocery bill by more than 4% of household income. That's a lot of money if your budget is tight.

So if you live in a poorer neighborhood and you want to eat healthier, your food budget goes up for two reasons: food is generally more expensive and healthier food is even more expensive.

▌ Poor Access to Quality Stores

If you live in a suburban environment, it's hard to imagine that people living in inner cities and in rural areas don't have access to affordable quality fruits and vegetables (especially out of season), but they don't.

In an inner city or in a rural area, your neighborhood store is most likely a mini-market selling a fine selection of processed foods in bright attractive packages. Any fruits and vegetables will be expensive and sad-looking. You may want to buy better food for your family, but how can you afford to pay $2 a head of wilted iceberg lettuce or 50 cents for one brown and bruised apple?

If a supermarket is available, it's likely to have a more limited selection and be more expensive than suburban supermarkets. Stores, for whatever reason, don't like to enter the inner city.

My personal experience backs this threat up. I live in the San Francisco Bay Area in California, which produces an amazing amount of lovely fresh fruit and vegetables. On my trips to other areas of the country, I have been shocked at the lack of quality fruits and vegetables. I would go into a store and see very little choice and that choice was low quality and very expensive. Nobody in their right mind would pay so much for so little, especially with such tempting alternatives available.

It's not as easy as you would like to think to replace a diet of soft drinks and fast food with home-cooked meals, fresh fruits and vegetables.

....

⚠ Threat 44. The Shopping Trap Threat

An endless number of tricks are used to influence you to buy goods you don't necessarily want or need. The real trick is that almost all of these tactics operate below your conscious awareness.

How often have you walked into a store and come out with more stuff than you planned on buying? This happens to me all the time at Costco. Costco is a big box retailer with excellent prices on all sorts interesting gear I didn't know I needed before I walked in the door!

But when you buy food you don't need, it usually means weight gain and a broken diet. Few people actually buy more lettuce on impulse. You buy chips, candy, soda, and all the other goodies. Retailers spend millions of dollars on consumer research. They are experts at getting you to buy things you don't need.

Product placement is an important trick stores use to get us to buy more goods. The more visible a product is, the more we'll buy. It happens all the time—or it used to happen all the time—that I would see something at the end of isle display and drop it into my cart. Simply putting a product on display at the end of an isle increases sales of that item by 40%.

That's the idea behind putting impulse items at check-out counters. They know we'll see it, want it, and probably buy it.

People spend a lot of time deciding on the brand they want to buy, but they don't spend much time thinking about how much of an item they want to buy. This means stores can use all kinds of gimmicks to trick you into buying more.

People are very influenced by numbers displayed at the point of purchase. The first number becomes our reference number for deciding how many items to buy, because we don't think about this before seeing the sign. Researchers have found two interesting examples.

People purchase up to 30% more when retailers use multiple-unit pricing: a sign says something like 5 for $5 versus 1 for $1. The price per item is the same, but you will still buy more when the point of purchase sign says 5 for $5 because the number 5 becomes the reference point for how many items to buy.

When a sign says, "Soup, no limit per person," people on average will buy three or four cans. Change the sign to say "Soup, limit 12 cans per person," people will then purchase seven. That's a huge unconscious increase in the quantity purchased with essentially no difference between the signs. There is not even a sale going on. But in the 12 cans per person sign the base line for making a purchase becomes the number 12.

Colorful oversized packaging, especially for kids' products, is yet another ploy stores and manufactures use to increase sales.

Retailers employ an almost endless number of tricks to get us to buy goods we don't necessarily want or need. But the real trick is that almost all of these tactics operate below our conscious awareness.

. . . .

Threat 45. The Pestering Kid Threat

The impulses of children end up driving the food choices for the whole family.

How? By being kids of course! And it works.

Seventy-five percent of unplanned food purchases can be traced to a nagging child. One out two mothers will buy food because a child requests it. As kids don't usually demand to eat more broccoli, the foods the family ends up eating are nutritionally poor and fattening. You as an adult may be having weight problems because of the food your kids demand. And the food isn't doing your kids any good either.

▌ Kids Do Not Have Adult Minds

It's easy for adults to treat kids as small adults. Many kids look physically grown up and may act very worldly and mature, but it's all an act. Brain researchers have found that the human brain doesn't fully mature until about age 25!

The front part of the brain is the last to mature. This area, the prefrontal cortex, is responsible for rational thought and provides skills like organizing thoughts, weighing consequences, assuming responsibility and interpreting emotions. It's the part of your brain that helps you do the harder thing when you are ready to do the easier thing.

Kids simply don't have the brain power to seek delayed gratification or to predict the far-reaching consequences of their actions. Kids are not trying to be moody, reckless, and irrational. Rather it's just that the part of their brain controlling these skills is still under construction.

This helps to explain all the stupid things we did as kids and whatever stupid things your kids may be doing now. Kids in the company of their friends are far more likely to engage in risky behaviors. Kids seek out immediate rewards and excitement, avoid stress and seek out easy situations.

What does this mean? You can't trust your kid to decide what your family should eat. They aren't mature enough to make those decisions. If you let them then your whole family will suffer.

. . . .

Threat 46. The Restaurant Threat

Eating away from home is associated with weight gain.

It's estimated that any meal you eat away from home has 197 more calories than the same meal you would have had at home. As nearly half of all money spent on food is spent away from home, this adds up to a lot of calories. What's the difference?

Meals eaten away from home are larger and contain more fat and sugar. That's what people want, so that's what restaurants provide. Foods available in fast food restaurants are estimated to be 2 to 5 times larger than 2 decades ago. And as we have talked about in other threats, larger portions lead to more eating more and more eating leads to more weight.

The Center for Science in the Public Interest surveyed restaurants and you might be surprised at how many calories you might eat in one:

- Chef's Salad: 930 calories
- Patty Melt and French Fries: 1,350 calories
- Chicken Fajitas: 840 calories
- Kung Pao Chicken: 1,620 calories

If you add to your meal a side dish, an appetizer, a drink, and a dessert then you could easily eat a whole day's calories in one restaurant meal. And you most likely won't even realize you have eaten so many calories.

It matters where you eat too. Half of all meals eaten away from home are now fast food meals. Increasing fast food visits by 3 a week was linked to an average weight gain of 4.75 pounds in African Americans and 3.5 pounds in Caucasians.

It all adds up.

. . . .

Threat 47. The Social Eating Threat

The more people you eat with, the more you will eat.

In a fascinating finding, John de Castro, a University of Georgia State University psychologist, found that you will eat more when you eat with other people. And the amount you eat increases as you add more people.

Meals eaten in large groups were over 75% larger than when eaten alone. When you eat alone you will eat 44% less than when you eat socially.

Why might you eat more socially? When you eat with other people you talk, you argue, you laugh. It's fun. All that social interaction takes time. The more people you eat with, the longer your meals take to eat. And **when your**

meals take longer you eat more because you eat through the whole meal. Watch yourself the next time you find yourself lingering around a table filled with leftover food. As you talk, you will inevitably reach over and pick food off the table. The calories add up quickly and you won't even be aware you're eating them.

Another possible explanation from an interesting study on the effects of subliminal messages might help explain at least part of why we eat more in social situations. Subliminal messages are messages your brain picks up but you aren't consciously aware of. This study found **subliminal smiles caused thirsty people to pour and drink more** of a beverage. Subliminal frowns caused the opposite effect. If you are eating in a group it's likely there are lots of smiles that could unconsciously affect how much people eat and drink.

You will eat even more when with family and friends. Perhaps you are more relaxed so you don't control what you eat as well.

Eating in groups doesn't always encourage you to eat more. You tend to eat less when eating with coworkers and mere acquaintances, probably because you aren't comfortable with them.

De Castro also found that **women eat more when they are with a man,** somewhat less when they are with another woman, and still less when they eat alone.

De Castro's research revealed something else quite amazing: **social eating may have a genetic component.** How? How much you like to be with people is part of your personality and is inherited.

If you like to be around people, it means you will probably eat with bigger groups and if you eat with bigger groups you will eat more! This is how your environment can be, in part, created by your genetics.

. . . .

Threat 48. The Man Threat
Men are bad for women's waistlines.

"Men are very bad for women really," said Dr. David Haslam, Clinical Director of the National Obesity Forum. Dr. Haslam said research shows that women tend to gain weight if they live with men and begin to share meals with men who naturally have higher energy needs and therefore appetites.

We also see *The Social Eating Threat* kick in when women eat with men. Haslam said, "If you are eating with a partner, the evening meal is a **social event** and it's no longer just filling a gap. You may eat more and maybe more extravagant stuff."

Couples could also be more frequent victims of *The Restaurant Threat* as they may go out to restaurants more often than single people.

....

 Threat 49. The Air Conditioning Threat

Air conditioning may contribute to weight gain.

Air conditioning helps you to gain weight through two mechanisms: you eat more and you burn fewer calories maintaining your body temperature.

▌ You Don't Eat in the Heat

A report published in the International Journal of Obesity says that you eat less when you are overheated.

"Restaurateurs report that when their air conditioning goes out, they lose business. People don't want to eat a lot in the heat," says David Allison, the leader of the study team and a professor of biostatistics at the University of Alabama at Birmingham.

This idea is backed up by research by John de Castro. He found **people eat more as the weather cools.** People's daily intake is 200 calories per day greater in fall than in the rest of the year. With air conditioning, every day is a fall day.

Interestingly, residential air conditioning started becoming more common in 1980, and obesity rates have steadily risen since 1980. Just a coincidence?

▌ You Don't Burn as Many Calories

Air conditioning and heating help keep you in "the thermoneutral zone," a temperature range where you do not have to regulate your body temperature.

When your body is above or below this zone, you need to burn calories to maintain your body temperature at the right level.

You might think this isn't a lot of calories, but an adult 154 pound male burns an average of 75 calories per hour to maintain his normal body temperature. Over the years, reducing that amount by even a little can add up to a lot of extra calories and weight.

· ·

Threat 50. The Free Market Threat

Free market forces will forever create environments that make it easy to gain weight and hard to lose it.

The beauty of the free market is that there are millions of people tirelessly trying to make available the exact goods and services you want.

What you seem to want is: tasty food, cheap food, and convenience. Tasty food usually means fat and sugar. Cheap food means large portions. Convenience means we'll be even less active in the future.

All these forces combine to help ensure that our environment will always be one in which it is easy to gain weight and hard to lose it.

Is it bad that the free market caters to your every whim? Not at all, but it does mean that the need to control your weight won't ever end and it will only get harder as time goes on.

Chapter 10

The Hodgepodge Threats
Threats 51–60

This chapter is a collection of threats that didn't fit nicely in any of the others. Sometimes a threat belonged in too many chapters so I gave it a home here. Other times a threat simply wasn't a match for any of the power threats. Whatever the reason a threat is here, it's bound to give you some insight as to why staying on a diet can be so hard.

. . . .

Threat 51. The Average Joe's Diet Threat

The average person's diet is worse than you think.

How bad do you think the diet is for the average American? It may be worse than you imagine. Researchers found that nearly one-third of our calories come from junk food and alcohol. One-third!

Soft drinks, alcohol and sweets account for more than 25% of calories. When fruit drinks and salty snacks are added, the figure rises to 30%.

Why are soft drinks such a diet killer? Dr. Frank Hu at the Harvard School of Public Health was lead on a report that found **a single can of soda a day can add up to 15 pounds in a single year.** Researchers think the evidence strongly suggests that this sort of increased consumption is a key reason that more people have gained weight.

This isn't surprising. The average American now gets an amazing 21% of their calories from beverages, and soft drink consumption has increased 135% from 1977 to 2001. People are now getting between 75 and 150 more calories a day from soft drinks and fruit drinks than they did 30 years ago.

The problem is soft drinks add a lot of calories and no nutrition. And even worse, liquids aren't real food. **Liquids won't make you feel full** so you won't eat any less. Liquids just give you extra calories that will cause you to gain weight.

Wow! People are eating a lot of calorie-dense foods that provide next to no nutrition. People are both overfed and undernourished at the same time.

If this sounds like you, then you can immediately make big differences in your life. Just don't be like Average Joe.

....

Threat 52. The Want it All Now Threat

Lower your expectations of how fast you should lose weight.

People aren't patient when it comes to weight loss. They want to lose it all now and if they can't, they just won't try. Worrying only about weight loss won't create your perfect diet. You can lose weight on any diet. They real goal is keeping on your diet for the rest of your life and you simply can't do that if you lose weight too fast.

Let's run some numbers. Some people want to lose a lot of weight fast so they'll cut back by 1,000 calories a day. At that rate you would lose 2 pounds a week or 104 pounds in a year. That's fast track weight loss for sure.

The problem is eating 1,000 fewer calories a day has a good chance of triggering your starvation response. Your body dials up your hunger level and starts conserving calories by lowering your metabolism. You soon fall off your diet because you won't be able to resist the call to hunger. You gain weight and the scenario starts all over again.

Another way to get to your 1,000 calorie deficit is by exercising more. Can you exercise 1,000 calories off everyday? That's walking about 10 miles each day. If you can, excellent. Whatever works. That's too much exercise for most people.

Your next choice is to split the 1,000 calories up somehow between eating less and exercising more. Maybe you eat 500 calories less each day and exercise 500 calories more. That's still hard, but at least it sounds doable.

But you have another option: **lower your expectations of how fast you should lose weight.**

High expectations set you up for repeated cycles of failure, disappointment, and self blame. You will blame yourself for not reaching your high goals because you still feel it's possible not to slip-up. At some point you will simply get depressed and give up. Don't let this threat get you.

Accept that **losing weight slowly is OK.** The tortoise beat the hare, remember? Don't be in a hurry. Your weight took a long time to put on. It'll a take a little while to lose as well. If you think you can beat the system by losing weight fast, you'll probably fail. The odds are against you.

If you follow a go-slow approach, you will still lose a lot of weight in just a few years. And better yet, you'll keep it off for the rest of your life.

 ## Threat 53. The Going Off Plan Threat
How you handle failure is what really matters.

There are an unlimited number of ways to fail on your diet and we all handle failure differently. Some people are prone to go into a cycle of depression that throws them off their diet. Other people react to one mistake as if their whole diet attempt is a failure. They then use that mistake as an excuse to go off their diet and back to their old habits.

How you handle going off your eating plan is one of the most important skills you can learn as a person. We all fail. It's how you handle failure that really matters. Several strategies will talk about how to prevent a lapse from becoming a collapse.

The ease with which bad habits reestablish themselves is yet another reason that relying on willpower doesn't work. Very few people can fend off bad habits by willpower alone. That's why the strategies in this book don't depend on willpower to work.

 ## Threat 54. The Frog in the Pot Threat
Weight gain happens so gradually most people don't realize they have become overweight.

They say that if you put a frog into a pot of boiling water it will leap out right away to escape the danger. But, if you put a frog in a pot of cool water and then gradually heat the pot until boiling, the frog won't notice the threat until it is too late.

We are the same with our weight.

After a couple of years, a lot of people suddenly notice they have gained 40 pounds. Over two years that's only 200 extra calories a day. A small increase in what you're eating combined with a slowdown in exercise can easily account for 200 calories.

Perhaps you changed your routine a little bit and you no longer take that daily walk. Perhaps you started adding cream to your coffee or you started super-sizing your fries. It doesn't take much.

Weight gain happens so gradually that most people don't realize they are overweight until they try to squeeze into a pair of jeans or go swimsuit shopping. By then it's too late. We need to get constant feedback about our weight so we know as early as possible when we are starting to gain weight and we can do something to stop it.

A study from Cornell University found that monitoring weight on a daily basis can help prevent this silent weight gain. Women who weighed themselves every day and emailed their weight to researchers lost almost 2 pounds during the study. Women who didn't weigh and send email daily gained up to nearly 7 pounds. That's a big difference.

· ·

Threat 55. The Bad Estimation Threat

People are bad at estimating their health, how much they eat, how much they exercise, and about their risk of dying.

We underestimate how much we eat, we overestimate how much we exercise, and we underestimate the health risks from obesity. We are a very optimistic bunch!

Poor estimation skills matter, because if your estimates are wrong, you are making decisions on bad information. If you eat more than you think and exercise less than you think, then you aren't likely to take action to eat less and exercise more.

▍ We Are Bad at Estimating How Much We Really Eat

Most people underestimate their daily calorie intake by 25%. You may think you are not eating too much, but you are probably eating more than you need to. I'm actually surprised we aren't off by more than 25%. Portion estimation is difficult, especially when you haven't learned how. It's easy to be off by a lot.

There are many possible reasons for your calorie estimates to be wrong:

1. Calorie estimation is difficult. You don't learn it in school and you never learn it out of school either. So how are you supposed to know how to do it?
2. You may be nibbling during food preparation.
3. Portions may be larger than you think.
4. You don't know how food is prepared so your food may have more calories than you realize. It only takes an extra bit of butter to raise the calories in a meal a lot.
5. Estimating small meals is easier than estimating larger meals. People are pretty good at estimating a 300 calorie meal, but people underestimate a 1,500 calorie meal by 30%.

Even dietitians, people who you think would be good at estimating how many calories are in a dish, aren't that good at calorie estimation. In a study by Pierre Chandon and Brian Wansink, dietitians estimated that a 1,000 calorie fast food meal had 857 calories while non-dietitians estimated the meal at 664 calories.

Both estimates are pretty bad for your waistline, and not just for the obvious reason. Poor calorie estimation can lead to **portion creep** in meal sizes. You may look at a meal and think it has a certain number of calories, and then you think to yourself "Hey, that meal only has 500 calories so I can get the next bigger meal with no problem." What you don't realize, because you misestimated both meals, is that the larger meal really has 1,500 calories. By selecting the larger meal you've just blown up your calorie intake for the day with one decision on one meal.

If you ever catch yourself complaining that you aren't eating much, but aren't losing weight, you are probably a victim of *The Bad Estimation Threat.*

▌ We Are Bad at Estimating How Much We Exercise

People aren't good at estimating how hard they have exercised either. In one study, only 15% of the people who thought they exercised moderately hard actually did exercise moderately hard. Only 11% of those who thought they exercised strenuously really worked that hard. You may not be exercising as much or as hard as you think you are.

▌ We Are Bad at Knowing How Obesity Impacts on Our Risk of Dying

People don't seem to have an accurate feel for how obesity increases their risk of dying. To be fair, there have been a lot of arguments about how dangerous obesity actually is to your health, so we have some reason to be a bit confused.

In one study, they asked a group of obese people what they thought their chances of living to 75 and 85 would be. People were very optimistic and underestimated their risk of dying by between 17% and 22%. Heavy smokers were the most optimistic about their survival.

I have no idea how any of us would know when we are likely to die. It's not like the information comes in fortune cookies. I wonder if people would change their behavior at all if they had a hard estimate of when they were likely to die given their current health, habits and genetics.

....

Threat 56. The Fructose Threat

Fructose may trick you into thinking you are hungrier than you should be. Fructose is in many processed foods like soft drinks, jellies, pastries, ketchup and table sugar.

University of Florida researchers have identified fructose as one possible reason for rising obesity rates.

"There may be more than just the common concept that the reason a person gets fat is because they eat too many calories and they don't do enough exercise," said Dr. Richard J. Johnson of the University of Florida. "And although genetic predispositions are obviously important, there's some major environmental force driving this process. Our data suggest certain foods and, in particular fructose, may actually speed the process for a person to become obese."

High-fructose corn syrup is a form of sugar used to sweeten foods, especially soft drinks. The industry switched in the 1970s from using refined sugar, known as sucrose, to using fructose as a sweetener because fructose is more economical. The switch to fructose may be partially to blame for the rapid increase in obesity in recent years. Certainly, at the time nobody knew fructose might be something other than an economical sugar replacement, but recent research has shown fructose might boost calorie consumption by encouraging overeating.

It's not that fructose is inherently bad. In small quantities it's fine. The sweetness in fruits comes from fructose, for example. The trouble is, because fructose is such a good sweetener, its use in all types of foods has jumped and we are eating more of it than ever.

People get about 132 calories a day on average from fructose, with many getting far more. Most processed foods contain fructose, though most calories are consumed in beverages.

Since the late 1970s, soft drink consumption has doubled while the number of people with metabolic syndrome has more than doubled worldwide, to more than 55 million in the United States alone. Metabolic syndrome is a group of conditions that happen together, increasing your risk for heart disease, stroke and diabetes.

Couldn't we just make food less sweet? Not likely. Making products less sweet isn't a popular option with consumers. "Our research confirms that consumers are not willing to sacrifice taste in order to reduce caloric intake," says Graham Hall, president of Nutrinova Inc.

The problem is that your body is more likely to convert fructose into fat than is the case for sugar. Fructose doesn't stimulate insulin production, increase leptin production, or suppress the production of ghrelin, all of which control hunger.

You end up eating more than you otherwise would when eating and drinking foods high in fructose.

....

Threat 57. The Self Denial Threat

Many overweight people think they don't have a weight problem.

Dr. David Schutt, from the health care research firm Thomson Medstat, performed a survey of over 11,000 people, of whom 3,100 were obese or morbidly obese and another 4,200 were overweight. He found some surprising responses about the eating and exercise habits of Americans.

Here are some of the study findings as reported in the news media:

1. Over 75% of obese Americans say they eat healthy.
2. About 40% of obese American said they do "vigorous" exercise at least three times a week.
3. Twenty-eight percent of obese Americans said they snacked two or more times a day, only slightly more than 24% of normal-weight people who said they did.
4. About 29% of obese people said they eat out at restaurants three or more times a week, compared with 25% of normal-weight people.

5.   About 41% of obese compared to 31% of normal-weight people said they always ate all the food served at restaurants.

When you look at the results this way what pops out is how similar are the habits of normal, overweight, and obese people. There doesn't seem to be a giant difference between how people eat and exercise.

This has prompted Schutt to say, "There is, perhaps, some denial going on. Or there is a lack of understanding of what does it mean to be eating healthy, and what is vigorous exercise."

And this is the spin the media gave the survey. Article after article gushed at how obese people must be in denial. They are in denial because they think they are eating right, they think they are exercising. They think they are doing all the right things, but because they are obese they must be fooling themselves.

But a different picture emerges if you look at the actual study results. The answers are actually fairly well slotted by weight classification (normal, overweight, obese, morbidly obese).

If you look at the question "How healthy would you consider your eating habit?" most morbidly obese people say their eating habits are "not healthy" and they are least likely to say their eating habits are "very healthy." To me, true denial would give a different result. Someone in denial would say they are eating very healthy, but that's not what people are saying.

You see the same sort of distribution for the exercise question. About exercise they were asked: "During the last month, have you personally engaged in vigorous physical activity for at least 20 minutes a day, three or more times per week?"

In response, the normally weighted people thought they exercised the most (55.3%), the overweight people thought they exercised the next largest amount (53.3%), then it's the obese people (40%), followed by the morbidly obese people who thought they exercised a lot less then the other groups (24.8%).

So who's in denial?

The conclusion section at the end of the survey does a good job of summarizing the issues:

Sometimes is a very dangerous word.

While very few respondents in any of the BMI categories consistently ate super-sized fast foods for the majority of their meals, snacked recklessly, or even characterized their eating habits as poor, several high risk behaviors have combined to become part of the average American's weekly routine. Through a combination of occasional fast food meals, moderate snacking, not quite enough exercise and the belief that these habits are "somewhat healthy," Americans are rationalizing themselves into ever-expanding waistlines.

I don't agree that people are necessarily "rationalizing themselves into ever-expanding waistlines," though that could be part of the problem. There are other ways to look at the survey results that don't involve people lying to themselves.

In *The Lost Exercise Threat* we talk about how exercise doesn't use as many calories as most people think. People could easily be doing the amount of exercise they say and not be losing or maintaining their weight. They didn't say they were running a marathon a day, they may just not know that more exercise is needed for weight loss.

It is interesting how the answers between the weight groups are not wildly different. Rather than denial, I think this points to a lack of understanding of how few extra calories a day you need to eat to slip into obesity.

The small differences found in the survey could very well be all that is needed to move from a normal weight to being obese.

The strategies in this book are aimed and keeping all those small differences from adding up to big weight gains.

....

Threat 58. The Child Denial Threat
Parents don't realize their children are overweight.

With childhood obesity rates skyrocketing, some people might ask: why don't parents do something about how much their kids eat? Oddly enough, many parents may simply not recognize their children as having a weight problem.

Several studies have shown that parents don't always realize their children are overweight. In the November 2003 issue of *Obesity Research*, Debra Etelson, MD and her colleagues reported only 10.5% of parents with overweight children perceived their child's weight accurately. Parents of overweight children always underestimated their children's weight.

Why do parents make this mistake?

One thought is that being overweight is now the norm, so it may not stick out as a problem. Another explanation is denial. Parents have their heads in the sand and don't notice. Other parents might think being chubby is cute.

I also think it's just hard to notice changes in people you see every day. A child gaining weight won't seem to have changed to a parent because parents see their children on a continuous basis. An outsider will notice it right away, but we become blind to what we are familiar with.

When a parent does notice their child is overweight they might think their kid will grow out of it. That's what I heard growing up. But most kids are now growing out more than they are growing up.

Parents are also concerned that if they push too hard on the weight issue, they might create a weight disorder in their kids, or they might just turn their kids off completely.

Other parents just view being overweight as a cosmetic problem, not a health problem, so they think there's nothing to worry about.

Another problem is that you can't always look at a child and know how overweight they are. A child may have a lot of fat yet not appear that big.

This is a very serious threat because the health risks for overweight children are so severe.

. . . .

Threat 59. The Trans Fats Threat

You gain more weight on a diet rich in trans fats.

Trans fats are the worst kind of fats. They are bad for several reasons: they cause you to gain weight, the weight you gain is around your belly, and they increase your levels of "bad" cholesterol (LDL), which increases your risk of heart disease.

Trans fats are everywhere. You can find trans fats in: margarine, shortening, fried foods, fast foods, french fries, fried chicken, doughnuts, potato chips, corn chips, cookies, pastries, waffles and crackers. If the food is manufactured, trans fats could be in it.

Why do food manufactures use trans fats if they are so bad for you? Because food manufactures have a problem. A lot of food recipes call for oil, but oil spoils quickly on the shelf. Trans fats on the other hand have a long shelf life, so food made with trans fats will last a long time.

OK, so trans fats are bad for you and they are everywhere. How do trans fats affect your weight?

It is often said a calorie is a calorie, that it doesn't matter what food you eat. But some recent research shows you'll gain more weight when you eat food made using trans fats.

This shocking effect was shown in a study at the Wake Forest University Baptist Medical College, which investigated the effects of trans fats on monkeys.

Here's what they found: male monkeys who were fed a western-style diet containing trans fat had a 7.2% increase in body weight when compared to a 1.8% weight increase in monkeys who ate monounsaturated fats (like olive oil). That's a whopping **5.4% weight gain just by eating food made with trans fats!** The study lasted over 6 years and the monkeys were all given the same amount of daily calories, with 35% of the calories coming from fat.

"We conclude that in equivalent diets, trans fatty acid consumption increases weight gain," said lead researcher Dr. Kylie Kavanagh. You could be doing a good job, checking the total number of calories you are eating, but if you are eating a lot of calories from trans fats, you'll gain weight anyway.

This isn't just a weight problem. The trans fat eating monkeys had about 33% more fat around their bellies. "You can see white gobs of fat in these guys", said Kavanagh. This is significant because belly fat is associated with a higher risk of diabetes and heart disease.

Many people recommend a diet with zero trans fats.

If you eat a lot of fast food, you could have trouble reaching a goal of zero trans fats. Fast foods are usually fried in trans fats so the cooked food ends up having a lot of trans fats in them too. As an example, a meal from KFC including three pieces of extra-crispy chicken contains 15 grams of trans fat and a single pot pie contains 14 grams.

The FDA now requires the amount of trans fat to be listed in the nutrition facts panel on all foods. The restaurant industry is exempt however. And there's a loophole.

The regulations allow labels to say "zero trans fats" if there is 0.5g or less trans fats per serving. Some products have a very small "serving size," so you need to be careful. You could unknowingly eat a lot of trans fats from products that are supposedly free of them.

. . . .

Threat 60. The Distraction Threat

Distractions make you more likely to follow your emotional impulses and give in to temptation.

The modern world throbs with distractions. We multitask between work, home, play, TV, cell phones, games and the Internet. We barely get a moment to think. And it's those distractions that may tempt us onto the path of overeating.

Baba Shiv, in a fascinating University of Iowa study, asked one group to memorize a two-digit number and a second group to memorize a seven-digit number. Before the groups were asked to recall the numbers, Shiv offered them a choice between a healthy bowl of fruit salad and a piece of mouth-wateringly delicious chocolate cake.

What choice should the people make? On the one hand your rational mind is saying, "We should choose the fruit salad, it is healthy and tastes pretty good too." On the other hand your emotional mind is saying, "That chocolate cake looks awesome!"

Which way do you go? The answer is: it depends. It depends a lot on how distracted you are. You see, the memorizing the digits task was just to see how a distraction would affect people's choices. Memorizing a longer number is hard so it is more distracting than memorizing a short number.

Were people's choices affected? Oh yes. Sixty-three percent of the people who were trying to memorize the longer number chose the cake and only 41% of the people memorizing the shorter number chose the cake.

What's happening? Like we talked about in *The Two Brain Threat,* the rational part of your brain is busy on the memorization tasks. So, it was more likely people would follow their emotional impulses. **In an environment where you face continual distraction, it's easy for your rational mind to be involved in fewer of your food decisions.**

Shiv has also found thoughts of death made people choose the cake more often than the fruit salad, even for people who normally had very strong self-control over their eating. Thinking of your own death can be a big distraction.

Traditionally, we like to think people are rational like a computer is rational. The computer calculates all the factors and spits out the optimal solution. But people aren't like that at all. Once emotions kick in, people can easily make decisions that go against their best interests.

Chapter 11

The Weird Threats
Threats 61–62

This chapter is a collection of surprising threats I hadn't expected to find when I started my little adventure of trying to understand why staying on a diet is so hard. What I discovered is that the world is a wild and crazy place. You might just agree when you read these threats.

 Threat 61. The Bacteria Threat

Some obesity may be caused by bacteria.

You are not alone. Your digestive system is home to between 10 and 100 *trillion* bacteria, 10 times the number of cells in your body. Those are mind numbingly large numbers. It's kind of spooky to think about all these little guys in your stomach. Bacteria are single celled organisms and are among the earliest forms of life. They can "eat" everything from sugar and starch to sulfur and iron.

What do all these bacteria do? We don't really know, but some of them help digest your food. The bacteria make a nice home in your stomach and in exchange they help you extract nutrients and calories from the food you eat.

Dr. Jeffrey Gordon, director of the Center for Genome Sciences at Washington University School of Medicine in St. Louis, thinks that people with certain communities of bacteria may get more calories from food and that those extra calories are stored as fat. Gordon has already shown this to happen in mice.

It's fascinating to think that each of us could eat exactly the same meal and each of us would extract a different number of calories, depending on the bacteria we had in our stomach. Your bacteria could be highly efficient and eek out every calorie. Your friend's bacteria could be inefficient and let a lot of potential calories go unconsumed. You would have a much better chance of surviving famine than your friend, but your friend would be thinner, just from having a different mix of bacteria.

How might this work? Let's say that every day your bacteria extract 20 additional calories from the food you eat. Over a year that's two pounds of weight gain and over 10 years that's 20 extra pounds. So the numbers can be significant.

Gordon thinks that it may be possible to make you thin by manipulating your bacteria. After all, if the bacteria can help make you overweight, they should be able to help you lose weight too.

This science isn't in on this threat yet, but I thought it was interesting enough to include.

. . . .

Threat 62. The Virus Threat
Some obesity may be caused by a virus.

Amazingly, a virus may cause you to gain weight. Even more stunning is that this virus is highly contagious and is transmitted by direct contact and through the air.

In the mid-1990s at the University of Wisconsin-Madison, Dr. Richard Atkinson and his colleague, Dr. Nikhil Dhurandhar, started studying the connection between viruses and obesity. In animal studies they discovered a virus, adenovirus-36 (Ad-36), that caused obesity in monkeys, mice and chickens.

Later tests on humans appeared to support the same conclusions as the animal studies: you can catch obesity like you can catch the flu—through a virus.

If you get this virus your chances of being overweight are between 70 and 100%, which is pretty high. In a test of 500 people, about 30% of obese test subjects were shown to have the virus, compared to only 10% of non-obese people. Those with the virus were an average of 50 pounds heavier than those without it.

Many people don't like the idea of a virus contributing to obesity, because they want obesity to be caused by a lack of personal control. But the world is weirder than that.

Interestingly, the virus doesn't work by making you hungry, but by making your body convert more of the calories you consume to fat. So you could be eating the same amount of food yet mysteriously gain weight.

And this is exactly what has been happening since about 1980. Since 1980 food intake has gone up slightly, but physical activity has gone up enough to make up for increased calories. Yet obesity rates have jumped from 15% in 1980 in the U.S. to 31%.

What happened? Maybe the virus? The virus was isolated in 1978, and given how fast it spreads, it's possible it could be making a significant contribution to obesity in America. Clearly not all obesity is caused by viruses, but viruses could be one of the causes.

This research is still relatively new and there's more work to be done, but it's very interesting to think about. Hopefully scientists will be able to create a vaccine. Currently there are three known obesity causing viruses, but there could be close to 50 of them, so it might be a while before a vaccine can be developed.

I've included this threat as both a **shock** and **warning.** The shock is that we don't know everything about how our bodies work yet. Not by a long shot. There's much yet to learn. The warning is for people who just know the only solution is to eat less and exercise more. It's not always that simple.

Chapter 12

The Strategies—How to Stop the Threats

After reading dozens and dozens of reasons why controlling your weight is so hard, it's natural to wonder how you can overcome the threats. The threats seem overwhelming and inescapable. Take heart, there is a way to defeat almost every threat. The ways of defeating threats are called strategies.

A strategy is a counter move to one or more threats. If you have a problem controlling your portions, there are strategies for helping you learn portion control. If you naturally move less, there are strategies for helping you naturally move more. You will be able to find a way to control your weight.

In all the chapters that follow, we'll talk about the different strategies you can use to defeat the threats. The strategies in this book have been specifically structured to help you stay on your diet, eat in moderation, and naturally exercise more, all without having to rely on willpower.

Please don't interpret "not relying on willpower" to mean you don't have to do anything. You'll have to do a lot of work, but it will be worth it because you'll see measurable results in your life.

▌ Just Knowing about the Threats isn't Enough

You might think that just knowing about the threats is enough to control your weight. Unfortunately, it's not. Most of the threats operate at an

unconscious level. You won't even know when they are attacking you. So simply being aware of the threats won't help you stop them.

Imagine you are watching TV and a commercial comes on advertising a tempting food. It looks delicious. You can taste it. You can smell it. You want it. And soon you find yourself in your kitchen looking for a treat to eat.

When you see the commercial, knowledge of the threats won't help you. The path from stimulus, wanting, and getting something to eat is automatic. Unless you develop strategies for coping, you will mysteriously find yourself eating without realizing how it happened.

That's what knowing the threats is good for: helping you to create strategies for stopping the threats. In the next four sections of this book, we'll talk about the strategies for defeating the threats:

- **The Designer Way.** In this chapter you will learn a complete process for losing and maintaining your weight that works no matter how crazy your life becomes.
- **Learn the Art of Joyful Eating.** In this chapter you will learn how to eat in moderation and prevent diet-crushing cravings by turning eating into a peak pleasure experience.
- **Put the Brake on Automatic Eating.** In this chapter you will learn how to physically retrain your brain into healthier, more effective behaviors and away from bad habits like automatic eating.
- **Weight-Proof Your Life.** In this large group of related chapters you will learn how to create protected areas in your life in which you naturally achieve your weight loss goals without relying on willpower every minute of every day.

Taken together, these strategies help to make up for weaknesses in your genetics and environment by showing you how to eliminate the slip-ups that cause you to fall of your diet. They do this by recognizing, building on, and taking advantage of the way humans work in real life. You use your intelligence to outwit and outlast the ancient part of yourself that drives you to survive.

Using the strategies puts you in the best position to succeed at controlling your weight. The world is full of threats. Fortunately, you are full of strengths too, many of which you aren't even aware of yet because you've never been fully exposed to all the strategies you may be good at. You'll learn how to counter the threats by finding your strengths. The result is a safe space where you are no longer a victim of the unconscious processes behind the threats.

This book covers many strategies, and there are many more on our website, but there are still a lot more strategies for you to discover for yourself. This book is not the end. It's just the beginning of a wonderful process that will hopefully result in your losing the weight you want, maintaining the weight you need, and staying on your diet for the rest of your life.

Chapter 13

The Designer Way
Strategies 4–16

I magine you are taking a road trip, driving cross country with a group of friends. How do you plan your trip? Do you plan every turn of the steering wheel? Do you insist on knowing every pot hole or detour ahead of time?

No, that would be absurd. It's impossible to know all that before you start. And what good would it do anyway? It'll all changed by the time you get there and you know how to drive so you'll miss most of the potholes anyway. And your car is more than strong enough to absorb a few bumps along the way.

Even if a detailed plan were possible, which it isn't, you wouldn't need it. You'll get where you are going because you know the process of how to take a successful road trip. You know how to drive, follow a map, deal with problems, work with friends, ask questions, and find new places to visit. At the root of all these amazing skills is your ability to achieve your goals by learning how to overcome obstacles.

The problem is you probably haven't learned a similar process for controlling your weight. Not many people have, because it's never been necessary before. We learn how to take road trips because we've taken them with our parents and friends. We've read about road trips in books and watched them in the movies and on TV.

When do we learn the process for controlling our weight? We don't. What we learn are marketing slogans like "eat less and exercise more" or "eat right and get plenty of exercise." That's like telling someone asking how to plan a road trip to "drive safely." It's worse than useless. It's frustrating and demeaning and makes you just want to give up.

You need to know exactly how to control your weight. The process I created for controlling weight is called the Designer Way. We were introduced to the Designer Way in *The 10 Designer Principles* chapter. For a gentle introduction to the Designer Way, please reread that chapter again.

What does the Designer Way teach? If your journey toward permanent weight loss is a road trip, then the Designer Way shows you how to make the best decisions to get you there. The secret is learning how to continually improve your diet by making **small changes** in direct response to real events in your life. Over time these changes add up to amazing differences in your weight, and powerful changes in your life.

How you make changes to improve your diet is explained in loving detail in this chapter. Let's start with a simple step-by-step description of the Designer Way.

▌ The Weekly Spin

To deliver on my promise of showing you exactly how to control your weight, I've developed a simple step-by-step process I call the *Weekly Spin*, which is diagramed on the next page. Please take a look and for the rest of the chapter we'll learn how to apply it.

Let's go over its major components. Don't worry, we'll cover it in a lot more detail on everything later, I am just trying to give you an overview of all the pieces right now.

First, exactly what does "Weekly Spin" mean? The *weekly* part means it's a schedule of activities you perform during the week to control your weight. The *spin* part means you don't just do it for one week. You keep going round and round performing the same activities every week for the rest of your life.

There are three steps in the Weekly Spin:

1. **Start Spin.** A time for reflection. Every week, take time to check if you are meeting your goals, set new goals, and update your plan on how you want to meet your goals. A spin normally starts on Sunday, but you can start your spins on any convenient day.
2. **Daily Check.** A time for quick response. Every morning, perform a quick check to see if you unexpectedly gained weight. If you gain weight, quickly respond by adjusting your strategies.

Start

←— Weekly

Sunday	Monday	Tuesday	Wednesday	Thursday	Friday	Saturday
⃠	⃠	⃠	⃠	⃠	⃠	⃠
Ⓜ	Ⓜ	Ⓜ	Ⓜ	Ⓜ	Ⓜ	Ⓜ

Weekly —→

Start Spin: Ask yourself:

1. Did I meet my spin goals for last week?
2. What is standing in my way of meeting my spin goals?
3. What are my new spin goals for the upcoming week?
4. How will I meet my new spin goals?

Daily Check: Every morning adjust strategies immediately on any unexpected weight gain.

Make a Move: Always look for opportunities to prevent slip-ups, exercise more, eat to your diet and find more joy.

3.   **Make a Move.** A time for immediate action. Always look for opportunities to prevent slip-ups, exercise more, eat to your diet and find more joy you in your life. Take any opportunity to implement a strategy.

The Designer Way is really just that simple. It works for two reasons: 1) continual learning and improvement, 2) quick response to any weight gain.

You are continually trying new strategies and learning which work for you and which don't. Keep the successful strategies and toss the rest. Over time, these small improvements help you control your weight.

It's like improving at any skill. Practice makes perfect. By following the steps, you are always practicing at getting better and better at your diet. You are continually fine tuning your existing strategies and introducing new ones that increase your chances of losing and maintaining your weight.

A crucial part of the improvement process is figuring out when a strategy doesn't work. If it doesn't work you'll gain weight, but because of the steps, you'll notice the weight gain immediately. This allows you to try new strategies to get your weight back down again. By never letting your weight get too far out of control, you are always making forward progress toward your weight loss and weight maintenance goals. It's far easier to correct a problem when it's small than it is to fix a problem after it grows too big.

The Weekly Spin becomes a steady rhythm in your life. You continually look for moves that will help you lose weight. Every day you improve by making adjustments to your strategies. And every week you create a plan for doing better next week. It becomes a pattern you follow. Every week you do something. Every day you do something. And every moment you do something. The process pulsates like a drum beat. Every strike of the drum is the sound of your diet improving.

The result is beautiful music. You control your weight by following this simple process. You never gain too much weight before you notice and take steps to lose it again. And you are always learning and improving your diet.

This is what it means to control your weight. You adapt to what is really happening in your life based on how the strategies really work for you. That puts you back in control of your weight. You don't have to let your weight spin wildly out of control again and you don't have to try random diets only to notice it's been six months and you haven't kept your weight off again. With the Designer Way that doesn't happen. You are in control.

Now let's talk about each activity—Start Spin, Daily Check, and Make a Move—in more detail.

▌ Start Spin–A Time for Reflection

The Designer Way divides time into a continuous series of **one week periods** called **spins.** Each week, usually on Sunday, you start a new spin. This is a time for reflection, evaluation and planning. Take a moment to see how you are doing, and think about how you can improve on the last spin. It's essentially a **meeting with yourself** to plan how you can control your weight better this week.

Gaining weight is very easy if you don't take this time. What use is it to notice that you have gained weight during the past couple of months? That's too late. Checking your progress every week gives your strategies a chance to take effect so you can notice if they are working or not. If your strategies aren't working, you can make changes to improve them.

Yes, the start of a spin is **taking time for yourself.** You can do that, you know. ☺ You don't always have to work, or be helping other people. Take some time to think about your progress. Your chances of staying on your diet are poor if you can't set aside even a little time for yourself. Remember, you are worth it.

If Sunday isn't a good time for you to start a spin, then pick any other convenient day. All you need is a little private time to carry out all the start spin steps. To begin your weekly spin, find a comfortable place where you'll have some relatively uninterrupted time.

Think about running your weekly spin with a friend who is also using *Your Designer Diet.* You can help each other to carry out all the steps, talk to each other, support each other, and give each other ideas.

▌ Ask Yourself Four Questions

Every spin starts by asking yourself the same four questions:
1.   Did you meet your spin goals for last week?
2.   What is standing in the way of meeting your spin goals?
3.   What are your spin goals for the new week?
4.   How will you meet your goals?

The end result of asking and answering these four questions is a plan for what you want to do this week and a reasonable idea of how you are going to get there. In creating your plan, you've looked at your life and you've learned from experience. Every week you adapt to changes in your circumstances, and you get better at losing weight and staying on your diet. It's this consistent focus that puts you back in control of your weight.

Let's look at each question.

Question 1: Did you meet your spin goals for last week?

A spin goal is something you would like to accomplish or do during a spin. It could be a strategy you want to implement, a goal like losing one pound, or a goal like walking 2,000 extra steps a day. A spin goal is anything you want to do that you think will help control your diet.

The point of this question is for you to evaluate your progress on your spin goals. Are your strategies working? You need to know this so you can decide if they need to be dumped, adjusted to work better, or if new strategies are needed to meet your goals.

To determine how well you did on your previous spin goals:

1.   Go through each spin goal you'd set in your previous spin.
2.   Use your feedback system to see how well you met each goal.

These two steps show if your strategies are helping to control your weight. They do this through **feedback.** Feedback is **information about responses to your actions.**

Let's say your goal during the previous spin was to lose one pound. How might you get feedback to determine if you've achieved this? You would probably weigh yourself. OK, calling weighing yourself a "feedback system" sounds a little grandiose, but feedback is a general concept and weighing yourself is just a good example.

Weighing yourself is a pretty easy form of feedback, so let's tackle a more difficult problem. Let's say you adopt a spin goal of walking 2,000 more steps each day. How would you know if you reached your goal? That's tough because it's not likely you can count your steps in a day. I've tried and it doesn't work.

It turns out there's a device called a pedometer you can wear on your hip that counts your steps as you walk. Using a pedometer, you can figure out how many extra steps you take in a day. If you created a spin goal of walking more steps, you could use a pedometer as a feedback mechanism for determining if you met it.

The knowledge of how many steps you actually took in a day would let you know if your strategies for taking extra steps were working or not. If you reached your 2,000 step goal then your strategies are working and you don't need to do anything. If you didn't reach your goal, you'll have to figure out why not and then plan how you can improve. That's the critical value of feedback: you learn when changes need to be made.

So, for each spin goal you need to create a feedback system that will tell you if you have successfully reached your goal. We'll talk about how to create a feedback system for your weight in the *Use Feedback to Control Your Weight* strategy. Whatever feedback system you create for each of your spin goals, use it here when answering this question.

Question 2: What is standing in the way of meeting your spin goals?

The point of this question is to help you remove any roadblocks that stand in the way of you meeting your spin goals. Sometimes a few little problems hold you back and once you clear them up, your progress races ahead.

Think over your week. How did you do in the spin? What worked well? What didn't? What changes can you make to improve your results? How can you remove the obstacles keeping you from reaching your goals? How can you make this spin a bit more successful?

Answering these questions helps you to continually improve your diet.

Question 3: What are your spin goals for the new week?

Now it's time to take your answers from the first two questions and turn them into *spin goals* for this spin. Your goals can include anything, for example which strategies you want to implement and how much weight you want to lose in the spin.

There's a lot to think about when setting your goals. If you didn't meet your goals in the last spin, how might you meet them this week? If there were forces standing in the way of meeting your goals, how might you work around them? What new strategies do you want to try?

A goal for almost every spin is **how much weight you want to lose in the spin.** At the start of a spin, think about how much weight you want to lose and which strategies you can use to reach that goal. We'll talk about picking a spin weight loss goal in the *How Much Do You Want to Lose in a Spin?* strategy.

You may have **other goals** too, like increasing the amount you bench press, or trying a new walking trail, or buying a set of smaller plates. **A spin goal can be anything you think will help you control your weight.**

Where can you get **ideas for new spin goals?** All over the place. You have all the strategies in this book to choose from. You can create your own. You can get ideas from magazines, the Internet, or your friends. Maybe there was a spin goal from the last spin you didn't get to and you can move it forward to this spin. **Make a goal of anything you think will help.**

At the beginning of a new spin, you have the opportunity to think about **new strategies** you might want to implement. Some strategies are simple and you can just adopt them without much thought or preparation. Others are more complicated and will take some planning.

Take some time now and look at which strategies you might like to adopt in this spin. In *Design Your Weight Loss Plan* strategy, you'll create a **strategy list** so you'll have a variety of strategies available to try when you're ready.

Once you select a set of goals, **write them down** so you can remember them for the next spin. In the first question, you'll have to check if you met your goals and that's hard to do when you don't remember them.

Question 4: How will you meet your goals?

The point of this question is to make your goals real by ensuring you have some idea of how you will accomplish them. After you decide on your spin goals, create a plan of how to achieve them. The amount of necessary planning can vary from none to lots.

Let your own nature guide you in your level of planning. I am not a big planner, so my plans tend to be simple without a lot of detail. I don't worry too much about it. Plans are life for other people, and they like every detail to be well thought out and scheduled. Either approach is fine, do whatever works for you.

Part of a plan is creating a feedback system for determining if you've reached your goal or not. We talked about feedback systems in our discussion of the first question, so you might want to reread it. Here's where you think about and decide how to implement your feedback system for each goal.

▮ Example Goal Plan: Buying a Treadmill Machine

Let's say one of your goals is buy a new treadmill machine. This allows exercise at home and you think that will give you more time to exercise. This might be too big a goal for one spin. We don't want spin goals to become another source of stress in our lives. So perhaps you might want to divide this goal into two goals, one for each of two weeks.

This week you might want to research which machine is the best for you. Your feedback system is to check if you've actually made a decision of which treadmill to buy.

Next week you might want to actually buy the treadmill, take delivery, and set it up. Your feedback system is that the treadmill is ready and waiting for use in your house.

Has this spin goal actually done anything to control your weight? No, because all you have is another piece of exercise equipment taking space in your house. To control your weight you actually need to use the equipment and that needs to be a spin goal in the next spin.

To move forward on your weight loss journey, a spin goal must result in a strategy that helps control your weight. Not all strategies work. That's OK. But a strategy must make some progress toward controlling your weight or it's not worth doing.

▌ Daily Check—A Time for Quick Response

Waiting a week in between spins means it could be a whole week before you deal with any weight gain. You can do better. A Brown Medical School study has convincingly shown **the quicker you notice and respond to small weight gains** the more likely you are to be able to maintain your weight loss.

That makes sense doesn't it? It's harder to lose a lot of weight than it is to lose a little. If you notice a small weight gain, you can take immediate action to lose it. Tackling a potential weight gain before it becomes a big problem is a better way to control your weight.

This is the idea behind the Daily Check. Make a quick check every morning to see if you unexpectedly gained weight. If you have, then make adjustments to your strategies to bring your weight back down. You don't usually have to make large adjustments. Maybe you exercise a little more, tighten up on your portion sizes, or reverse a habit you recently started. The idea is to notice quickly and just **do something.**

▌ How do you notice a little weight creep?

You notice weight creep using what we call your Daily Feedback System. You'll learn how to create one in the *Use Feedback to Control Your Weight* strategy.

For now let's say your daily feedback check is to **weigh yourself every morning.** Personally, I just use the fit of my clothes to see if I am gaining weight, but most people are probably more comfortable using a scale.

So let's say you've weighed yourself and you find you gained weight unexpectedly. Why worry only about unexpected weight gains? Because not all weight gain is a surprise. If you are a woman menstruating or you drank a lot of water, you could expect weight gain. A small amount of weight fluctuation is normal. You might want to ignore small weight increases until you become convinced it is a real problem and not a normal part of life.

When you notice an unexpected weight gain, **take action.** Make immediate changes to bring your weight back down again. You can make any move you think will help. If your weight doesn't come back down, then wait for the start of the next spin to give it more thought.

▌ Make a Move—A Time for Immediate Action

A move is **applying a strategy** to your life. Making moves is something you do all the time. It's not something you just do at the start of spin or at your daily check. You are always looking for opportunities to better control your weight. **When you see an opportunity** to make a move–**take it.**

A common example of a move is making the decision to take the stairs instead of the elavator. Chances for taking the stairs just pop up during the day. You couldn't possibly know at the start of spin that you'll have the chance to take the stairs on Thursday; it just happens. So when there's an opportunity, take the stairs because the extra steps will burn more calories.

Over time you make thousands of these "little" decisions. Little is in quotes because they are not little decisions at all. They add up to huge tidal waves of positive change.

The smallest of changes may seem trivial when you first make it, but the force of a thousand changes over time is awesome. A lake fills up one rain drop at a time. You lose weight one small move at a time. You don't have to make big changes to make a difference. Choosing to make a move instead of doing the easier thing is the most powerful weight control strategy.

Here's how you make moves:

1.   Continually pay attention to your life and be on the lookout for a strategy you can apply that will accomplish one of the following goals:
     ❖   Eat to your diet.
     ❖   Exercise more.
     ❖   Add more joy.
     ❖   Prevent slip-ups.
2.   Set the extreme-o-meter. Decide how extreme you need to be when applying a strategy. We'll talk more about setting your extreme-o-meter later.

3. Continually learn, create, and adjust strategies you can apply
    to your life. Use your knowledge of the threats to help you. If a
    strategy doesn't work, then drop it and move on to another one.
    Something will work.

Some moves are made once for one **specific situation.** If you are at a
wedding, for example, you'll have to decide how much of the rubber chicken
and delicious cake to eat. That's a one time move because you'll never be in
exactly the same situation again.

Some moves are made for **longer periods** of time. If you work at a company
offering a cafeteria, for example, you could decide to implement a strategy of
eating the salads every day for lunch. That strategy will last as long as you work
at the same company. If you change jobs, you have to change strategies too.

Some moves you make for **your entire life.** A good example is deciding
to walk more each day by parking far away from any building entrance. You
can use this strategy all the time.

Other moves are more **planned.** You may notice that your company has
vending machines stocked with junk food and you want to do something
about it. You may want your company to lower the price on healthy foods in
the cafeteria. You may want to move to an area of the country where you'll
naturally get more exercise. You might notice these opportunities at any time,
but they don't happen automatically.

At the heart of the move is simply being involved with your own life.
Often, life just seems like it happens to us. By making moves, you are continually engaged and active. Nobody else can make moves for you and nobody
else can tell you when to make a move. A move happens because you see an
opportunity and take it. That's truly being in control of your weight.

▌ Weight Gain is Information About What Doesn't Work, it's Not Failure

You will gain weight from time to time. Gasp! Don't get depressed or freak
out. Gaining weight is not the end of the world. It doesn't mean you should
just give up. It doesn't mean you are a horrible person. It doesn't mean you
are a failure. It means you have **learned something.**

Gaining weight is a learning opportunity. Weight gain is simply information telling you that something you are doing isn't working or your situation
has changed. Your job is to try and figure out what isn't working and fix it by
adjusting your strategies.

Figuring out what went wrong isn't always easy. Perhaps you've picked up a new routine of stopping by a coffee shop in the morning and ordering a shockingly high calorie coffee drink. Or maybe you stopped taking your daily walk at lunch.

Whatever the eventual reason for the weight gain, you need to try different strategies to meet your spin goals. Fortunately, with a new spin starting every week and your daily check, you can never gain too much weight before you notice. You will always have the time and the ability to adjust.

Don't let a little weight gain get you down. Use what you've learned to do better in your next spin.

▌ You are Always Seeing Progress

The Designer Way seems like a lot of work, especially when compared to doing nothing. Why follow it at all? First, in actual practice it takes very little time. Second, you will see results and seeing results is exciting. Seeing results is better than fun–it's a blast! Life becomes more joyful when you see your control over your weight continually getting better and better.

Using your Daily Feedback System, you'll see how your weight is progressing. Sometimes your weight will go up and that's fine. It just means it's time to make a move. Sometimes your weight will go down. Congratulations! A move you made must have worked. And sometimes your weight will stay the same. Excellent! Your weight staying the same is actually a huge accomplishment, yet many people see it as a failure instead of the amazing achievement it is.

If your weight is staying the same then that means your weight isn't going up! Think about that. **Your weight isn't going up.** That's a big deal. Most people's weight goes up steadily throughout their lives. But your weight is holding steady. That's great. Any move you make at this point will help you improve. That's a wonderfully powerful position to be in.

▌ Example: Weekly Spin Session

All this talk about spins, daily checks, and moves may seem a little abstract. Let's go through a few example spin sessions so you can get a better idea of how it all works together.

Spin 1, August 13th, Sunday

This is your first spin. You need to create your initial weight loss plan. That's covered in the *Design Your Weight Loss Plan* strategy. In creating your plan, you'll learn important information like which threats impact you most, which strategies you want to try, how extreme you need to be, your initial spin goals, and much more. You'll be able to use all this information during this first spin.

Even though you haven't created your plan yet, we'll show a few example spins anyway. It's more important that we run a few spins than it is to go into all the gory details.

For now, let's say my plan is:

1. **Spin Weight Loss Goal:** lose one pound this week. I plan to do this by eating 250 fewer calories and burning 250 additional calories from exercise. If I lose 1 pound a week that's 52 pounds a year! That's a good attainable weight loss that will make a big difference to me.

2. **Weekly Feedback System:** weigh myself. I weighed myself so I would know my starting weight.

3. **Daily Feedback System:** feel the fit of my clothes.

4. **Strategies to Implement:**

   ❖ Walk on the treadmill for 30 minutes four times a week. I figure that will burn about 400 calories for each session. For my feedback system I'll just remember that I exercised. You may choose to keep a journal instead.

   ❖ Find more steps to take each day with a goal of reaching 2,000 extra steps a day. For my feedback system I bought a pedometer to count my steps. I'll establish my baseline average number of steps this week and start looking for more steps next week.

   ❖ Watch my portion sizes and cut out one piece of junk food a day. For my feedback system I'll just check my weight to see if I've been successful. You could use a food journal for a more rigorous check. I'll just keep it simple until it's clear whether what I'm doing is working.

For your first spin, choose strategies you feel comfortable with or feel excited about. It's up to you. These are just examples. Keep it simple though, as I tried to do. Start simple and add more strategies as you feel comfortable.

For example, I don't count calories, even though it's a powerful and useful strategy. I'll just watch portion sizes and see how well that works. If it doesn't work, I can always add calorie counting a little later. You may want to use a computer program or journal to help track your weight and count your daily calories. Many people find this extremely useful, especially when starting out.

One goal of your first spin is to figure out your own way of running spins. Some people like a more formal approach with a lot of structure. They will want graphs, spreadsheets, lists, and accurate calorie counts because that's what helps them succeed. Other people will want to just wing it. Either way will work. As always: do whatever works for you and be as extreme as you need to be.

Let's assume I've followed my plan for a week and it's time to start the second spin.

Spin 2, August 20th, Sunday

I start each spin with a big cup of hot coffee, early on a quiet Sunday morning. To prepare for your spin you might want to collect any journals and charts you've kept, as these might help answer the four questions.

At the start of a new spin we always answer our four questions:

1. **How did you do on meeting your spin goals for last week?**

    Not so good. My weekly feedback system is to weigh myself, so I did that first. My spin weight loss goal is one pound and I ended up gaining a pound! I did reach my exercise goal of walking on the treadmill for 30 minutes four times for the week, so that was good. And I did figure out my base line average number of steps taken each day.

2. **What is standing in the way of meeting your spin goals?**

    Where did the weight gain come from? That was a bit of a shock. I must have eaten too much. I don't keep a food journal, so this is only guessing, but I went through a lot of changes last week, so I may have eaten more than usual.

    I changed jobs last week, which threw me off. I need to make some changes to make up for my different environment. Where I worked before, we had good cheap salads for sale in the cafeteria. In my new job, we don't even have a cafeteria. And in my old job I had to walk a lot. In my new job I don't have to walk at all.

    I was lazy and I didn't use the daily check last week. That wasn't smart. If I had performed a daily check I would have caught the weight gain earlier and responded faster.

3. **What are your spin goals for the new week?**

    I am still going to try to lose 1 pound during this spin. There's no reason to try and lose more. I'll just keep doing the right things and once I find the right mix of strategies the weight loss will happen.

    I'll check my portion sizes very carefully.

    I'll add in another exercise session and go 5 minutes longer on my existing exercise sessions.

    I need to find a way to eat a better lunch.

    I need to find some moves to walk more at work.

    I want to find some smaller plates and some tall thin glasses to help me maintain my portion sizes better (see the *Use Smaller Plates and Bowls* strategy).

    Oh, and now that I know my baseline number of steps, I'll try finding 2,000 more steps each day.

    Every morning I'll implement the daily check step.

4. **How will you meet your goals?**

    I am going to read *The Honest Calorie Estimation Method* strategy to help develop my portion control skills. All the other goals are pretty simple and don't need a plan.

August 21, Monday

Daily Check: No change in how my clothes fit.

This morning I figured out a new move! This is always exciting.

Every morning I wake up and refill the water bowls for the dogs. We have two dogs so we have two bowls. Every morning I walk to the dog room to get both their bowls, walk to the kitchen to fill them both with fresh water, and then I walk back to the dog room and set the bowls down. I have done this for years and the dogs have never once said thank you!

Of course, I always want to be as efficient as possible, so I make one trip. The drive for efficiency is almost always a bad move.

It dawned on me today that I was missing an opportunity to make a quality weight loss move. If I made two trips, one for each bowl, I'd naturally get more exercise.

You might say "big deal, that's nothing." Well, it's actually twenty extra steps a day. So I would be getting 20 extra steps per day, and there are about 2,000 steps in a mile, so over 100 days I would be walking an extra mile. Walking a mile burns about 100 calories. Over 10 years I would burn off one pound worth of calories because a pound is about 3,500 calories. Don't worry about the math; we'll cover all this later in more detail.

But you are still probably saying "big deal, a pound over 10 years, that's nothing." Well, alone it's not much. But what if I can make 100 such tiny moves? That would be 10 pounds over 10 years! Now that's a big deal, especially when you are trying to maintain your weight loss.

And that's how the Designer Way works: continually searching out and making small improvements that add up to big results.

August 22 Tuesday

Daily Check: No change in how my clothes fit.

Driving to my new job, I have to pass by a really nice donut shop. I couldn't take it anymore. The temptation to drop by on the way to work was too much. So I made a move. I found another route to work that didn't go by the donut shop. That's an easy 1,000 calories a week saved.

August 23, Wednesday

Daily Check: Clothes feel a little looser.

I found a grocery store within walking distance from work. I kill two birds with one stone with this one move. The grocery store has a nice salad bar so I can get a good lunch and I walk a quarter of a mile.

You might say "big deal" again, but you can't only search for big wins, every move counts, no matter how small.

August 24, Thursday

Daily Check: No change in how my clothes fit.

I tried some of the ideas from the *Volumetrics* book at dinner tonight (see the *Pump Up the Volume* strategy). I added more vegetables to the sauce, which made the meal more filling and it has fewer calories than my old recipe.

August 25, Friday

Daily Check: No change in how my clothes fit.

I got one of those computer programs to remind me every hour to get up, stretch, and take a little walk. That adds another 500 steps to how much I walk every day.

I also stopped by the store to buy some smaller sized dishes.

August 26, Saturday

Daily Check: Clothes feel a little looser.

I checked my spaghetti dinner portion sizes and they had crept up again. So did my salad dressing portion size. I always seem to add more as time goes by.

I think I'll make the move of prepackaging my spaghetti into the correct portion sizes again. This worked before, but I just drifted away from doing it. And I'll also use a measuring spoon when putting dressing on my salad.

Spin 3, August 27, Sunday

Let's go through the four questions:

1. **How did you do on meeting your spin goals for last week?**

   Better. My weight loss goal for the spin was 1 pound and I lost 1.25 pounds. I reached all my exercise goals, including walking an extra 2,000 steps. I got the smaller dishes, but I haven't had a chance to really use them, so I'll have to make that goal in the next spin.

2. **What is standing in the way of meeting your spin goals?**

   I think most of my issues with my new job are worked out. Nothing else this week, just the usual trying to outwit and outlast the power of food.

3. **What are your spin goals for the new week?**

   I will aim to lose 1 pound this spin too. In fact, I think that will be my goal every spin.

   I'm going to start using my new dishes.

I'll keep the same exercise goals and give the previous changes another week to work. I think that will give me the results I'm looking for.

4.   **How will you meet your goals?**

Nothing really to plan. I'll just implement the strategies from question three and we'll see how they work. If I lose another 1.25 pounds next week, I'll drop the extra exercise session and drop the extra 5 minutes too. I am getting tired of it and it's really more exercise than I'll be able to keep up over the long run. If I don't meet my goals after those changes, I'll just have to figure out something else.

August 28, Monday

Daily Check: Clothes feel a little looser.

Today we are having a party at work to celebrate a new product release. There will be a lot of people and lot of wonderful tasting food at the party. I think I'll reread the *How to Eat Joyfully in Different Situations* strategy. And I'll also read the *Put the Brake on Automatic Eating* chapter again to review some strategies that will help me not overeat at the party, which I usually do.

August 29, Tuesday

Daily Check: No change in how my clothes fit.

At 7:00 PM I only had about 200 calories in activity for the day and my goal is 250 calories from activity. I decided to take a walk to the mailbox to add another 50 calories.

I noticed a new threat. We bought a new sugarless whip cream last week and I was using way too much of it. That's not good. Because I wasn't consistently able to stop myself from placing a frothy dollop of cream in my coffee, my best move is to throw away what I have left and not buy it anymore. Is that too extreme? Not for me. I can always make whip cream from scratch for the times I really need it.

August 30, Wednesday

Daily Check: No change in how my clothes fit.

I was just browsing *Your Designer Diet* last night and I read in one of the strategies about how getting support can help you be a lot a more successful at staying on your diet. I think I'll go to the *http://YourDesignerDiet.com*

website and see what their support is like. Maybe that can help me with some more ideas.

Let's stop the example here.

▍ A Little Post-Example Discussion

We've run through a couple of spins in the example, and I hope you started to get a feel for the rhythm of the Designer Way process. You make moves, check your weight every day, and every week you try to do better. The result is powerful and supremely simple.

This process takes very little time, and the example may not have made this clear. No time is wasted in the Designer Way. If it was, you wouldn't follow it for very long. Every step can be as quick and simple as you need it to be.

I know this process sounds deceptively simple. It may sound like all I am saying is, make some goals and create a plan to reach your goals. I am saying that, but that's not what I'm really saying. That sounds too much like a marketing slogan.

Remember the deep underlying wisdom behind the Designer Way: pay attention to your life and react to it as you are living it.

Everything else just helps you do better.

The Move is the heart of the Designer Way: look, plan, try, and learn. By making moves you are always finding more and better ways of eating less and exercising more. If you can only do one thing then do the Move.

The Daily Cycle is the next most important part. Getting daily feedback on your weight means that your weight can never fall too far out of control. If you can only do two things, then do the Move and the Daily Check.

The crowning jewel of the Designer Way is the Weekly Spin. It helps you develop perspective and see a little farther into your future. If you can do all three parts of the Designer Way, you are creating for yourself the most powerful weight control process possible.

▍ Did I Fulfill My Promise?

Earlier I promised I would show you exactly how to control your weight for the rest of your life. I think the Designer Way fulfills that promise. You've learned a simple, clear, and powerful step-by-step process for creating your perfect diet. Through each step you learn how to fit your diet to your nature and your life. The result is a diet designed just for you. And because of that finely tailored fit, you'll finally lose weight and keep it off for the rest of your life.

▌ What's Next

We've covered the core of the Designer Way in enough detail that you can get up and see results immediately. But there's a lot more you can learn about the Designer Way. The rest of this chapter explores strategies for helping you get the most possible benefit out of the Designer Way.

. . . .

 ## Strategy 4. How Extreme Do You Need to Be?

Every strategy has an *extreme-o-meter* you can dial up or down, according to your need.

On a scale of 1 to 10 how easy is it for you to gain weight? A setting of 1 is if you were let loose in Willy Wonka's chocolate factory, you would end up losing weight. A value of 10 means even the thought of a chocolate factory adds 5 pounds.

Your honest answer matters, because you have to decide for yourself which strategies to choose and how extreme you need to be in implementing them.

Every strategy has an **extreme-o-meter** you can dial up or down according to your own unique nature and what you wish to accomplish. For some strategies, I dial the extreme-o-meter high because I know I have a particular problem in that area. For other strategies I dial the extreme-o-meter lower because it's not as big a problem for me.

How extreme you need to be for a particular strategy is something you need to figure out for yourself. Think of the extreme-o-meter as a **knob you dial up or down as your life changes.**

▌ Everyone Has Their Own Unique Way of Being Overweight

You are unique in all the world. Nobody is exactly like you. Your genetics are unique, your life experience is unique, your talents are unique, your place in your life is unique, and the environment in which you live is unique.

What being unique means is that nobody can look at you and know why you are overweight. We simply don't know if you have fewer dopamine receptors, a higher weight set-point, problems with your hormone system, if you have fewer taste buds, the inability to get good results from exercise, a system more sensitive to stress or the lack of sleep, or a whole host of other issues that could contribute to your being overweight.

▌ Who You are Matters: Are You a Morning Person or a Night Person?

One way to think about your own uniqueness is to consider another very personal point about yourself: are you a morning person or a night person?

Do you jump out of bed in the morning singing "zippity-do da zippity-ay" or do you hide your head under the covers hoping your alarm explodes? Over the years it has probably become obvious to you which type of person you are.

It may surprise you that being a morning person or night person is genetically based. We can look at your DNA and figure out which kind of person—morning or night—you are likely to become. DNA determines what is likely to happen. You could turn out differently than your DNA specifies, but if I were a betting man I would bet on your DNA.

This doesn't mean that a night person can never get up early or that an early person can never stay up 'til dawn. What it does mean is you'll probably end up living your life toward one edge of the extreme.

What happens if you try to go against your nature? What if you are a night person who works the early shift? What if you are an early person working the night shift? Unhappiness. Either way you'll walk around like a zombie in *Night of the Living Dead* because it just doesn't work. You are what you are. Through extreme discipline you can make it work for a while, if you have to. But you won't be as happy as you would be if you were living with your nature instead of against it.

Nobody tells you if you are a morning person or a night person. You figure it out for yourself through trial and error. You just know what works best for you. People will believe you if you say you are a morning person. They won't say something absurd like if you just had more willpower you could be a night person. They'll understand because they are a particular type of person too.

In the same way **you are a particular type of overweight person.** Nobody can tell you which kind, because there are so many ways of being overweight. Only a few people share your kind of being overweight, so most others won't understand when you say something doesn't work for you.

▌ I am an 11 on the 10 Point Scale

My family has obviously survived many a famine. I've found I have to be extreme on many strategies to be successful. For the most part I don't feel bad about this. Someone will always be faster, stronger, smarter, and better than I am at something. I accept this is how I am. It's a fact. I have to deal with the facts by understanding the threats and being creative on how to counter them.

For example, one of the strategies we'll talk about later is to avoid stocking extra food in your house. This means, for example, not buying 20 boxes of crackers at a time. You'll eat more when have more food available than if you had the right amount.

This is so true for me, so I don't stock food anymore. I know I had to adopt this strategy and be as extreme about it as I can. Honestly, if I could, I'd have no food in the house at all and I would have a Star Trek Replicator prepare a perfectly portioned and nutritious meal on demand.

Would better willpower solve the problem? A little. But remember, only a few slip-ups a week leads to weight gain. My willpower hasn't been that good in a lot of areas, but it's surprisingly good in others. Of course, as always, your mileage may vary.

▌ What's the Best Way for You Personally to Lose Weight?

Whatever works. That's my favorite saying of all time. Find what works for you and do it. Nobody can tell you which strategies will work for you. Nobody, not your doctor, not your partner, not your best friend, not the media. Nobody can know how you feel inside or how your body will respond to different strategies. **Believe in your own experience to figure out what works for you.**

You'll have to **experiment** with different strategies and how extreme you have to be in each strategy. Don't feel bad if a strategy doesn't work; keep trying and be creative. Something will work.

Everyone is similar enough that we can share ideas on what works or not, but we are dissimilar enough that what works is different for each of us. One size does not fit all. The support website at *http://YourDesignerDiet.com* can be a big help in your journey of trying to find what will work. You can also help others by sharing your successes.

▌ The Nibble Example

Here's a good example of the extreme-o-meter in action. Many people are tempted by food in close nibble distance. They keep eating even when they are "done" eating. The hand automatically reaches for the food and places it in the mouth. No thinking required.

If you are one of these people, then move the food away, pack it in a to-go box, or hide the food from sight. Out of site out of mind. Using this strategy you really protect yourself from overeating.

Some other people may be tempted by the food, but not enough to keep nibbling. For them, the Lifeguarding strategies we'll talk about later in the book may be enough.

And still other people won't give the food a second thought. They get to do nothing, blind to the food-generated torment many of us experience.

Be as extreme as you need to be when threatened. Don't worry about how you think you should feel or how other people react to the same tempting food. Do what you need to do to help you deal with the immediate threat. And then take pride and satisfaction in knowing that you both noticed the problem and took action to solve it. That's good stuff. That's how you control your weight, being as extreme as you need to be.

▌ The Secret is to Experiment and Find What Works for You

Experiment. If something isn't working then try a little more, try a little less. Make a little change. Imagine in your mind how it might be made to work for you. Ask people for their advice. And in the end if a strategy doesn't work for you then toss it and move on to the next one. Something will work. **It's not a race.** It's OK if finding the right strategies takes a little time.

A fantastic example of the incredible power behind this idea is shown by a study at Children's Hospital Boston. It clearly demonstrates that paying attention to your personal biology is critical for controlling your weight. They put some people on a low-fat diet and others on a low-glycaemic diet. A low-glycaemic diet says you should limit the amount of quickly digested carbohydrates. Quickly digested carbohydrates like white bread and refined breakfast cereals spike your blood sugar and insulin levels. They found that some people naturally already produce a lot of insulin. When on the low-glycaemic diet, these people lose almost six times more weight than when they are on a low-fat diet!

The low-glycaemic diet controlled their insulin levels better. If you already produce a lot of insulin, should you really be on a diet that encourages you to produce even more insulin? But you'll find people pushing both types of diets—low-fat, low-glycaemic—like they'll work for everyone equally well. And then when it doesn't work they put the blame on you, implying you just lack willpower. What you really need is a simple oral glucose test to see how much insulin you produce so you can choose a diet that works with your biology, not against it. That's the general idea behind the Designer Diet. There are thousands of similar ways in which you are overweight and the Designer Diet helps you find them and stop them from hurting you.

Yes, everyone has weaknesses, but everyone has strengths too. **Search out your strengths and use them to your advantage.**

Strategy 5. Design Your Weight Loss Plan

Create a plan for controlling your weight that is as unique as you are.

Your goal here is to create a **strategy list**—a priortized list of strategies you would like to implement in the Designer Way. The first few items in the list are the strategies you might consider implmenting in your first spin.

Let me guide you through a series of questions that will help you create your strategy list. The questions help you set goals. They help you figure out where you are in your life and where you want to be. In short, they lead you through a process of introspection. The end result of all this hard work is a very personal and practical list of strategies for controlling your weight. And later, as you discover more strategies you would like to try, you can add those to the list too.

You may not consider a strategy list as a real weight loss plan. A typical plan is a detailed set of instructions on what you should do in every situation. That's the exact opposite of what I mean by a plan.

The chance of anyone following a complex plan over any length of time is about the same as me setting a new world record in the marathon and playing the lead in major motion picture—all in the same year. Not likely.

Even if you could create and follow a detailed plan, it would never work because your life is always changing. You will change jobs. Your body will change. Your favorite coffee shop may invent a new irresistible calorie bomb of a dessert. You may have children or your children may leave the nest. You get older. You may get married or divorced. You may move or your neighborhood may change around you. You may get injured or sick. You may heal from an old injury that has been holding you back.

A set plan can never keep up with your life. People think they can fix plans by making them more and more complex to handle more and more situations. But making plans increasingly complex always fails in the end, because a plan can never be as complex as real life.

That's why the Designer Way will never fail you. It is simple yet always changes. It always responds to what's happening in your real life as it unfolds.

▌ Strategy List Interview Questions

It's time to gather all the information you need to create your strategy list. Please follow these steps:

1. **What is your reason for losing weight?** Getting in touch with why you really want to lose weight could be a big help in staying on your diet. See the *Why do You Really Want to Stay on Your Diet?* strategy for some help.

2. **Decide which threats apply to you.** Take a look at the threats again and make a list of those you marked as threatening to you. Knowing your most dangerous threats should give you a better idea about which strategies might help you the most.

3. **What is your target daily calorie budget?** If you plan to count calories as a strategy, you'll need to know this information. You'll also need it to calculate your calorie deficit. See the *How Many Calories Can You Eat Each Day?* strategy and the *Weight-Proof Your Portion Control Safe Zone* chapter for help.

4. **What is your target calorie deficit?** You'll need to figure out your calorie deficit before you can run your first spin. It will help you decide how many fewer calories you need to eat and how many more calories more you need to burn, which is information you need to know before you can select which strategies to implement. See the *How Much Do You Want to Lose in a Spin?* strategy for help.

5. **What is your feedback system?** You'll need to know the result of your strategy efforts so you can evaluate their effectiveness at the end of each spin. See the *Use Feedback to Control Your Weight* strategy for help.

6. **Which areas in your life need a Safe Zone?** Perform a slip-up survey in each zone. Figure out how you can make each zone safer for your diet. See the *Weight-Proof Your Life* chapter for help.

7. **Visualize solutions to your automatic eating scenarios.** Confronting any problems you have with automatic eating will help you decide which of the strategies might be useful to you. See the *Visualize Your Own Automatic Eating Scenarios* strategy for help.

8. **How extreme do you need to be?** You'll need to decide how extreme you need to be when implementing any particular strategy. Having a feel for how hard losing weight is for you will help you select which strategies to try. See the *How Extreme Do You Need to Be?* strategy for some help.

Thinking about all these issues was probably difficult. Many of these questions touch on subjects we would often rather avoid, but they do provide a solid foundation for creating your strategy list.

▌ Create Your Strategy List

After completing the interview process, you should have a pretty good idea about your goals and your greatest threats. Look over all the strategies in the book and use any insights you've learned from answering all the interview questions to decide which strategies make sense for you.

Make a list of all your selected strategies. Sort the list so your highest priority strategies are listed first. When trying new strategies, it makes sense to implement the most important first.

You are under no obligation to try a strategy on the list. You can always remove them. Be as detailed or as simple as you would like when creating your list. You can always add more strategies as you learn more, but you need to start somewhere.

Keep your strategy list up to date with any new discoveries and goals. As you find new strategies you would like to try, add them to your strategy list.

▌ Start Running Weekly Spins

With this list of initial goals and strategies, you are now in the perfect position to start running your first Weekly Spin. This is a really exciting time because it's the spins that really help to control your weight.

....

Strategy 6. What Do You Do if Your Plan Isn't Working?

Don't panic.

From time to time your plan will stop working and you'll gain weight. **Don't panic.** Gaining weight is perfectly normal. Controlling you weight is not easy. In fact, the design of your body purposefully makes it hard.

The threats never go away. Your environment will always be full of wonderful and cheap high calorie foods filled with fat and sugar. The smell, the thought, and even the sight of food will always make you hungry. You will always be tempted to eat more than you should because food will always taste so good. Your brain will always want to make short-term emotional decisions. Your body will always want you to survive by gaining weight. Life will always give you hard times and temptations. Industry will forever bombard you with advertisements and create new tasty foods for you to love. It will always be easier to sit around and do nothing than to be active. And as you get older, your metabolism will slow down.

With all that, how could you always control your weight?

That's why **learning to forgive yourself is so important.** You will go through periods where you gain weight and then lose it again. Hopefully your feedback system will keep the amount of weight gain low, but it will happen. Don't let it make you give up and quit. Expecting adversity means you won't be shocked when problems happen and that puts you in a better position to respond without panic. We can do some pretty stupid things when we panic.

What can you do, or think about, when your plan isn't working?

1. **See your doctor.** Maybe something has changed with your body and you just don't know what it is yet. Please reread the *See Your Doctor Now* strategy for some thoughts on this subject.

2. **Are you running your weekly spins?** The Designer Way helps you to continually get better at staying on your diet. If you aren't using the Designer Way you are ignoring a major weight loss strategy.

3. **Has your life changed recently in such a way that you need to update your plan?** If it has, take a look at the *Changes in Your Life Means Changing Your Plan* strategy for some help.

4. **Are you eating more calories than you think?** Revisit how many calories you are actually eating, using the *How Many Calories are You Really Eating?* strategy. You may not be counting foods that add a lot of calories to your diet. I once found that my innocent-looking snack of a handful of peanuts had 800 calories! A friend found she was drinking 400 extra "hidden" calories a day from the milk in her coffee. You never know where calories might hide.

5. **Is your calorie target correct?** Maybe your daily calorie target calculations from the *How Many Calories Can You Eat Each Day?* strategy is off. Try recalculating the numbers. Your body may be different now. If you've lost weight you may need fewer calories than you did before. You can also try gradually lowering your calorie target in 100 calorie increments to see if it makes a difference.

6.   **Reexamine your daily routine.** Keep a daily activity log for a while. This is where journaling is helpful because you can look it over for clues. Where are your Safe Zones letting you down? Where are you slipping up? Where are you eating extra calories? Where aren't you getting exercise? Talk it over with your support group. Then ask yourself which strategies you can add to create Safe Zones that will prevent any problems you have found. Take a look again at the strategies in this book and also see if you can think of any new ones that fit your life.

7.   **Are you always hungry and thinking about food?** Maybe your calorie target is too low and you aren't eating enough. Keep your calorie deficit small so you can keep the starvation response away. Take a look at the *How Much Do You Want to Lose in a Spin?* strategy for some help.

8.   **Are you getting enough exercise?** Perhaps you can add a few more exercise-related strategies to see if that makes a difference.

9.   **Do you have any new automatic eating scenarios you aren't dealing with?** Take a look at the *Put the Brake on Automatic Eating* chapter for some help.

10.   **Are you following the strategies?** Are you creating Safe Zones where it is hard for you to slip-up? Try some new strategies, even if you don't like them at first. Take a look at the *Daily Reminders* strategy; it can really help.

11.   **Are you extreme enough?** Can you dial up some of your existing strategies a notch or two? Walking at faster pace, for example, really burns a lot more calories. Maybe there are other strategies where you can be more extreme.

12.   **Is the diet you have selected appropriate for you?** Maybe the diet you are following isn't working for you and you need to pick another one.

13.   **Are you visiting your support group?** Participating in a support group is one of the most important strategies for keeping you on target. I know it seems like you can blow it off, but it really does help.

14.   **Are you working Joyful Eating into your life?** Joyful Eating can be the fun that helps keep you on plan. Don't ignore Joyful Eating. Diets don't work if they are just about denial. You need joy in your life too.

15. **Reexamine your reason for wanting stay on a diet.** Maybe getting in touch with why you are working on your weight might help. Redo the exercise in the *Why Do You Really Want to Stay on Your Diet?* strategy.

16. **Maybe you are just going through a rough patch?** Weight loss is frustratingly unpredictable. You go weeks without losing weight, and then one day 5 pounds just disappears. Maybe that's what you are going through. Wait it out a while longer. Keeping using the Designer Way and keep doing the right things. Don't give up.

17. **Could you be destined to be big folk?** If so, don't get sucked into thinking it's the end of the world or it is some deep personal flaw. You can still be fit and big and live a great life. See Big Folks Health FAQ at *http://www.faqs.org/faqs/fat-acceptance-faqs* for more information.

18. Visit *http://YourDesignerDiet.com* for more help, support, and inspiration. Maybe somebody at the site can help you figure out what's going on.

Hopefully all these questions and suggestions will give you ideas on how to handle the inevitable weight gains and plateaus. It's helpful to consider, what else are you going to do? Do you really want to give up and start doing all the wrong things again? You know that won't work. Be patient. Let the process work. It will in the end.

Strategy 7. Changes in Your Life Means Changing Your Plan

When your life changes it's also time to take another look at your plan to see if it needs changing too.

Life changes so quickly. It's easy to catch ourselves with the wrong plan in a new life situation.

Your feedback system is often the first warning of a previously unnoticed life change. Your weight will start increasing for no reason you can think of and then pow! You'll remember you changed jobs or some other life-changing event happened. It's time to take another look at your plan.

▌ Dealing with the Monster Flu

I remember when I had a monster flu that just wouldn't go away for months and months. I would start feeling better, start exercising a little, and then wham, I was sick again. I finally decided to stop exercising to give myself a chance of getting better.

You might think I would see feeling sick as a life change and that I should adjust my plan and create a new Safe Zone for myself. You might think that, but I didn't. A week or so later I noticed I was gaining weight. At first I blamed it on the flu. But then I remembered, duh! I stopped exercising. That would do it.

A new situation requires a new plan. I had to adjust my plan and create a new Safe Zone for my new life situation. I decided to dial up the extreme-o-meter on several strategies so I could maintain my weight. That was really, really hard. I count on exercise to keep my weight in check. Without exercise I had to eat a lot less. So here's what I did:

❖   Take easier walks. Easy walks didn't seem to interrupt my healing and I still got some exercise.

❖   Dial down my portion sizes to lower my daily calorie total. I made less food and put less on my plate so I would eat less. By exercising less I figure I had to eat 400 fewer calories a day.

❖   I made doubly sure that there were no foods in my Safe Zone that I would eat automatically.

❖   I tried more *Volumetric* recipes (see the *Pump Up the Volume* strategy) so I could up the amount of food I ate, but still kept the calories low.

❖   I was extra vigilant in applying my automatic eating strategies.

Nothing really difficult or dramatic. But it worked. Eventually I got better and then I went back to my old plan. When you notice a life change early you can react immediately. That's the value of setting up and using your Daily Feedback System.

▌ A Tale of Two Changes at Once

My wife Linda had two life changes at once, and of course we missed them both! Life changes are tricky that way. They just sort of happen and you only think about them later when you are gaining weight.

Linda's seasonal work of doing taxes ended for the year. She had created a Safe Zone at work and that helped her stay on her diet. Once her work ended, she was back at home and nothing took the place of the Safe Zones she had been using. When you don't consciously think about creating your Safe Zone, you fall back into old bad habits and that weight starts coming back. Fortunately, Linda's feedback system told her she was starting to gain weight and she adjusted her Safe Zones to compensate.

Soon after her job ended, Linda was selected to be on a jury for a trial that would last 6 weeks. She realized a few days into the process that she was gaining weight and that she needed to create a new Safe Zone for the court house. She decided to bring lunch and healthy snacks to court. And because Linda was sitting so much, she also decided to take a walk during her hour and half lunch break.

Again, nothing magic, but Weight-Proofing your life isn't about magic, it's about creating your own Safe Zones to bring about your personal goals. Nobody said it had to be difficult.

▌ Life Changes that May Change Your Plan

Any change in your life may require changing and creating a new Safe Zone. Here's a list of some common life changes:

- ❖ Going on vacation or traveling for work.
- ❖ Jury duty.
- ❖ Changing or losing your job.
- ❖ Changing schools.
- ❖ Changing seasons.
- ❖ Becoming sick or injured.
- ❖ Moving to a new house.
- ❖ Having visitors over to your house.
- ❖ Having a baby, or a child leaving home.
- ❖ Getting older or starting menopause.
- ❖ Some particularly happy or sad event like a wedding or a funeral.
- ❖ Any time you go someplace new that isn't inside your Safe Zone.

The list is endless. Any change in your life can upset the tightrope you walk while trying to control your weight.

▌ How do You Handle Life Changes?

When your life changes, you can follow the steps under the *What Do You Do If Your Plan Isn't Working?* strategy. The process works for life changes too.

In general though you have three options:

1. **Dial up the extreme-o-meter** on your existing strategies.
2. **Add new strategies** that fit your new world.
3. **Remove strategies** that don't work and put your efforts elsewhere.

Some set of strategies will work for you. Stay creative. And most of all, even though it is hard, do your best to anticipate changes in your life so you don't have to be reacting all the time. Be proactive when you can.

Strategy 8. Why Do You Really Want to Stay on Your Diet?

Do you really want to lose weight? Or do you just think you should?

In *The Two Brain Threat* we talked about how important motivation is in decision making. The decision not to eat tasty food goes against almost every instinct you have and that's why most people slip-up. The parts of your brain dealing with short term and long term rewards compete when making decisions.

For your brain to reliably choose the long term reward of staying on a diet over the short term reward of food, you need to create in your mind a really valuable long term reward for staying on a diet. **Finding a really strong and valuable long term reward for staying on your diet will help your brain make the decision not to give in and eat the tasty food it so desperately wants.**

Don't worry if you can't find a reason, the strategies in this book assume from the start that you can't always stay motivated enough to prevent the slip-ups. But life will be a lot easier if you can find a powerful reason to control your weight.

Let's see if you can find a reason to control your weight. Imagine for a moment you are the main character in a play about your life. What do you think motivates your character to lose weight and stay on a diet?

Spend some time now and think about why you want to lose weight and stay on a diet. Block out some quiet-time for yourself and think about your life. Ask yourself why? Why do you really want to lose weight and stay on a diet?

Here are some potential reasons for staying on a diet:

1. **Health.** We'll see in the *Know Your BMI* strategy all the nasty health consequences related to obesity. Overweight people have an increased risk of high blood pressure, diabetes, heart disease, infertility, joint and pain problems, and other illnesses. And you probably won't just have one problem, you'll have several.

2. **Well-being.** Being lighter generally makes you feel stronger, more energized, and more mobile. You will be able to move without pain and take part in fun activities.

3. **Beauty.** Maybe you want to look hot. Perhaps you want to fit in your clothes better. Or maybe you feel pressured by society to conform to an unrealistically thin ideal.

4. **Money.** Being sick is very expensive. The healthier you are the less you'll spend on medical costs and the more money you'll have left over to spend on other things.

5. **Your Children.** Even if you aren't concerned about yourself, you might be very concerned about your child's health. There is an alarming growth rate of Type II diabetes in children as young as 10 years old. Statistics show that one in three children born today will develop diabetes in their lifetime. **Children with obesity-related diabetes face a much higher risk of kidney failure and death by middle age than people who develop diabetes as adults.** Plus, with uncontrolled Type II diabetes, your child will look forward to constant pain from neuropathy, going blind, having limbs amputated, and dropping dead of a heart attack. Sorry to be so brutal here, but this is serious business.

6. **Maintaining Independence as You Age.** If you want to be fit and play with your grandchildren rather than prematurely enter a nursing home, controlling your weight is a good plan. Being heavy is hard on your knees, hips and ankles. If you maintain a lower weight you may be able to live independently longer as you age. One study found that extremely obese people, those who are 80 or more pounds overweight, are over twice as likely as normal-weight people to stay in hospitals longer or end up in nursing homes after an illness.

7. **Special Events.** People can get motivated to lose weight for important events like weddings, vacations, and reunions. But after the event is over, you also lose your motivation. Special events are not a persistent source of motivation.

8. **Help the Economy.** A recent study found that each one year increase in life expectancy was worth an average of $1.2 million per person to the economy. It seems the longer you live the more productive you are, which adds to the wealth of the nation.

Can you think of any others? Perhaps there is some deeply personal reason that is meaningful to you?

It appears that the reasons for staying on a diet primarily center around health, yours and your family's, and how you look.

Are these highly motivating reasons to lose weight and stay on a diet? It depends on who you are and where you are in your life. For a lot of people, the clear answer is **no.** These aren't really motivating reasons to control your weight. Otherwise fewer people would be overweight.

The reason why there are few compelling reasons to stay on diet is clear: **food has power.** Food tastes better than being thin feels. Most pledges of "it will be different this time" melt under the unrelenting reward of food.

That is, until you get a wake up call like a stroke, a heart attack or diabetes. Contemplating your death can motivate a lot of people, but even death is not enough to motivate you every moment of every day for the rest of your life.

You've probably seen sad images of people still smoking through the wracking coughs of emphysema. They have every motivation not to smoke, yet they still do. The addiction is that strong. Food can also compel you to go against your own best long term interests.

Fear of a serious medical problem isn't the only motivation though. Maybe one day you just can't stand who you see in the mirror anymore. Or maybe you miss playing sports like you used to. Or maybe you think that you need to make an effort to attract a person of the appropriate sex.

Base at least some of your reasons for staying on your diet **on joy** not fear. Even people facing the threat of open heart surgery don't make lasting changes in their life. Fear alone won't work. **Why would people be motivated to live longer when they are miserable?**

A lot of people simply aren't happy enough to want to live longer and they don't want to give up the few sources of happiness they've found. It would be like someone bobbing up and down in the ocean after a wreck giving up their life preserver. You would never give up your life preserver. You would cling to it with every ounce of energy you had left. And that's what people do with food. They cling to food because it makes them happy and they can't see anything taking the place of food in their lives.

That's why you need a vision of your life that includes joy. Being happy is a reason to control your weight. What if staying on your diet would give you pleasure and make you happy? What would be worth living for?

Hopefully you have found some really powerful and meaningful reasons for you to control your weight. But, unfortunately, even that's not enough.

We've seen in *The Gumption Threat* how your motivation can wear down. We've seen in *The Distraction Threat* how easy it is for you mind to lose focus. We've seen in *The Power of Slip-ups Threat* how few slip-ups it takes to gain weight. And we've seen the power of food.

Clearly, you can't rely on motivation alone. *Your Designer Diet* helps you to win despite not having perfect motivation. In the times when you are really motivated and more in your logical mind, you will be able to set up the strategies that work for the times when you lose motivation.

Strategy 9. Know Your BMI—Are You Overweight and What Does It Mean for You?

Knowing your BMI helps you figure out your weight-related health risks, but BMI doesn't always tell fit from fat.

Almost every report you hear about obesity and health also talks about BMI. Just what is BMI and why does it matter?

▌ What is BMI?

BMI stands for Body Mass Index and it is recognized by the National Institutes of Health and The World Health Organization as the best standard to judge obesity. Not everyone agrees with this judgment, and we'll talk about that disagreement later.

BMI is a quick and easy calculation to estimate how much fat you have. Mathematically, which you shouldn't worry too much about, BMI is defined as your body weight divided by the square of your height.

The idea is, the higher your BMI the more fat you probably have. And the more fat you have the less physically active you probably are. And the less physically active you are and the more fat you have then the less chance you have of being healthy.

BMI is popular because it's easy to calculate. All you need to know is your height and weight, which are both easy to measure. And that's the source of the problem with BMI too. We all know people can be the same weight and height and look totally different. One person can be mostly flab and another person can be solid muscle, and they'll have the same BMI.

Researchers looked at how various BMI ranges were related to disease and death. They found certain BMI ranges were associated with better health, and certain BMI ranges were associated with worse health. They assigned weight ranges into categories based on projected health risks.

Here are the BMI categories the researchers came up with:

❖ Underweight: less than 18.5.
❖ Ideal: greater than or equal to 18.5 but less than 25.
❖ Overweight: greater than or equal to 25 but less than 30. This is approximately 10% over your ideal body weight.

❖   Obese: greater than or equal to 30 but less than 40. This is approximately 30 pounds over your ideal weight.

❖   Morbidly Obese: greater than or equal to 40. This is approximately 100 pounds over your ideal weight.

These relationships were figured out by statistics, which means they were calculated using data from lots of people. It doesn't say anything about how you in particular will turn out health-wise. But statistically, to be in the healthiest group, you should have a BMI in the ideal range, between 18.5 and 25.

To help you get a feel for how height, weight, and BMI are related, here are the BMI ranges for someone who is 5' 9" tall:

Weight Range	BMI	Weight Status
124 lbs or less	Below 18.5	Underweight
125 lbs to 168 lbs	18.5 to 24.9	Normal
169 lbs to 202 lbs	25.0 to 29.9	Overweight
203 lbs to 269 lbs	30 to 39.9	Obese
270 or more	40 or higher	Morbidly Obese

▌ What are the Historical Obesity Rates?

In the US, the percentage of obese adults varied little from 1960 to 1980. Obesity increased considerably between 1980 and 1991, from 13 to 21% among men and from 17 to 26% among women. This trend continued. In 1999–2000 obesity increased to 28% of men and 34% of women.

Imagine a movie of how obesity rates have changed over time on a state by state basis. According to the Centers for Disease Control (CDC) statistics, in 1990 only 4 states had obesity rates between 15–19% and no states had rates above 20%.

Move the calendar ahead 10 years to 2000 and a lot had changed. All 50 states had obesity rates of 15% or more. Thirty-five states had obesity rates as high as 20% or greater.

Flip the calendar ahead another 5 years to 2005. Only 4 states had obesity rates less than 20% and 17 states had obesity rates of 25% or greater. Three states—Louisiana, Mississippi, West Virginia—had obesity rates greater than 30%.

This isn't just an American problem. Worldwide obesity rates are climbing fast too.

▍What are the Current Obesity Rates?

Here are the general obesity rates in the US as of 2002–2004:

- ❖ Over 66% of adults are overweight or obese.
- ❖ Over half of the adults are overweight.
- ❖ Nearly one-third of adults are obese.
- ❖ 17% of adolescents ages 12–19 years old are overweight.
- ❖ 19% of children ages 6–11 years old are overweight.
- ❖ Nearly 3% of men are extremely obese (having a BMI of 40 or more).
- ❖ Nearly 7% of women are extremely obese.

Obesity varies a lot by race/ethnicity and by age as of 2002–2004:

- ❖ About 30% of non-Hispanic white adults are obese.
- ❖ About 45% of non-Hispanic black adults are obese.
- ❖ Nearly 37% of Mexican Americans are obese.
- ❖ Nearly 29% of adults between 20 to 39 years old are obese.
- ❖ Nearly 37% of adults between 40 to 59 years old are obese.
- ❖ 31% of adults 60 years or older are obese.

A RAND study found the percentage of Americans who are extremely obese—about 100 pounds or more overweight—increased by 50% from 2000 to 2005. That's twice as fast as the growth of moderate obesity.

US obesity rates may be even worse than they appear. These numbers are gathered via a telephone survey in which people volunteer their own height and weight numbers. It has been found that people aren't completely honest about their height and weight, which could lead to a **significant under-reporting of obesity rates.**

According to the World Health Organization, worldwide there are:

- ❖ Over 300 million obese adults.
- ❖ Over one billion overweight people.
- ❖ Over 830 million undernourished people.

What we see now, probably **for the first time ever, is that more people are overweight than are hungry.** Most of the hungry live in the underdeveloped countries. Only an average of 300 calories a day stands between getting enough calories and hunger.

▮ What are the Future Obesity Rates?

As you can probably imagine, the future looks grim.

❖   The International Obesity Task Force (IOTF) estimates that nearly 287 million children worldwide could be overweight or obese by 2010, which is 85% more than a decade earlier.

❖   The overall obese population could possibly rise to more than 700 million by 2015, with nearly 2.3 billion overweight globally.

❖   In the US and Canada, it's thought that half of all adults are likely to be obese with only one in five people of healthy weight.

❖   One in three people born in the US today is expected to develop Type II diabetes. The rest of the world isn't far behind.

There's no sugar coating these numbers. They are what they are. I don't expect scary numbers to make a difference to people, but they are an interesting perspective on where the world is headed. We are going to have an avalanche of health problems coming down on us in the not so distant future.

▮ What Does this Mean in Real Pounds?

The BMI measurement can be a little abstract. What does a BMI of 27.5 look like? What does a high rate of morbid obesity really mean? It's hard to tell because they don't give out actual weight numbers in the statistical data. I was able to dig up some weight numbers that can help visualize increasing obesity rates.

In the 1960s and 1970s, average-weight of American adults increased only a pound or two in each decade. Then in 1980, the average adult in America gained 8 pounds. And in 2002, the average American weighed nearly 25 pounds more than they did in 1960, yet averaged only an inch taller.

Averages are still hard to visualize. In 2004, the International Health, Racquet & Sportsclub Association sponsored a nationwide survey to see what people actually weighed. Here's what they found:

❖   3.8 million Americans weigh more than 300 pounds, which is fine if you are 7 foot tall, but it's not so fine if you are of average height.

❖   More than 400,000 Americans weigh more than 400 pounds.

❖   1 in 9 adult men weighs more than 250 pounds.

❖   1 in 6 women weighs more than 200 pounds.

❖   The average adult male weighs 196 pounds.

❖   The average woman weighs 163 pounds.

I don't know if these numbers seem high or low to you, but using real weights instead of BMI numbers makes it easier to see what's going on.

▌ Why Should You Care About Your BMI?

You should care about BMI for two reasons:

1. A lot of medical conditions are related to your weight. Knowing your own BMI gives you an idea of your health risks.

2. BMI is frequently mentioned in studies and news reports. Knowing your BMI will help you make sense of new information as it comes in.

Being overweight may increase your risk of the following health problems:

* Hypertension
* Dyslipidemia (for example, high LDL cholesterol, low HDL cholesterol, or high levels of triglycerides)
* Type II diabetes
* Coronary heart disease
* Stroke
* Gallbladder disease
* Osteoarthritis
* Sleep apnea and respiratory problems
* Some cancers (endometrial, breast, prostate, and colon)
* "Man boobs," or pseudo gynecomastia
* Psychological problems (low self-esteem, depression)
* Infertility
* Knee joint, and other musculo-skeletal problems
* Skin problems

This time it's not just personal. People with a BMI over 40 are expected to have twice the health costs of normally weighted people. Moderately obese people (a BMI of 30–35) are expected to have increased health care costs of 25%. Obesity is a problem that affects us all in one way or another.

▌ Calculating Your BMI

There is a table you can use to look up your BMI on the following page.

The BMI calculation for children is more complicated because they are still growing. Please go to *http://YourDesignerDiet.com* to calculate the BMI for children (and adults too).

What is your BMI? Look in the following table. If you are overweight or above, take a look at section *Why Should You Care About Your BMI?* to see what problems you may have as a result.

BMI Table

			Ideal					Overweight					Obese										
BMI	19	20	21	22	23	24	25	26	27	28	29	30	31	32	33	34	35	36	37	38	39	40
										Weight (Pounds)													
58	91	96	100	105	110	115	119	124	129	134	138	143	148	153	158	162	167	172	177	181	186	191
59	94	99	104	109	114	119	124	128	133	138	143	148	153	158	163	168	173	178	183	188	193	198
60	97	102	107	112	118	123	128	133	138	143	148	153	158	163	168	174	179	184	189	194	199	204
61	100	106	111	116	122	127	132	137	143	148	153	158	164	169	174	180	185	190	195	201	206	211
62	104	109	115	120	126	131	136	142	147	153	158	164	169	175	180	186	191	196	202	207	213	218
63	107	113	118	124	130	135	141	146	152	158	163	169	174	180	186	191	197	203	208	214	220	225
64	110	116	122	128	134	140	145	151	157	163	169	174	180	186	192	197	204	209	215	221	227	232
65	114	120	126	132	138	144	150	156	162	168	174	180	186	192	198	204	210	216	222	228	234	240
66	118	124	130	136	142	148	155	161	167	173	179	186	192	198	204	210	216	223	229	235	241	247
67	121	127	134	140	146	153	159	166	172	178	185	191	198	204	211	217	223	230	236	242	249	255
68	125	131	138	144	151	158	164	171	177	184	190	197	204	210	216	223	230	236	243	249	256	262
69	128	135	142	149	155	162	169	176	182	189	196	203	209	216	223	230	236	243	250	257	263	270
70	132	139	146	153	160	167	174	181	188	195	202	209	216	222	229	236	243	250	257	264	271	278
71	136	143	150	157	165	172	179	186	193	200	208	215	222	229	236	243	250	257	265	272	279	286
72	140	147	154	162	169	177	184	191	199	206	213	221	228	235	242	250	258	265	272	279	287	294
73	144	151	159	166	174	182	189	197	204	212	219	227	235	242	250	257	265	272	280	288	295	302
74	148	155	163	171	179	186	194	202	210	218	225	233	241	249	256	264	272	280	287	295	303	311
75	152	160	168	176	184	192	200	208	216	224	232	240	248	256	264	272	279	287	295	303	311	319
76	156	164	172	180	189	197	205	213	221	230	238	246	254	263	271	279	287	295	304	312	320	328

Height (Inches)

What do you think about your BMI? Does it seem accurate to you? It may not be.

Problems with BMI

The BMI was calculated for many Olympic gold medal winners in swimming, rowing, wrestling, and sprinting. If anyone is healthy it would be gold medal winners, wouldn't you think? Well, many of them were found to be overweight.

This almost comical finding points out a problem with BMI. It's not really all that accurate. Since muscle is heavier than fat, if you have more muscle, like our gold medal winners, your BMI will be higher and you'll seem to be overweight when you clearly are not. Yet at the same time, if you have a BMI of 39, you can be pretty sure it's mostly fat and not muscle.

It turns out there are a number of problems with BMI:

- Women tend to have more body fat than men.
- Older people tend to have more body fat than younger adults.
- Highly trained athletes may have a high BMI because they have more muscle which weighs more than fat.
- The location of fat is probably more important than the amount. Most methods of body-fat testing don't reveal how much fat is located in the abdominal area and how much elsewhere. Excess fat around your belly is linked to increased risk of diabetes, heart disease and other serious conditions. Excess fat around your hips and thighs may pose fewer health risks.
- BMI isn't all that accurate a measure of fat levels. For example, when using BMI as a measure it was found that 75% of middle class men in India were overweight. When using a technique that actually calculated the real percentage of body fat, they only found that 27% of middle class men were overweight.
- BMI is only one factor related to risk for disease. For assessing your chances of developing overweight- or obesity-related diseases, the National Heart, Lung, and Blood Institute guidelines recommend looking at two other predictors:
  1. The individual's waist circumference (because abdominal fat is a predictor of risk for obesity-related diseases).
  2. Other risk factors the individual has for diseases and conditions associated with obesity (for example, high blood pressure or physical inactivity).

It would be far more accurate to directly measure your fat percentage, but that would be too difficult to do for everyone because it is an involved and expensive procedure, so BMI is still the obesity measure of choice. Just keep in mind that BMI is not an accurate measure of whether you are overweight or obese, it's just an estimate.

▌ Is Your Waist Size a Better Predictor of Risk than BMI?

Your waist size may be a more useful predictor of disease risk than either BMI or body-fat percentage because, if you have excess fat you will rarely have a small waist.

Women with a waist size of more than 35 inches or men with a waist size of more than 40 inches may have a higher disease risk than people with smaller waist sizes.

Some experts feel that the maximum safe waist size is 37 inches for men and 32 inches for women.

Don't hold your breath to measure your waist size accurately! I know you want to. Then place a tape measure around your bare stomach just above your hip bone. Keep the tape parallel to the floor. Make the tape snug, but not so tight that it cuts into your skin. Relax, exhale, and look at the tape.

Getting a good waist measurement is harder than calculating BMI, so BMI will probably be around for a long while.

▌ Is it OK to be pudgy?

A controversial study by the National Cancer Institute and the Centers for Disease Control (CDC) found people who are overweight, but not obese, have a lower risk of death than those of normal weight. This would be good news because being overweight is an easier target weight range than the normal BMI weight range. But the good news didn't last long.

Not long after the CDC study was published, two new studies came out that found being even a little overweight can kill you. What did the studies find?

- ❖ Overall, people who were obese had an increased risk of death compared to normal-weight people. This risk was higher for Hispanics, Asians and Native Americans than for whites or blacks.
- ❖ Overweight people were 20–40% more likely to die prematurely than normal-weight people. The risk was 2–3 times greater for obese people.

❖ Overweight people had a 10–50% greater risk of dying from heart disease or cancer than normal-weight people.

The unavoidable conclusion is: being overweight is bad for your health and being obese is *really* bad for your health.

More evidence of the health risk of being obese is shown by a University of Pittsburgh study of over 90,000 women who were followed for 5 years or more.

The study found white women with a BMI 30.0–34.9 (about 60 pounds above a normal weight for a 5' 5" tall woman) have a 12% higher risk of death. Extremely obese women with a BMI of 40 and above (about 110 pounds above a normal weight for a 5' 5" tall woman) had a stunning 86% higher risk of death than their normal weight counterparts.

Let's say that again: there is an **86% higher risk of death for extremely obese women.**

In general, your chances of dying climb as you gain weight above a BMI of 30, as do your chances of getting heart disease, diabetes, and hypertension. The good news is that **losing as little as 20 pounds improves a woman's mortality risk.**

The problem is that **more and more people are becoming obese,** not just overweight. The rates of extreme obesity vary by race/ethnicity from 10% for black women, 7.9% for Native Americans, and 1% for Asian and Pacific Islanders.

▌ What I take out of all this is:

❖ The heavier you are the more important it is to lose weight. Losing even a little weight can help a lot.

❖ If you are obese, try to get in the overweight BMI range.

❖ If you are overweight, try to get in the normal BMI range.

❖ Target a waist size of 40 or under for men and 35 and under for women.

❖ Weight isn't everything, being fit matters a lot too.

You, of course, must draw you own conclusions. But when you are making long term goals for yourself, you have to pick something. These seem like reasonable goals to me. You may want to aim higher. You may want to aim lower. It's your choice.

I will take this opportunity to remind you **I am not a doctor** so I am not advising you to do anything.

▌ The Big Jump in Obesity Rates Caused by a Small Increase in Weight

Dr. Jeffrey Friedman, a famous obesity researcher, has made a couple of very interesting observations on the rise of obesity rates:

- ❖ The overweight are becoming even more overweight while thinner people have remained pretty much the same.
- ❖ The increase in obesity rates translates to a relatively modest weight gain of between 7 to 10 pounds, depending on height, compared to how heavy people were in 1991.

I don't know about you, but when I hear about the obesity rates skyrocketing I visualize people all around me blowing up like balloons. Now, some people are gaining a lot more weight, but not everybody.

In 1991, 23% of Americans fell into the obese category. Currently about 33% of Americans are obese, which is more than a 30% increase. But the average weight of Americans has increased by about 7 to 10 pounds since 1991. That relatively small increase was just enough to bump a lot of people from the overweight category into the obesity category.

The good news is that you may not have to lose that much weight to drop below the obesity level.

Strategy 10. How Many Calories are You Really Eating?

If you don't know how much you are eating you won't lose weight. Find out how many calories you are really eating.

IF YOU DO NOT KNOW HOW MANY CALORIES YOU ARE EATING THEN YOU WON'T LOSE WEIGHT. Sorry for shouting, but this point deserves to be shouted because it is so obvious people don't pay attention to it.

In *The Bad Estimation Threat* we saw that people aren't very good at estimating at how many calories they eat each day. You will be truly stunned once you start measuring. You will be shocked at your real calorie count. I know I was. As I've mentioned, my snack of a handful of peanuts turned out to have 800 calories! A small bag of croutons had 70 calories! What I thought was a normal-looking hamburger had almost 800 calories! A small package of salad dressing surprised me by having 350 calories. Oh my.

Calories are everywhere and you are probably eating a lot more calories than you think. If you aren't losing weight, even when you expect you should be, the most likely cause is that you are eating more calories than you realize. Once you get control over those hidden calories, you will start losing weight. This isn't magic. The problem is that most people simply don't know how much they eat each day.

So, you need to **begin by finding out where you are.** You have to start somewhere and that somewhere is by getting a handle on how many calories you are really eating.

Track the number of calories you really eat for one week. Many people find that continuing to do this helps them stay on their diet. If that's you, then please continue tracking your calories. Whatever works. If the thought of tracking your calories each day makes you want to jump off the top of a pile of day-old bread, don't worry, you don't have to count calories for long.

Counting calories is not practical for many people over the long run anyway. Later, you will learn to manage your weight by selecting the **correct portion size** to begin with and by using **feedback** to determine when you may be eating too much.

One unexpected problem may be to **remember what you have eaten.** You probably eat a lot of food you won't remember eating later. You may think I'm crazy, but I'm not.

Have a meal with several people and then ask each person what they ate. The results will all be different and usually wrong. If you have an omelet, how many eggs did you eat? Did you remember the sour cream you dappled on the top? Did you remember to add the cheese? How much cheese was that? Did you forget the bacon bits? How many ounces of soda or juice did you drink? It's so easy to forget that piece of toast with butter, but that will be 190 calories that won't show up on your total.

The key to success for this strategy is to **write down what you have eaten immediately.** If you wait until the end of the day you'll miss so many items that the whole exercise will be almost worthless.

Another interesting strategy is to **take a picture** of all the food you eat. Counting calories is easier when you can see the food rather than having to remember it.

Many **computer programs** are available now to help you track and count calories. You no longer have to break out a calculator and a giant food calorie book. Please visit *http://YourDesignerDiet.com* for a list of calorie counting programs and websites.

Tracking your calories accomplishes several goals:

1. It gets you to be honest with yourself about how much you are really eating.
2. It helps you build up in your mind the number of calories different foods have. This will be quite surprising in itself. Knowing the approximate calories in the foods you eat is a critical skill for portion control.
3. It helps you figure out which calories are easy to eliminate. **Calories are an investment that you need to spend wisely.** Don't waste calories on food that's not worth it. In the next few strategies, you'll be determining how many calories you need to hit your weight loss target. That means you will need to figure out how to reduce the number of calories you eat each day. Your job is much easier if you can figure out the junk calories in your diet. Save your calories for food you really want, don't waste them on food that doesn't matter to you.
4. You'll start to see the benefit of strategies that support portion control. It's very difficult to know how many calories you consume if you are always eating at restaurants or picking up food on the fly. Without counting, there's no way for you to know. By using strategies that help control portion sizes, you can know exactly how many calories you are eating and you can begin to control your weight and stay on a diet.

· ·

Strategy 11. Understand the Pound

One pound of body fat equals about 3,500 calories. One can of soda has about 150 calories. Walking one mile burns about 100 calories. Food has more calories than exercise burns.

A lot of people don't understand the relationship between calories and their weight. We talk about gaining or losing a pound, but how many calories are in a pound?

One pound of body fat equals about 3,500 calories. That means to lose 1 pound of weight you must somehow burn about 3,500 calories more than you eat. Or another way to look at it is you need to eat 3,500 calories less than you burn.

You may have noticed that walking a mile only burns a puny-sounding 100 calories and drinking a soda costs you a hefty 150 calories. A mile is a long way; it hardly seems fair! Would you walk a mile for a soda? This is why it's very difficult to lose weight by exercise alone. You can easily eat far more calories than you can exercise off.

I call this the **Exercise Problem.** You can exercise like crazy and only burn a few hundred calories. Eating a single bowl of ice cream can easily wipe out a day's hard work. Many people think they can eat more just because they are exercising. Unfortunately, it doesn't work that way. **Food has more calories than exercise burns.** One study found that people who ran more than 30 miles a week still gained more than half a pound every year. The number of calories you need to burn through exercise to control your weight is frustratingly large.

Still, it's not a good idea to lose weight just by cutting calories, because of the starvation response we talked about in *The Starvation Threat.* Safe weight loss and weight maintenance usually combine both eating fewer calories and burning more calories through exercise.

If you exercise enough to burn an additional 250 calories each day, and you eat 250 calories under your required calorie level, you will lose about one pound per week or about 50 pounds a year. That's a lot of weight!

It's clear that exercise combined with eating less is the most effective way to lose weight. But if you can't exercise, you can still lose weight by controlling your calories. The problem is being thin doesn't mean you are healthy. Without exercise you could be a TOFI: thin outside yet fat on the inside. Fat on the outside is fat stored under your skin, which is a relatively healthy place to store fat. The fat on the inside is called visceral fat, that's fat around your internal organs. It's the visceral fat that's thought to contribute to heart disease, diabetes, and metabolic syndrome. Sumo wrestlers ripple with fat yet they are healthier than many of their thin, less active spectators. Sumo wrestlers mainly carry their fat under the skin. They exercise enough to burn off the visceral fat, which is some of the first fat to go when you exercise. To get the best of all worlds, you need to work exercise into your life. All is not lost if you don't see yourself hitting the gym for an hour every day. Later we'll talk about a lot of ways to work exercise into your daily life without becoming a gym rat.

Let's say every day at breakfast you slather one pat of butter onto a piece of toast. A one teaspoon-sized pat of butter is about 35 calories. If you eat an extra teaspoon of butter a day, you gain about 3.5 pounds a year. That adds up over the years. Just eating that one extra teaspoon of butter a day could gain you about 18 pounds in 5 years!

As you can see, **your food choices matter.** Here's a table to give you an idea how calories and weight are related.

Weight Gained In a Year	Number of Extra Calories Per Day
1 pound	10 calories
5 pounds	50 calories
10 pounds	100 calories
20 pounds	200 calories
30 pounds	300 calories

This table answers the question: how much weight will you gain by eating how many extra calories each day? For example, a Lifesaver® has about 10 calories. If each day you eat an extra Lifesaver you will gain one pound a year. Over 10 years that's an extra 10 pounds of weight gain just by eating one very small piece of candy you probably wouldn't give a moment's thought about eating.

▌ Use the Divide by 10 Rule to Go From Calories to Pounds Gained in a Year

You can quickly calculate the approximate number of pounds you'll gain in a year from eating a certain number of calories every day by **dividing the number of calories by 10.**

The math works out so nicely because there are 3,500 calories in a pound and nearly 350 days in year.

▌ Ask yourself: How much will I gain a year if I eat this?

One way to evaluate your food decisions is to think about how much weight you would gain in a year if you ate this food every day. This simple question gives you perspective. It helps you better judge the impact of how your food decisions today will change your waist size tomorrow.

Let's say you have a choice between two cereals for breakfast. One cereal has 20 more calories per serving than the other. If you eat the cereal with 20 extra calories everyday for a year you will gain an 2 extra pounds a year. That's a big weight gain for one small choice.

Here's another situation: if I am strolling down the hall and I see a can of soda sitting on a table and it's free for the taking, should I drink it?

Let's see. I know a can of soda has about 150 calories. If I wasn't sure I would take a look on the can. We'll also develop some portion judgment related skills in later strategies.

Using the *Divide by 10 Rule* I think to myself that extra soda will mean about 150/10 = 15 extra pounds a year. That's a lot for just a soda. I probably wouldn't drink it. The soda isn't worth that much to me.

You might argue that you are just having one soda so it's not fair to say you'll gain 15 extra pounds a year when it's really only 150 calories. And you would be correct, but not necessarily right.

These "should or shouldn't I eat this" situations come up many times each and every day. You make hundreds of food decisions on a daily basis. So really this one decision will have an impact because you make the same type of decision every day.

If today you decide to have the soda because it only has 150 calories, then you'll probably make the same decision tomorrow, and the day after that, and the day after that. Over a year that adds up to a year's worth of calories. That's why its more accurate to make a decision on what you should eat today based on how much you'll gain over the whole year.

The Lifesaver is a good example of why this way of reasoning works so well. You might not think a second about having a Lifesaver because it has so few calories. But the calories add up over the year. **Thinking about the calories over a year shows the real impact each food choice has on your weight.**

▌ Just what is a calorie?

We toss the word calorie around a lot, but few people have any idea what it actually is. It doesn't help that the scientific definition of a calorie is very technical and hard to understand, so it's often easier for us to act like we know what we are talking about, even when we don't.

A calorie is simply the measure of the amount of energy available in a food. The more calories in a food, the more energy it has. This means you can do more work from eating the food. And the more work you can do the better chance you have of surviving.

The energy is in a different form, but energy in food is the same idea as energy in the battery you use in a flashlight. Without the battery—energy—the flashlight doesn't work. Same with your body. It won't work without energy from food. And because your body demands a constant supply of energy, finding and eating food is the highest of all priorities for your brain. That's why you think of food so much of the time.

Here are a few examples to help give the idea of calories some meaning. A gallon of gasoline contains about 31,000 calories. It takes about one Big Mac to drive a car four miles. And there is enough energy in 5 pounds of spaghetti to brew a pot of coffee. Yet you can walk a mile using only 100 calories. Humans are pretty efficient users of calories.

Fat is the highest calorie density food at **9 calories** per gram. Density is the number of calories that are in the same amount of food, in this case a gram.

In the US, at least, we don't use grams very often, so it would help to get a better feel for what a gram is. A paper clip weighs 1 gram. A US nickel weighs about 5 grams. Find a nickel and hold it in the palm of your hand for a little while. Get a feel for how much it weighs. You might be more familiar with M&Ms. One M&M weighs about a gram. And 30 grams is equal to about 1 ounce.

Protein and carbohydrates both contain 4 calories per gram. Alcohol has 7 calories per gram. Water contains no calories at all. If you eat food made up of fat, then you'll be eating a lot more calories than if that food contained water. We'll use this fact in a later strategy as a way to eat fewer calories while still getting full.

Fat is such a good source of energy that your body has developed a special relationship with it. Your brain is constructed to love fat because sources of fat were scarce in humanity's past and your body wants you to hunt and eat as much fat as possible. Your love of fat is no accident. It is built-in to your body to help you survive.

 Strategy 12. What is Your Long Term Weight Goal?
Decide on a realistic long term goal weight.

Your ideal weight is almost impossible to calculate. Everyone is different, so plucking your ideal weight from a height-weight chart or by BMI or through some other means is difficult. Your ideal weight depends on how active you are, your fitness goals, how you want to look, your lean body mass, your genetics, and a host of other things.

So don't try to pick your ideal weight. For your long term weight goal, pick the actual weight you **can reach and maintain.**

At this point you should have a feel for what you think a reasonable long term weight is for you. You've thought about your BMI and looked at the health issues. You've looked at why you want to stay on a diet. And you've thought about how hard it is for you to lose weight and how extreme you need to be.

Pick a weight that is doable and reasonable. Don't try to be someone you are not, but don't sell yourself short either. Your long term weight goal is something you will keep in the back of your mind as a source of motivation.

The larger point is to **pick a target weight range you feel you can maintain** otherwise all these fancy numbers and calculations don't mean a thing. Let's get real here. If you think a lower weight is better for your health, but you aren't willing to do what it takes to get there, then why bother? We play too many games with ourselves. Be honest. It's your life, you get to make the trade offs. At the same time, don't be afraid to challenge yourself. We don't get anywhere without a goal. Like most grown up stuff, picking a target weight is a balancing act.

You don't need to say when you want to reach your goal weight because you can only lose weight safely at a certain rate. Losing the weight will take as long is takes.

▌ Reduce Your Expectations? Target Keeping Off 10 Pounds

This is something to think about. We've seen how an average weight gain of 10 pounds created a large jump in the percentage of people who are considered obese. Reducing your expectations and going for a 10 pound weight loss target makes a lot of sense. Medically it makes sense too. Even a 10 pound weight loss reduces your chances of getting diabetes and can significantly help with other medical problems as well.

Once you hit your 10 pound goal you can go for another 10 pounds. And after you reach that can go for another 10 pounds. There's nothing wrong with getting where you want to go 10 pounds at a time.

▌ What is your long term goal weight?

My long term goal weight was 260 pounds. I felt I would be satisfied if I ever reached that while maintaining my strength and muscle mass. I wouldn't be jumping for joy happy. I wouldn't have a washboard stomach. And I wouldn't be able to pose on the cover magazines. But at that weight I would help my diabetes and other health problems, look reasonably good in clothes, and feel better about myself. I also thought it would be a weight I could maintain for the rest of my life.

Don't worry about picking too high a goal. Once you reach your long term goal, you can always set another one.

Strategy 13. How Much Do You Want to Lose in a Spin?

Decide on a realistic spin weight loss goal by working backward.

A spin is a one week period during which you aim to meet a set of goals established at the beginning of the spin. One common goal is the amount of weight you want to lose in a week. How much weight should you lose per spin?

When you have reached your long term target weight, then the amount of weight you want to lose in a spin is a very nice looking zero pounds. You just want to stay at your current weight so there's no weight to lose.

If you haven't reached your long term weight loss goal, then you need to figure out an amount to lose per spin than makes steady progress, doesn't kick in the starvation response, and that you can successfully achieve given your nature.

How do you arrive at such a miracle number? By working backward.

First we figure out your daily **calorie deficit.** A calorie deficit is how many more calories you burn than you eat. Figuring out your daily calorie deficit will tell you how much weight you can be expected to realistically lose each spin.

▌Calculating Your Calorie Deficit—Using Fat for Fuel

The fat on your body is a form of energy storage. Calories you eat now that aren't used are stored as fat for use later. Fat is like a gas tank. When your body needs more energy it will dip into the gas tank. What does your body need energy for? Everything it does: thinking, running, building muscle, breathing, and a thousand other activities. In our ancient past we might have gone many days without eating, so being able to store fat was critical for survival. When food was plentiful we would eat all we could and store up fat for the lean times when food wasn't available, yet we'd still have to work to get more food.

Your fat came from eating more calories than you needed. That's called a *calorie surplus*. Only in our modern world, the lean times may never come so you have to artificially arrange the lean times by creating your own *calorie deficit*.

Two questions need to be answered about your calorie deficit:
1. How big a calorie deficit do you need?
2. How do you create a calorie deficit?

▌ How big a calorie deficit do you need?

We don't usually gain weight by eating thousands of calories extra a day. Instead, **we slowly accumulate one to three pounds a year by eating 10–30 extra calories a day.** Over ten years that's an extra 10 to 30 pounds, made one slip-up at a time. From *The Bad Estimation Threat,* you can see how easy it is to eat a few extra calories a day. Once you start counting your calories for a few weeks, you will definitely see how you are eating the extra calories that add up over time to obesity.

Dr. James O. Hill, Professor of Pediatrics and Medicine Director, Colorado Clinical Nutrition Research Unit, estimates that **90% of weight gain could be stopped by having a calorie deficit of 100 calories a day.** That's not that much really. It's one soda or a tablespoon of butter less a day.

Remember that a pound of fat has about 3,500 calories. If you create a daily calorie deficit of 500 calories, you will lose a pound week or about 50 pounds a year (remember the divide by 10 rule). A calorie deficit of 100 calories a day means a weight loss of about 10 pounds a year.

The goal of *America on the Move* (see the *Walk the Walk* strategy for more information) is to get people to have a daily calorie deficit of 200 calories. Some people might think losing weight at this level may be too slow, but slow weight loss is better. **The weight took a long time to gain, give it some time to come off.**

The **slower you lose weight, the less hard your body will fight to keep the weight on** because your body won't see the weight loss as starvation. Remember the slowly boiled frog? Slow weight loss may also minimize the intense cravings you'll get if you go faster.

Think back to the Minnesota starvation experiment. Eating too few calories slowed their metabolism down by 40%! So, by eating too few calories you can actually make yourself gain weight because your body thinks it is starving.

Many people suggest a maximum calorie deficit of 500 from reducing how much you eat. You can create a bigger calorie deficit by exercising more. The idea is to decrease your calories a little and increase your activity levels as much as you can.

A deficit of 1,000 calories just from eating less will almost certainly kick in your starvation response.

You'll have to decide for yourself which calorie deficit number is best. You can always start at 100 or 200 and work up. Whatever the number you pick is one you'll have to live with, so there's **no use lying to yourself** by picking a number that's too high.

▌ How do you create a calorie deficit?

Once you decide on your target calorie deficit, you need to come up with a set of strategies for implementing your goal. It's easiest to combine strategies that **reduce the number of calories you eat** and by **increasing your exercise level.**

Let's say your calorie deficit goal is 500 a day. People seem to like that number because it means they'll lose a pound a week which is a significant amount of weight to lose in one year. Now you need to decide how to meet this goal. Is it by eating less or exercising more?

Let's split it down the middle. Let's say you'll reduce your calorie consumption by 250 and you'll be more active for the remaining 250 calories. We'll call the 250 calorie deficit from eating less your *calories from eating less.* We'll call the 250 calorie deficit from being more active your *calorie deficit from exercising more.* You'll need to remember both numbers for use in the *How Many Calories Can You Eat Each Day?* strategy.

You may be asking, reduce consumption by 250 calories below what? Good question. You'll calculate the number of calories you should eat each day in the *How Many Calories Can You Eat Each Day?* strategy.

Creating a Calorie Deficit by Increasing Your Activity Level

Increasing your activity can mean something as simple as walking more. You need to add an extra 4,500 steps a day to burn an extra 250 calories. Later we'll talk about lots of strategies for increasing your number of steps.

Be careful when calculating your **calories burned** from exercising as everything may **not be as it first appears.** Walking a mile is typically said to burn 100 calories. So if you walk 35 miles you would think you should lose a pound of fat because there are 3,500 calories in a pound. But it doesn't quite work that way.

You burn a lot of calories from just sitting around, even if you don't walk. So that number has to be subtracted from the 100 calorie figure used for walking to get a more accurate number. Once you subtract the calories used by sitting, it turns out that walking really only burned an extra 54 calories per mile.

The 100 calorie per mile number is just an approximation anyway. **A heavier person will burn a lot more calories** than a lighter person. If you exercise on a treadmill or other equipment, the **mechanical advantage** provided by the machine means you don't burn as many calories either.

If you are losing weight slower than you think you should, then your calorie deficit from exercise calculations may be inaccurate. You'll have to exercise a bit longer or with greater intensity to make up for the fudge factor.

Creating a Calorie Deficit by Eating Less

Reducing the calories you eat can mean just switching from regular soda to diet soda. Stop eating that extra donut. It doesn't have to be traumatic. As you read on, you'll see a lot of strategies that will be able to help you reach your calorie deficit goal.

▌ Your Calorie Deficit isn't Related to Your Target Weight

Notice how your calorie deficit isn't tied to what you may consider your ideal weight. It doesn't matter if you want to lose 10 pounds or 100 pounds. You can only lose weight as fast as your calorie deficit will let you.

This has been my approach. I try to create a calorie deficit with the strategies and use the feedback techniques to fine tune my weight.

. . . .

Strategy 14. How Many Calories Can You Eat Each Day?

How many calories do you need each day to both live a healthy life and meet your weight goals?

The number of calories you can eat determines your portion sizes and portion sizes determine your weight. That's why you need to figure out how many calories you should eat each day.

Let's say you are sitting down to breakfast. How much can you have? Then it's lunch time. How much can you have? You feel like an afternoon snack. How much can you have? It's dinner time. How much can you have? Hey, dessert looks really good. How much can you have? You would like another glass of wine. Can you?

To answer all these "how much" questions, you first need to know how many calories you can eat each day. Eat more calories than you should and you'll gain weight.

The formula—I know, I don't like formulas either—we'll use to calculate how many calories you should eat each day is given by:

calorie budget = calories for living – calorie deficit from eating less

The calorie deficit from eating less is the number you decided on in the *How Much Do You Want to Lose in a Spin?* strategy. In that strategy you determined your daily **calorie deficit** target. The calorie deficit had two parts: the **calorie deficit from eating less** and the **calorie deficit from exercising more.**

When calculating your **calorie budget,** we only want to use the calorie deficit from eating less.

▌ Calculate Your Calories for Living

What I call **calories for living** is usually called your maintenance calorie level: how many calories you need to breathe, heal, think, digest food, and everything else your body does to keep you alive. You need to know this number before you can calculate your daily calorie budget. It doesn't include calories supporting any exercise you may perform.

I know this sounds a bit complicated. But you probably have no idea how many calories you should eat each day. I know I certainly never did. The problem is, if you don't know how many calories you should eat then you don't know how much food you should eat.

The average maintenance level for women in the US is 2,000 calories per day. For men it is 2,500 calories per day. These are only averages. Very active people will need a higher number of calories. Some triathletes need as many as 6000 calories a day to maintain their weight.

Rather than write a long sequence of boring instructions on how to calculate your maintenance calorie level, please use the calculator tool at *http://YourDesignerDiet.com* to perform the calculations instead. It's a very complicated calculation that's confusing and complex when explained. Using the website is much more practical.

In this book, we'll use 2000 calories for women and 2500 calories for men in all the examples. If you don't plan to run the calculation, you can use these numbers too.

▌ Finally: Calculate Your Daily Calorie Budget

Now we have all the information we need to calculate your daily calorie budget. Let's take a look at the formula again:

calorie budget = calories for living – calorie deficit from eating less

We decided for example purposes to use 2,000 calories as the *calories for living* and 250 as the *calorie deficit from eating less.* Plug in your own numbers, of course.

So our daily calorie budget is:

calorie budget = calories for living – calorie deficit from eating less
1,750 = 2,000 – 250

If you eat 1,750 calories a day and burn an additional 250 through increased activity, you will have a calorie deficit of 500. So, you should lose one pound a week or over 50 pounds a year.

That's really a lot of weight loss for what is a pretty doable calorie deficit for many people. Don't worry if your calorie deficit causes slower weight loss, it just means it will take a little more time, and more time is fine.

The daily calorie budget you have just calculated tells you how much food you can have in a day. We'll use this information later when determining the portion sizes of foods you can eat.

The American College of Sports Medicine (ACSM) recommends that calorie levels should never drop below 1,200 calories per day for women or 1,800 calories per day for men. Even these numbers may be too low. If you find yourself targeting a calorie budget in this range, you should rethink your goals.

▌ The Calorie Budget is Not Too High, Others are Too Low

After you calculated your calorie budget, are you thinking that the number of calories you are supposed to eat is too high? Are you thinking you'll never lose weight if you eat so many calories?

Lots of weight loss programs want you to eat a pitifully small 1,200 calories a day. And you may think "I gotta go low to lose weight. I'll just go for it and get the weight loss over sooner."

That's a losing strategy. A 1,200 calorie diet is semi-starvation for a lot of people. Keep the men in the Minnesota starvation experiment in mind. They were on a semi-starvation diet. Do you want to end up like them? Please read that threat again. Very few people can stay on a diet with their body constantly driving them to eat because they aren't eating enough.

Less is not more. You aren't in a race to see who can lose weight the fastest by starving themselves. You are not just trying to lose weight. People lose weight all the time and gain it right back again. The **goal is to stay at your target weight for the rest of your life.** You'll never manage to stay on a starvation diet. It's too hard and even if it wasn't, starvation doesn't work as a weight loss strategy.

Your body can't tell the difference between a diet and starvation. As soon as you start eating too few calories, your body will go into starvation mode and you'll stop losing weight. That's why low calorie diets are a sucker's game. They don't work for the same reason your ancestors were able to survive all those generations. Your body is looking out for you.

If you do "go for it" by starting a low calorie diet, you'll drop a lot of weight fast, you'll be losing more muscle than fat. And that's not what you want. Muscle burns calories. Lose 5 pounds of muscle and your daily calorie burn plummets by about 250. Over a year that's 25 pounds of weight gain. And once you go back to a more normal diet, your weight will bounce right back even higher than it was, because you have less muscle and burn fewer calories.

You have to work with your body. **You seduce your body into losing weight.** You can't pound your body into shape with an ultra-low calorie diet.

▌ Adjust Your Calories Down Slowly

If you try the *How Many Calories are You Really Eating?* strategy, you should get a good idea about how much less (or possibly more) you need to eat to meet your calorie budget.

If your calorie budget is substantially higher or lower than your current calorie intake, then you may need to adjust your calories gradually over a period of a few weeks to allow your metabolism a chance to adjust.

▌ Are You Thinking of Food All the Time?

If you've cut back your calories to match your calorie budget and you are starting to think of food all the time, it could be a sign of the starvation response. First, recalculate your calorie budget. Perhaps there was a mistake in the calculations.

Second, try increasing your calorie budget a hundred calories or so and see if the constant hunger thoughts go away. Try this a few times. I won't say increase your calorie budget until you stop feeling hungry, because for some people it's possible they may never feel full.

You have to understand that eating too few calories is not the way to lose weight. I know this idea may go against every impulse you have. Your brain may scream that you mustn't eat. Your brain may yell that you are eating too much and your calorie budget is too high. Ignore those thoughts. The only way you can stay on a diet for the rest of your life is to eat enough to keep your body from thinking it is starving.

▌ Do You Have to Count Calories Forever?

No, you don't need to count exact calorie totals forever because that's too difficult. You just need to become calorie aware. You can do a good job at maintaining your calorie budget by just knowing about how many calories you have eaten and about how many calories you have left to eat. That's all the information you need to make better eating decisions.

▌ You Need to Recalculate Your Calorie Deficit

Some estimates show that for every 20 pounds of fat you lose, your daily calorie burn drops by 100 calories. So, as you lose weight or gain muscle, you'll need to recalculate your calorie requirements.

Many people hit a weight loss plateau because they don't realize that fat requires calories and once you lose some fat you need fewer calories to live. If you don't reduce your calorie budget, then you stop losing weight. You hit a plateau. But there are deeper reasons why you'll need to recalculate your calorie budget.

All the numbers you have calculated are simply estimates. They can all be wrong. All the estimates for the number of calories you are eating will be wrong too. That's why you need to be patient and figure out what you need to do over time. Using the feedback techniques we'll cover in the next strategy, you can figure out what adjustments you need to make. Using feedback to adjust the number of calories is important for your success over time. But you have to start somewhere.

If you are sure you are eating to your calorie budget and you are sure you are getting your goal amount of exercise then something must be wrong. Recheck everything. Check your portions. Check the activities you are doing. But in the end, if you aren't losing the weight you expect, then you have to adjust something. You can either lower your calorie budget, increase your exercise levels, or some combination of both.

What matters is **making adjustments to what's really happening in your life,** not what some estimated numbers say should happen.

Strategy 15. Use Feedback to Control Your Weight—Know When to Take Action

No one will tell you when you need to lose weight. Creating a feedback system lets you know how you are really doing with your weight, so you can take corrective action sooner rather than later.

Weight gain happens so gradually that it's easy to miss the pounds as they pile on. Imagine for a moment that you could notice almost immediately when you started gaining weight. Do you think that would help you stop? Do you think you could make some moves to lose what little you had gained?

That's the idea behind creating a feedback system for yourself. Your feedback system alerts you to when you are gaining weight so you can immediately make counter moves. If you don't know you are gaining then you can't do anything about it, or at least you can't act soon enough to prevent more.

People won't tell you are gaining weight. You have to figure it out for yourself. Who would want to go up to another person and say: "Hey, I think you are gaining weight, you might want to watch that." Not me!

Most of us have been very successful at cutting out all feedback about our weight. We know how to ignore all mirrors. We know how to explain away larger clothes sizes. We know how to justify eating just one more helping.

Without feedback, one day you'll just wake up and notice how much weight you have gained. You might be genuinely surprised at the amount of weight gain because you've been ignoring it.

▍ What does feedback mean?

Feedback is information that tells you how you are doing on your diet and other goals.

Step on a scale every day and you have feedback on how your diet is doing. If your weight is just right, then nothing needs to be done. If it's too high then something needs to be done. Once you get feedback that you are losing control of your weight, you know it's time to take some sort of action to bring it back under control.

Weight isn't the only or even the best form of feedback. If you gain muscle then your weight may go up. By only paying attention to your weight, you could be missing out on a lot of the excellent progress you are making.

▌ Feedback Works, Please Don't Skip It

You may be tempted to skip using feedback. It's not very pleasant to think about your weight. You would probably just like to ignore it. The problem is, **feedback works.**

A University of Minnesota study showed, over a two year period, **daily weighers lost twice the weight** than those who weighed themselves weekly. This was 12 pounds on average compared to 6 pounds. Those who never weighed themselves *gained* 4 pounds on average.

In a study at Brown University Medical School, researchers found that people who have lost 10% or more of their body weight are more likely to avoid regaining 5 pounds or more if they weigh themselves regularly, especially daily. Sixty-one percent of those who weighed themselves daily maintained their loss within a 5-pound range after a year and a half. Most dieters, according to the researchers, regain a third of their loss within a year, two-thirds within two years.

So, feedback works. Feedback acts as a psychological barrier you must break through before you can regain weight. While your preferred form of feedback may not be the scale, your chances of staying on your diet are much better if you create some form of a feedback system for yourself.

▌ Creating Your Feedback System Step-by-Step

The steps to creating your feed back system are:
1. Select your feedback strategies.
2. Track your progress.

▌ Step 1: Select Your Feedback Strategies

There are quite a few possible forms of feedback. The options are divided into *daily, weekly,* and *as-needed* strategies.

Daily Feedback Strategies

The daily feedback strategies need to be as quick and painless as possible or you won't do them. Choose one you can do easily every day with minimal effort. They are like an early warning system. If you detect a weight gain with these strategies, then you can immediately take corrective action rather than wait until the next spin.

Some possible feedback strategies are:

❖ **Clothing size and the fit of your clothes.** When your clothes start to get tight, it's a good clue you are gaining weight.

❖ **Look at yourself the mirror.** This feedback strategy works best if you're naked. By looking at yourself you can usually tell if you are gaining weight. It's easy enough to do right before you take a shower.

❖ **Try on a belt.** If you usually wear lose fitting clothes then you can try on a belt every morning when you get up. If the belt doesn't fit well, then you know you are gaining weight. One study found people who tied a cord around their waist were successful at keeping their weight off because the cord would become tighter as they gained weight, which would alert them and they could make changes.

❖ **Total body weight.** This is weighing yourself on your home scale. Please see the entry under Weekly Feedback Strategies for the complete explanation.

❖ **Weight Angel.** Researchers have found that if you weigh yourself every day, email in your weight, and then get advice and feedback on how you are doing, you are far more likely to maintain your weight loss. It turns out, the more you bug people and keep them thinking about their weight, the more likely they are to keep the weight off.

As long as your approach is quick and easy, you can use it as a daily feedback strategy.

Weekly Feedback Strategies

Feedback strategies are in the weekly category because they are either a lot more work or they might be too psychologically counterproductive to perform daily.

Some possible weekly feedback strategies are:

❖ **Total body weight.** This is weighing yourself on your home scale. Your weight changes so much on a day-to-day basis that it can be very depressing for a lot of people. Weighing weekly may be less traumatic. If weighing yourself daily isn't something that would bother you then you can make a daily weigh-in part of your daily feedback strategies.

- ❖ **Photograph.** Taking a picture of yourself allows you to see yourself as others see you. I know, I didn't want to see myself either, but it is a very powerful form of feedback. A picture is worth a thousand words. These days with digital cameras, taking pictures has never been easier.

- ❖ **Body Measurements.** Total body weight can hide your progress with your weight lifting and cardio program efforts. To get a different perspective on how your body is doing, take regular measurements of your chest, waist, hip, bicep, thigh, forearm, and calf. The downside of this choice is that taking measurements the same way every time is hard for a lot of people.

- ❖ **Weight lifting and cardio workout results.** Keep track of the pounds, repetitions, and sets you are performing in your workouts. Even if you aren't losing weight as fast you hope, you may still be getting stronger and healthier.

- ❖ **Body fat percentage.** This is a measure of your actual body fat percentage. Tracking this figure helps you know if your weight is going down slowly because you are gaining muscle. When you don't see the scale moving, this can be comforting information. There are a number of ways of calculating your body fat percentage: looking at yourself, measuring tape, BMI, bioimpedence, calipers, hydrostatic tank, and DEXA scanning. We've talked about some of these methods already, but many are too complex for us to cover here. You can find out more information on calculating your body fat percentage at *http://YourDesignerDiet.com.*

Many of the weekly feedback strategies would work great with a personal trainer. Every week you could meet with your trainer who could do all the hard work of measuring your body fat percentage and weighing you. You could then talk about nutrition, exercise, and anything else that might help you.

As-Needed Feedback Strategies

Implement these feedback strategies when you think the time is right. Each different strategy explains when the time may be right for you.

- ❖ **Count calories consumed.** Track exactly how many calories you eat each day. This is as-needed because counting calories is a lot of work. It's used when you are trying to learn your portion sizes or when checking if you are meeting your calorie deficit from eating less goal.

❖ **Count calories burned from exercise.** Track exactly how many calories you burn each day from exercise. It's used when checking if you are meeting the calorie deficit from exercise goal.

❖ **Other people's opinions.** It's unlikely, but is there someone you would trust to give you feedback on your weight? Just don't hold it against them if they tell you the truth!

Which strategies look good to you?

If you don't have any strong opinions, I recommend a mix of feedback strategies like:

1. Daily weigh-in.
2. Look at yourself in the mirror.
3. Track weight lifting and cardio workout results.
4. Count calories consumed and calories burned from exercise when necessary.

This combination of strategies gives you a wide range of feedback on how you are doing. If you just use weight alone, then you risk getting down on yourself when your weight doesn't change even when you are doing everything right.

You are not a machine. Even if you do everything perfectly, you can't guarantee a certain amount of weight loss every day or even every week. Weight is just weird that way. Sometimes you may not lose weight even though you have created the mathematically correct calorie deficit. It's incredibly frustrating because it's at these times you start doubting yourself, start thinking you can't lose weight so why bother?

Hang in there and keep using the Designer Way and you will eventually see progress with your weight. It's not easy. Those horrible and unexplainable weight plateaus are brutal on your self-confidence. Have some faith. You will make progress if you do the right things, constantly adjusting your strategies to get better at sticking to your diet, eating less, and preventing slip-ups.

Using several forms of feedback helps you deal with those periods when your weight is not going down like you think it should. If you are taking body measurements, perhaps your weight is steady but your waist is getting smaller. Or perhaps you see that you are using heavier weights or you are walking at a higher level on your treadmill.

All of these are examples of positive feedback. You can still be doing good things even when your weight stays the same.

Daily Weigh-ins Aren't For Everyone

Some people simply can't handle daily weigh-in sessions. A bad number on the scale in the morning can ruin the entire day. If you are one of these people, you may want to go extreme and stay off the scale.

People are psychologically looking for big changes in their weight when they step on the scale. The problem is, because they've been doing everything right they often expect a big weight loss, but instead they see a big weight gain. This can be extremely frustrating and demotivating.

Your weight fluctuates daily due to changes in water retention and menstrual cycle. You can gain between 2–5 pounds in a day just from water retention. And every pound gained on the scale doesn't mean you've gained a pound of fat.

Your weight will go up sometimes, go down fast at other times, or sit at a plateau for what seems like forever. If you can't handle the roller-coaster ride of the scale then you may want to consider using other forms of feedback.

People struggling with depression are often advised to stay away from the scale, because it can be a source of even more negative thoughts.

People with eating disorders are also advised to stay away from the scale because they often weigh themselves compulsively, obsessing over every small change in weight.

You don't need to weigh yourself daily to be successful. Other feedback options will work well too, as I've already said is my case. If you are going to weigh yourself daily, **be very sensitive to your weight loss patterns.** If your goal is to lose one pound a week, probably no one in the world will lose 0.15 pounds a day. You'll lose it in clumps. Some people will lose weight in smaller, more frequent clumps. Some people will lose their weight in larger, less frequent clumps.

How do you lose weight? Be sensitive to your particular pattern and don't get down on yourself when your weight loss isn't happening as fast or in the way you would like it to. We all want our weight to come off predictably, but that's not the way weight loss works. Maintain your calorie deficit by using the Designer Way and the weight will come off. Keep in mind that as you get closer to your target weight, you start losing weight more slowly. Don't get down on yourself then either. Just keep up the good work and good things will happen.

Tips for Weighing Yourself

For you to be able to compare your weight from day to day and week to week, you need to weigh yourself the same way every time. Here are a few tips:

❖ Only weigh yourself first thing in the morning after using the toilet.

❖ Use the same scale at the same time of day, wearing exactly the same clothes.

❖ You can't weigh yourself after each meal to see how much weight you've gained or after exercise to see how much weight you've lost. It takes time for changes to be seen in your body.

❖ Put the scale on a flat, hard surface to get a good reading.

❖ If you are using your scale's built-in body fat calculator, then be sure to input all the information it asks for (height, sex, etc.). Body fat calculations from scales aren't very accurate. They can fluctuate just like weight. Use them merely as a general trend of how you are doing. Don't expect the number to be your true body fat percentage.

▌ Step 2: Track Your Progress

A lot of people encourage you to keep detailed records on your weight so you can create all sorts of nice graphs and charts. If that's what you want to do then please go ahead. There are many good software programs available to help you.

But I don't recommend you keep a record of all your feedback data. Why not?

Collecting and tracking information is a hassle. And the more hassle a process is, the less likely you are to do it. I don't want the spin to be a hassle. I want you to feel that the small amount of effort you need to put into each spin is worth the results.

Detailed records of your weight are great when you are doing well and your weight is falling. **But when weight goes up, those graphs can cause a lot of heartache** and bad feelings. You may not want to risk possible depression by looking at your weight history if the history doesn't help you enough to justify collecting it.

Here's all the information you need:

❖ Feedback data from the beginning of the spin.

❖ Feedback data at the end of the spin.

That's it. **With just one week's worth of information, you can make plans for what to do in the next spin.** You don't need a lot of history. You just need a one week view showing how you are doing this week compared to last week. If you can keep getting better and better each week, then you will eventually reach your long term weight goal. It's pretty simple.

Definitely use a software program when counting calories. Calorie counting is a complicated job that is made much simpler that way. You probably won't be counting calories for the rest of your life. Calorie counting becomes less important once you learn proper portion sizes.

Feedback strategies must be simple and quick, because you'll use them for your entire life. If you like detailed records and they work for you then please use them. Some people feel they must track every detail or they aren't doing it right. I just want to let people know you can do perfectly well with a much simpler approach. Remember, whatever works.

▌ People are Sources of Ideas, Not Points of Comparison

Imagine you are talking with someone and they gush over a new diet they are on and they aren't hungry at all eating only 1,200 calories a day. And you remember how you were thinking of food 25 hours a day when you were only eating 1,200 calories a day.

What should you do? Should you:

1. Suck it up and eat a lot fewer calories because someone else can do it?
2. Turn bitter and jealous over their good fortune?
3. Do nothing. They are different from you so you can't expect what works for them to work for you.

If you answered (3) then congratulations, you are right...and unfortunately you only win the warm glow of self-satisfaction. If you didn't get the right answer here's why doing nothing is the right answer when something works for another person and not for you: **everyone is different.**

If you get down on yourself because you are hungry and someone else isn't, then that's the same as being depressed because you aren't as tall or have a different hair color from them. Does that make any sense? No, it doesn't.

That's why: people are sources of ideas, not points of comparison. If someone is using a strategy that looks good to you, then give it a go. If it works for you, great! If it doesn't work then no harm done. Just move on to the next strategy. But if a strategy doesn't work for you, it doesn't mean you are broken and the other person is a hero. It just means that this strategy doesn't work for you. Some strategies will work for you and that's all you need to succeed.

By creating a feedback system, you are taking advantage of a powerful and proven method of controlling your weight. Just keep your system simple and quick. It will reward you by helping you control your weight until the day you die.

. . . .

 ## Strategy 16. Darrell's Classic Weight Loss Move

Can you be as creative as Darrell Nelson in creating your Safe Zones?

Darrell Nelson could win an award for the most creative strategy of the century. What did Darrell do? He created a new weight-loss strategy of offering to mow people's lawns for free! That's thinking outside the box and is a wonderful example of doing **whatever works** and being as **extreme as you need to be.** I know I'm impressed.

Darrell, weighing in at 258 pounds, knew he should lose weight. He tried dieting and joining a gym, but like for many, they did not work. Did Darrell give up? No he didn't.

Darrell was aware of his strengths and weaknesses and tried to come up with a strategy that took advantage of his strengths and minimized his weaknesses. A classic weight loss move.

He was always good at keeping his work-related commitments. So he figured if he could turn his exercise into work he would have a lot better chance of sticking with it.

Brilliant! Some people might say Darrell should just be disciplined enough to go to the gym. But that doesn't work for him and rather than worry about what he can't do he figured out what he can do.

So Darrell hatched a plan of mowing lawns for free. You get a lot of exercise mowing lawns and because mowing lawns is a job, Darrell felt like he couldn't go back on his commitment. Blowing a commitment to yourself to go to the gym is easy. Not showing up to mow a lawn after promising a family you would is hard, at least for Darrell.

Then Darrell took it even one step further. His old push-model mower couldn't keep up with the work. Rather than spend money for a new mower, he sought out a sponsor. Toro agreed to provide him a new mower as long as Darrell lost 50 pounds! Now Darrell had double the incentive to keep up the work.

Isn't Darrell just lying to himself? He's mowing lawns for free so nobody could say anything if he didn't show up. I don't think he's lying to himself at all. He's being smart. Darrell is using his rational mind to provide himself the little bit of structure he needs to succeed. He knows himself well enough to know what works for him and he's taking advantage of it.

What matters is what works for you. Don't worry about what other people think or about useless questions like are you "lying" to yourself. Do whatever works.

How is Darrel's strategy working for him? He lost 18 pounds in two weeks.

What works for Darrell may not work for you. What you can learn from Darrell is his creativity, his insight into his own nature, and his courage in acting on what he thought was right.

Chapter 14

Learn the Art of Joyful Eating
Strategies 17–21

Joyful Eating is an exciting new tasting technique I developed for experiencing peak pleasure from every glorious bite of food. It's based on a great deal of research in how our sense of taste works and, as you might imagine, a lot of very fun experimentation!

Earlier I talked about how Joyful Eating helped me stay on my diet when I was about to give up. How could a method of tasting food make such a big difference in my life?

Most weight loss diets feature denial as their key element. To lose weight you are supposed to deny yourself certain foods—usually those you love the most—forever.

The problem is it's tortuously hard to stay on a diet over the long run by denying yourself the foods you love. Food is fun. Food is a great source of joy in life. The loss of joy is one of the biggest reasons diets fail. For many it simply isn't worth it. **Being thin doesn't feel better than how food tastes.** That's why so many people would rather feel the pleasure of food than stick to a denial-based diet.

Following a diet isn't the only reason people deny themselves the foods they love. Many people are on **health-restricted** diets as part of their treatment. As a diabetic, for example, I avoid high carbohydrate foods. People with heart conditions, high blood pressure and many other diseases must watch what they eat too. Many feel like outcasts when they can't eat what other people are eating. It's often easier just to give in and eat everything.

How could you have the best of both worlds? How could you fully enjoy food while sticking to your diet? That's what Joyful Eating does for you. By reveling in the power of food, Joyful Eating allows you to eat as little as one bite and feel satisfied. That's why Joyful Eating—tasting to its fullest—is one of the **secrets of eating in moderation.** You can feel more satisfaction from perfectly tasting a few bites of truly excellent food than from mindlessly eating a truck full of junk.

Now clearly, if you have an allergy or your doctor says you should never eat certain foods, then don't use Joyful Eating for those. But maybe you can use Joyful Eating for others.

I will never eat a full piece of cake for the rest of my life. It would send my blood sugar numbers to the moon. But I can safely eat one glorious perfect bite of cake. The trick is learning how to extract enough pleasure from that one bite so that I will feel satisfied enough not to eat more. Joyful Eating teaches you how to make one bite enough. One bite of anything won't have too many calories or other bad things, so it should be safe. And if you can stop eating after one bite, you will lose weight.

Joyful Eating works for any food. Use it for eating dessert, bread, potatoes or whatever else you must be careful about eating. You can eat one, two, or even three bites and feel satisfied.

The reason this approach works so well is because your sense of taste is designed to make it work. Your brain encourages you to eat a wide variety of foods by dialing down the taste after a few bites. You actually stop tasting a flavor after just a few bites.

So why eat more than a couple of bites when you won't taste it? Why not spend your calorie budget on foods you can enjoy? If you can learn how to extract the most pleasure from those few bites then you've learned how to eat any food in moderation while still feeling satisfied. You've maximized pleasure while minimizing calories.

This is incredibly powerful, potentially life changing stuff. At least it was for me. You can eat all the foods you love in moderation using Joyful Eating. You can go anywhere with anyone and not feel like an outcast. You don't have to abandon your health-restricted diet to feel like a real person again. And you will enjoy yourself more than you ever have before.

Strategy 17. Joyful Eating Step-by-Step

Learn Joyful Eating using this tutorial and open your taste buds to the pleasure available from food.

Wine lovers make a big deal out of learning how to taste wine because they have specific techniques that really bring out the best taste experience from each sip. In the same way, Joyful Eating helps bring out a peak taste experience from all the food you eat.

Joyful Eating works by adding a little bit of ritual to eating. Savoring great food deserves a ritual. The ritual of Joyful Eating leads you through the tasting process using a series of carefully considered steps. The steps work by adding emotional vibrancy, beauty, drama, and visual excitement to eating in order to create a more intense experience. Feeling and eating meld into one fully integrated adventure.

Joyful Eating is a **whole new kind of eating experience.** Perhaps for the first time in your life, you will have completely tasted food with all your senses, including your most important sensory organ: **your mind.**

The Joyful Eating practice has been carefully constructed to maximize the available sensory information to your brain. The more stimulation you get from your senses, the more satisfying any food will be. The more satisfying a food is the less you need to eat of it. This is why there is such an emphasis on getting all your senses, including your mind, involved in the tasting process.

A little demonstration will help to show how bland and boring your normal way of eating is. **This will blow your mind because food will have never tasted so good.**

For this demonstration please get a raisin. If you don't have a raisin you can try any other small edible snack.

This demonstration also serves as the template for how to eat any food joyfully. In the instructions, please mentally replace the word *raisin* with the name of whatever food you are eating.

Follow these instructions for any food you eat joyfully, making any obvious adjustments as needed. A raisin, for example, is a food eaten with your hands. If you are eating food with a fork or spoon, you'll want to change the parts where you are holding the raisin between your fingers.

Please take your time. Pay attention. Allow yourself to be in the moment. And focus just on eating. Let's begin.

▌ 6 Steps to Joyful Eating

Here are the six steps to follow when eating joyfully.

Step 1: Clear Your Palate and Your Mind

1. Clear your taste buds by taking a drink of room-temperature water.
2. Wait at least 90 seconds for any previous tastes to fade away. While waiting, you can perform the following steps:
    ❖ Clear your mind of any preconceived ideas of how the raisin should taste. Discover the taste anew every time you eat.
    ❖ Give thanks for the raisin you are about to eat. Truly appreciate how special is the opportunity to be alive to eat this raisin at this time.
    ❖ Take a deep breath. On a long exhale, let all the tension flow out of your body.
    ❖ Give yourself permission to enjoy yourself. Allow yourself to have fun.
    ❖ Bring to mind any pleasant memories from similar situations in the past.
3. Actively seek out new tastes and experiences with both your mind and senses as you eat. Find something new in every bite.
4. Take your time. Don't rush.

Step 2: Get to Know Your Food with Your Senses

We'll explore how to taste using your sense of sight, touch, and smell.
Using sight...

1. Place the raisin in the palm of your hand.
2. And as you become aware of the weight of the raisin in your hand, carefully look at it, as if you have never seen a raisin before.
3. Ask yourself, what does the raisin look like? How does it compare to other things you have seen before? Appreciate its color and texture.
4. Become aware of the different colors in the raisin. Are some rich? Are some light? Are some dark?
5. And as you are feeling the raisin, hold it up to a light. Become aware of how the light shines on the raisin. Notice the highlights... the darker hollows and folds...explore every part of the raisin...as if you had never seen a raisin before.

Using touch...

1. Become aware of how the raisin feels.
2. Turn the raisin over between your fingers.
3. And as you feel the pressure of the raisin on your fingers, explore its texture using your fingers and your entire hand.
4. Ask yourself, what does the raisin feel like as it touches your fingers? Does it feel wet, dry, sticky?
5. How does it compare to other things you have felt before?

Using smell...

1. Now bring the raisin close to your nose and take three short sniffs.
2. What do you smell? What does the raisin smell like?
3. How does it compare to other smells you remember?
4. How powerful are the aromas? Are they faint or bold?
5. Become aware of how your body is responding to the smell. Your body may go on sensory alert in anticipation of eating. Savor this anticipation.
6. Are you starting to salivate?

Step 3: Food Enters Your Mouth

1. And now slowly put the raisin in your mouth. Don't bite it just yet.
2. And as you are placing the raisin in your mouth, notice how your hand, arm, and mouth know exactly how to do this.
3. Become aware of the sensations of having the raisin in your mouth. Explore the feelings generated in your mouth.
4. And when you are ready, with awareness, slowly bite into the raisin. As your teeth gently sink into it, notice the taste as it releases.
5. Notice the sensations as your teeth enter the raisin. Does it feel smooth or crunchy or something else?
6. Ask yourself, what does the raisin taste like? How does it compare to other foods you have tasted before?
7. Let the raisin warm up by spending some time in your mouth. Are there any changes in flavor?

Step 4: Chewing

1. Breathe in and out through your nose as you taste.
2. And when you are ready, slowly start chewing the raisin. Chew 10 or more times to mix the flavors and textures and bring the odors to your nose.

3. At this point you may want to close your eyes so you can focus just on the tasting.
4. When you are ready, roll the raisin around in your mouth. Let it hit all the taste buds on your tongue, mouth, and the roof of the mouth.
5. On the first chew or two, if you feel comfortable, draw air through the raisin by pursing your lips and sucking in air, as if through a straw. Suck in air for about 3 seconds. Then close your mouth and breathe out through your nose. Notice any flavors and aromas.
6. Let your taste buds speak to you. Try to hold back from translating experience into words for a while until you have captured the flavor.
7. Hold the raisin in your mouth long enough to register an impression. You will be confronted by a lot of different sensations. Now try to put your impressions into words. Concentrate on one thing at a time.
8. Try to distinguish all of the different tastes: sweet, bitter, sour, salty, fat, and savory.
9. Does your mouth feel like puckering? Does it feel tingly or dry? Do you detect any acidy or bitter flavors?
10. Become aware of how the sensation of the raisin develops after the first impression.
11. Notice if the taste changes and deepens, or whether it becomes weaker or flatter, or whether it sweetens and softens, or hardens.
12. Become aware of the texture of the raisin in your mouth. Is it harsh? Oily? Fizzy? Smooth? Rough? Buttery? Silky? Watery? Creamy? Thick? Thin?
13. Does the raisin have a rich, interesting, satisfyingly full taste?
14. Is the flavor complex or simple?
15. Is the flavor balanced? Does any one flavor overwhelm any of the others?
16. Are there any flavors missing that you were expecting to taste?
17. Continue to taste as the raisin cools. Some characteristics reveal themselves most clearly in cooler food.

Step 5: Swallowing

1. See if you can detect the intention to swallow as it arises before you actually swallow the raisin.

2.   And when you are ready, swallow the raisin…as you are swallow-ing follow the sensation of the raisin moving out of your mouth, down your throat, and into your stomach.

Step 6: Afterward
1.   Take some time to notice how you feel after eating the raisin.
2.   How long does the taste of the raisin stay in your mouth?
3.   Notice what you taste and feel in your mouth. Is it sweet? Acidy? Burning? Is it fading or strong? Is your mouth drying out?
4.   Wait a few moments so you can appreciate the aftertaste. Are there any lingering flavors or mouth-feelings?
5.   Notice any feelings of satisfaction.
6.   If the taste experience was exceptionally good, then try to anchor it in your mind so you can recall it later.
7.   Talk about the raisin with your friends. Talk about how it tastes and feels. Try to find words to express your experience. Use con-versation to heighten anticipation from the next bite and to gener-ally learn more about raisins.

By following the six steps in Joyful Eating, you will have extracted every bit of pleasure out of one single bite. You will have experienced far more pleasure from one single bite than you would have from eating a whole lot more.

▌ Write About Your Experiences in a Journal
Some people find it helpful to write down their experiences in a journal. Writing helps you think and reflect and learn from your experience.

▌ Do the Exercise with a Friend
Invite a friend to eat joyfully with you. Please perform the tasting exercise separately. Compare notes afterward. You might be surprised at how different the taste experience was for each of you.

▌ Practice, Practice, Practice
Practice the Joyful Eating of a lot more foods. You'll find an excellent list of food suggestions in the *20 Tastes to Try Before You Die* strategy. Try many different kinds of foods with different textures and tastes so you can compare the experiences.

Have the Joyful Eating instructions in front of you for the first ten or so times you eat joyfully. There are a lot of steps, but they become second nature after a while. Pay special attention to the steps that matter the most to you. Everyone is different. While practicing, figure out which foods, flavors, textures, and techniques optimize your taste experience.

Practice Increases Sensitivity

We are all born with differing taste and smell abilities. Yet all is not lost. You can learn to improve your senses with practice. Through repeated use, it has been shown that you can increase your sensitivity ten-fold. A little practice can go a long way.

▌ Example Joyful Eating Session

In this section we'll go over an example session of my eating a strawberry using all 6 steps. Each step will have its own section and the step number is included in the heading.

I have chosen a strawberry because they are coming into season now and I love strawberries.

Step 1: Clear Your Palate and Your Mind

This is a crucial step for me to remember. Too often I am in a hurry and I just toss food down my throat without first becoming receptive to the taste experience. I notice that I'm often not really engaged in eating. Eating is like something that is happening to me, not something I am doing. If I just slow down I get much more pleasure from the food.

How can you not give thanks for the strawberry? It's a wonderful, beautiful, life affirming miracle of nature. By giving thanks I feel it creates a special mood in me where I am capable of better appreciating what I am about to eat. I don't go easily into this mood and it doesn't happen all the time, but when it does it makes for an extra special experience.

The breathing step and the instruction to give yourself permission to enjoy yourself help you become actively involved in the current moment. That's when you can enjoy yourself the most.

The last strawberries I had were not quite ripe. I try not to let that bad experience negatively impact on my opinion of these strawberries. This is not difficult. Strawberries have a lot of pleasant associations for me. I usually take some time and remember them.

My grandma grew strawberries in her garden. I remember eating perfect big juicy sun-ripened strawberries standing in a garden bursting with life. The birds and the bunnies liked strawberries too, so I always had company.

I picked strawberries a few times as a kid. That always takes me back to the fun I had out in the fields, eating more strawberries than I got paid for.

These particular strawberries I bought at a farmers' market on a pretty sunny Sunday afternoon. Remembering that day brings back a lot of good memories as well.

With all these memories flooding into my mind, I am already halfway to having a peak taste experience.

Step 2: Get to Know Your Food with Your Senses

I think the humble strawberry is a work of art far surpassing anything made by human hands. And like with all such common items, we tend to forget how beautiful they really are. That's why it is important to try and get back to the beginner's mind when experiencing food.

The deep living red of the strawberry contrasted with the dark green top is always striking to me. I marvel at how beautiful the colors are individually and together. This strawberry looks fully ripe. I don't see any yellow or green patches on it.

Then my eye always wanders to the seeds. The lighter color of the seeds set inside small diamond pockets of the strawberry body add an amazing beauty and texture to the strawberry. A smooth strawberry wouldn't be the same.

Hold a perfectly ripe strawberry up to a light and slowly rotate it. You will see a constant play of shadow and light across the strawberry.

And a strawberry is no less interesting to the touch. The texture of the seeds is endlessly captivating. The gentle tapering curves are pure artistry. A good sized strawberry also has a pleasant heft to it. An individual strawberry stands on its own. During a strawberry fight you can throw a strawberry pretty far.

The aroma of a strawberry is pure captured sunlight. It has a bold distinctive aroma that can't be confused with any other food. Take your time smelling a strawberry. Enjoy it. Life is short.

There are few pleasures like a perfectly ripe strawberry. From just the smell I look forward to eating a strawberry all the more.

Step 3: Food Enters Your Mouth

I usually take a big bite from a strawberry. I think that concentrates the flavor more. When I bite into a strawberry I notice I have to put some pressure into my bite.

Strawberries are firm, not hard or soft. The first taste I notice is slightly sour followed by a little bit of sweet.

Strawberry is definitely a food you want to eat at room temperature. A cold strawberry doesn't fully release its aroma or flavors.

After taking a bite I always look back at the strawberry. The surface of the remaining strawberry glistens like a jewel in light.

Step 4: Chewing

I notice an immediate short puckering sensation that softens out into a longer sweet flavor. The texture of a strawberry is rough, thick, uneven and chunky. I always like that. I feel a lot of moisture from the strawberry. Later I notice a slight bitterness. After chewing for a while, the flavors tail off and the texture becomes smooth.

From the appearance of the strawberry I expected it to be sweeter. I was disappointed it didn't have that strong strawberry taste. I am not sure where these strawberries came from. It's still early in the season so I hope they will be better later.

I always think of a strawberry as having a simple flavor. There aren't a lot of competing components in a strawberry.

Step 5: Swallowing

I noticed after the taste had gone away, my body started to get ready to swallow, without my conscious thought.

Step 6: Afterward

There isn't a noticeable finish to this strawberry. After swallowing, the strawberry flavor is just gone. That isn't the case with other strawberries I have tasted. Some have a longer finish. Other times I have felt very satisfied and pleased after eating a strawberry. Not this time.

I do detect a slightly sour taste still in my mouth though. Interestingly, I feel slightly fuller from having the bite, even though it wasn't that big a bite. Not a special strawberry to the taste, yet it still smells wonderful.

Even though this wasn't the best strawberry in the world, by eating joyfully I still enjoyed myself and got the most pleasure possible out of that strawberry. Without Joyful Eating, even the world's finest strawberry wouldn't be memorable because you wouldn't take the time to experience and appreciate it fully.

I didn't have an opportunity to talk to anyone during this example, except for you of course. But even writing down the experience helped me explore it more than I probably would have otherwise. If you are able to talk to people about your meal while you are eating, you will multiply your enjoyment tenfold.

Several of the tasting steps ask you to put into words the impressions you are getting from the food. This can be hard because most people find it difficult to put an experience into words. It takes time and practice to learn how to give words to feelings. You'll find just the act of trying to explain what you are experiencing helps you notice more about what you are eating.

Choose to Eat Each Bite Joyfully

The ultimate evolution of Joyful Eating is to joyfully eat **every** bite of **every** meal. Joyful Eating all the time is very difficult. It takes a lot of discipline and concentration. Not everyone will be able to do it.

Start slowly. Every day, eat the first bite of one meal joyfully. Then add more bites and more meals as you feel comfortable.

Strategy 18. How to Eat Joyfully in Different Situations

Learn how to use Joyful Eating in real-life situations.

In the *Joyful Eating Step-by-Step* strategy, you learned how to joyfully eat a single bite of food. The next step is to learn how to use Joyful Eating in everyday real-life situations. It's not always obvious how to make the best use of Joyful Eating. To learn how, we'll first cover the steps used to apply Joyful Eating and then we'll run through several scenarios showing how to use them.

▌ The Four Steps for Using Joyful Eating

There are four steps to apply Joyful Eating in any situation:

1. Decide which foods you want to Eat Joyfully.
2. Decide on your portion size.
3. Eat Joyfully.
4. Stop eating on reaching your portion size.

One way I remember the steps is using the mnemonic "double DES" based on the first letter of each step. When you enter any new situation, you can follow these steps and you should be OK.

Step 1: Decide which foods you want to Eat Joyfully.

In every situation, decide exactly which foods you will eat joyfully. Is it pasta? Is it steak? Is it ice cream? Is it chocolate? Is it fruit? Is it bread? Is it a glass of orange juice?

Normally you will joyfully eat the food you have to be careful with. Typically these are high calorie foods like dessert; or as a diabetic I'll eat bread and pasta joyfully, but you can choose to eat any food joyfully. Just make a choice before you start eating or you will probably forget and end up eating too much.

Step 2: Decide on your portion size.

Now that you've decided what to eat joyfully, you have to decide how much you should you eat. Is it a spoonful of ice cream? A square of chocolate? Two bites of pasta? A serving of steak?

Without knowing how much you intend to eat, you won't know when to stop eating. How much should you eat? We'll talk more about portion sizes and calorie estimation in *The Honest Calorie Estimation Method* strategy.

Step 3: Eat Joyfully

Eat all the food you decided to eat joyfully by following the instructions in strategy *Joyful Eating Step-by-Step*. Here are a few points I like to keep in mind:

1. Really let myself enjoy the food. Often I am my own worst enemy by being in a hurry.
2. If I am eating more than one bite, I wait between bites and clear the taste buds with a sip of water. Both practices taken together ensure I get the maximum taste from each bite.
3. Make a special effort to smell the food. The majority of taste is in our sense of smell. Really smelling food kicks in our primal systems and can summon pleasant taste memories from the past.
4. Do the mental comparison steps. A lot of instructions ask you to compare sensations with your past experience. Don't skip these steps as they bring a valuable mindfulness to eating.

Step 4: Stop eating on reaching your portion size.

When you've reached your predetermined portion size, stop eating. When you are in the middle of eating, it is oh so hard to stop! This is where the Weight-Proofing strategies come to the rescue. They will help you put yourself in situations where it is hard to eat more than you planned. Your best bet is to only ever serve yourself the amount you intend to eat.

What happens when you don't want to stop eating? I examine the reason. Some common reasons I have found for wanting to eat more are:

❖ **Poor food selection.** Perhaps the food wasn't rich enough to be satisfying. Next time I'll try a different food.

❖ **Poor Joyful Eating technique.** Sometimes I hurry through the Joyful Eating steps and I don't get as much out of the food as I should. Next time I'll slow down and follow all the steps.

❖ **I am in a mood.** Sometimes no amount of food will satisfy. I could eat a moon full of cheese and that wouldn't be enough. I try to recognize these situations and just stop eating. See the *Put the Brake on Automatic Eating* strategy for more help.

❖ **I am still hungry.** If after dessert I am still hungry, then next time I have to make sure I am getting full by the time dessert rolls around. Getting full on dessert is a great weight gain plan, but that's not what we are going for here.

❖ **I am on a biochemical roller coaster.** Eating a lot of sugar can cause me to need a *sugar fix* to get me back up when I am feeling down. During the peaks and valleys of a sugar craving, I can't think about what I should be eating, or how much. I do my best to recognize these situations when they are happening. Then I get off the roller coaster by following my diet. This can be hard.

How much to eat is always your choice. You can always decide to eat more. But focus on making all your eating decisions consciously, don't accidentally eat more than you would like.

▌ Scenarios for Using Joyful Eating in Everyday Situations

Let's see all the steps for using Joyful Eating in action. To show them, we'll run through several common scenarios:

1. **Dinner Out.** This scenario will show how you can Eat Joyfully while dining out at a nice restaurant. This is one of the scariest scenarios because the temptations to overeat are so great. It is the longest and most complex scenario, spelling out each step in detail. The other scenarios are shorter and more informal.

2. **Reward.** You've done something worth celebrating! This scenario shows how Joyful Eating can help you control your weight while rewarding yourself with food.

3. **Birthday Party.** You are going to a birthday party or other social event. How can you use Joyful Eating to help you avoid temptation?

4. **Going to Grandma's House.** Social pressure to eat more than you want can be hard to ignore, especially when it comes from your Grandma! How do you deal with it?

The advice in all the scenarios is available to you at all times. You can mix and match strategies to handle any situation you face.

▌ Scenario: Dinner Out

Your relatives have come to town. One of the benefits of having visitors is you can splurge, so we decide to eat at a nice steak house. Good for me because I know I can easily eat low-carb at a steak place.

A fine dinner is a difficult situation. You face large quantities of wonderful food. How will you handle it? Before every "dinner out" situation, ask yourself: how will I stay on my diet?

My position is that to stay on a diet for the rest of your life, you need to think of food as a pleasure to be enjoyed, not a poison to be avoided. The **poison theory of food** leads people to suggest eating the most boring, safest food on the menu. You don't need to do that, unless you've determined that's how extreme you need to be.

Order a dish you will really enjoy. Don't order a boring old salad unless that's what you really want. Enjoy your meal. Take pleasure from it.

Isn't that dangerous? Won't you get fat? Won't the world end? It could, but it probably won't, especially if you eat joyfully. Let's apply the steps to your dinner out.

Here's what the steps would look like during dinner. Remember the steps using the "double DES" mnemonic.

Step 1: Decide which foods you want to Eat Joyfully.

After browsing the menu and thinking about what I want to eat, I decide that I'll joyfully eat bread, potato, and dessert. These are the high-carb items I love and are the foods I need to be most careful about. For dessert I also have to worry about calories, but Joyful Eating small portions naturally limits calories.

A large steak can have a lot of calories because of all the fat. I often try to pick a smaller steak. If I am not worried about calories that day, maybe because

I had a long cardio workout, I'll go ahead and order a large steak. I always eat steak joyfully because it just tastes so good that way. You can also divide the steak in half and put some in a doggy bag for later.

I can usually share my wife's potato and dessert. You may need to ask around at the table and see if anyone wants to share. If nobody will share, you can get a whole order and just eat your portion. Take the rest home or just leave it.

These days, I make a conscious effort to eat spicier foods. Being from the great Pacific Northwest, I was raised to consider salt and pepper exotic spices. Now spicy dishes excite me because they are an opportunity for a new taste experience. Plus, spices are low in carbs, fat, and calories. They add variety and excitement to your diet for almost no cost. A lot of people already know the secret of spice, but I thought slow people like me might want to give spicier food a try.

Step 2: Decide on your portion size.

After deciding what to eat joyfully, it's time to consider how much I'll eat.

If the bread doesn't look truly excellent, I'll usually decide not to eat it. I'd rather spend my carb budget on dessert or have a little more potato. One test for good bread is how it smells. A rich complex smell usually means a bread worth eating. If I did eat the bread I would make sure my one bite was covered in real melted butter. Yum.

I'll have one big spoonful each of the potato and the dessert. On a good exercise day, I may choose to have two bites each. This is actually a good part of the system because it encourages me to have good exercise days!

I love a fully loaded potato. I add sour cream, chives, butter, salt, and pepper. Joyful Eating is perfect for eating potato because potato has a very subtle flavor.

Choosing a dessert takes some real thought and that's part of the fun. A lot of desserts are just layers of sugar. As tempting as loads of sugar may sound, sugar-only desserts won't satisfy. Sugar is just one of our tastes. Combining other tastes into your meals, like bitter, sour, salty, and savory, enriches your taste experience.

Cheesecake with a strawberry topping is often my choice. I find the aroma of cheesecake uplifting. It has a smooth creamy texture with good mouth feel. Cheesecake is both sweet and sour, which gives it a complexity I like. Even a single bite of cheesecake can take a while to eat. If you add nuts in the crust or in the topping, then you also have a pleasurable contrast in textures. The fat in cheesecake gives it a rich deep taste. The flavor of cream cheese is mild and forms a good backdrop for a sweet topping. The contrast between the sweet strawberry flavor and the mild slightly sour cheesecake can be very pleasing. And because cheesecake has a lot of calories, eating just one bite keeps down the calorie count.

I think about all of these issues before I order. If I don't, I stand a good chance of eating too much and I can't afford the health risk. If you don't plan ahead it won't work. The temptations are too great.

Step 3: Eat Joyfully.

As each food is delivered I eat it joyfully, following the strategy *Joyful Eating Step-by-Step*. In this case the bread wasn't very good so I passed on it. The potato and dessert were excellent.

Step 4: Stop eating on reaching your portion size.

I served myself the foods I was going to eat joyfully using the Weight-Proofing strategies to make sure I only ate as much as I planned to eat.

I shared my wife's potato. I cut off the amount I wanted and brought it over to my plate. I had two big bites of potato because I didn't have any bread.

I also shared my wife's dessert. I served myself one big bite of her chocolate cake. Following the recommendation of the Joyful Eating steps, we talked about our experience of the cake as we were eating and I think that helped bring out the best taste from the cake.

▌ Scenario: Reward

In this scenario you've done something good and you want a reward. A lot of people say you shouldn't use food as reward because it's too dangerous, you might binge and fall off your diet. If this is a problem for you, then be as extreme as you need to be.

But if you think a food reward is OK for you then use Joyful Eating to ensure you'll get the most pleasure without overeating.

Before Joyful Eating, when it came time for a reward, I would eat too much. What the heck, I deserved it, didn't I? Inevitably, after eating far more than I ever should, I would manage to both gain weight and feel guilty. Some reward.

Use Joyful Eating to keep a reward a reward. Don't make it another opportunity for you to fail and feel bad about yourself.

Don't chase satisfaction. Dig deep inside and explore what is truly satisfying right now. It may not even be food. Settling for less than exactly what you really want will just encourage you to eat more.

The problem is knowing what you want. We don't normally know what we want because we don't listen to ourselves. Take some time and listen.

▌ Scenario: Birthday Party

In this scenario you are attending a birthday party or other social event. What can make you fall off your diet faster than a birthday party? Everyone is happy celebrating a milestone in a friend's or loved one's life. There's delicious-looking food everywhere. And unfortunately, little of the food conforms to your diet. Everyone around you is eating freely, unaware of your torment. It's likely that you'll feel frustrated and say what the heck, and start digging in. And here your diet ends and the weight gain begins.

But wait…it's Joyful Eating to the rescue!

At a birthday party I am not thinking woe is me, I can't have anything, my life sucks. I am thinking about what looks truly excellent to eat. I am asking myself, what can I have that will be worth eating joyfully? There's always something I like to eat. I am anticipating a pleasurable eating experience as part of a pleasurable event. I can have one bite of any food I want; I don't feel the cravings and the pressure I felt on denial-centered diets.

Of course, I would like to eat anything and everything, but I can deal with these feelings through Joyful Eating. What I couldn't deal with, in the past, was thinking I would never ever eat the foods I love again. My resolve would dissolve and I would eat and eat and eat. Now I can eat in moderation while still having fun.

▌ Scenario: Going to Grandma's House

In this scenario, you are going to Grandma's house. Soon after you take your shoes off and get comfortable, she says, "Here, have some apple pie. I made it just for you."

This is a tough one for me. Grandma makes me melt. So I eat a bite joyfully and then say that's all I can have. Then, if she makes me feel bad for not eating more, I just have to keep saying no. I explain to her it's not her pie, which it isn't because her pie is always excellent, but that for health reasons I can't have more.

Good luck!

Strategy 19. Tricks for Maximizing Your Food Pleasure

You can maximize the amount of pleasure you experience in your life by bringing it under conscious control.

There are certain tricks you can use to get more pleasure from a meal. Here are a few you might find fun to try.

▌ Save the Best for Last

What you experience last greatly influences how you think of your entire meal. Make the last bite great and you'll feel better about all of it.

▌ Eat a Greater Number of Smaller Courses

Your appetite and your pleasure increase by eating smaller selections of high quality food. You don't always need to eat large meals.

▌ Control Expectations

Having high expectations sets you up for almost certain disappointment. Go into a meal with an open mind and low expectations. Aim to be pleasantly surprised instead of knowingly dissatisfied.

▌ Space Out Experiences

You brain adapts to experiences if you have them too close together. Separate out how often you have a taste experience and you'll enjoy it more.

▌ Be Grateful

Don't talk about how much better the experience could have been. Look for the good in the experience you had.

▌ Forget What You Didn't Choose

Don't think about the attractive food options you didn't take. This only builds up regret. Focus on enjoying what you did order and forget what you didn't choose.

▌ Minimize Choices

Having lots of different choices builds up confusion and regret. If you order from a small set of excellent options, you'll be happier with your choice.

▌ You Don't Always have to Try New Things

If you are planning your meals for the next couple of weeks, you may be tempted to choose a lot of different meals because you think you will get bored if you have the same dishes every week. Surprisingly, this isn't true. You won't get as bored as you think. If you like something, as long as you don't have it all the time, you'll like it the next time you eat it too. If, for example, popcorn is a snack you love, then you'll still enjoy having it every day.

▌ Eat the First Bite of Any Dish Joyfully

Eat the first bite of every dish joyfully. You'll increase you sensory stimulation and get the most satisfaction from all your meals by following this rule.

▌ Keep Good Company

Eat with people who appreciate food and are willing to talk about the good points. It helps you appreciate food too.

▌ Share Food in a Group

If you are in a group, a perfect Joyful Eating practice is to order food as a group and share it. Pass your bread plate around the table and have people put different foods on it. Everyone will get a **small** portion of a lot of different tastes. And everyone will have a chance of tasting something truly excellent.

This trick works especially well for desserts. A full dessert, though very tempting, will usually be a lot more calories than you can afford. As a group, order a few desserts and share them. Then each person can eat one perfect delicious bite.

I've noticed comfort with food sharing is highly cultural. My Chinese friends are at first bewildered by the American practice of eating individual meals, even at a Chinese restaurant! I used to be one of these people.

You may need to be brave and overturn custom by suggesting that your table share food. Not everyone will want to share, but a lot of people might. The other people will soon see how much fun you are having and throw their food into the pot as well.

▌ Take Flavor Vacations

Not eating a flavor for a while revitalizes your ability to taste it. So take a 2 week vacation from sweet, salty, sour, or bitter flavors from time to time. Parting is such sweet sorrow, but the makeup tasting is great.

▌ Smell What You Love

Your sense of smell deteriorates with age. You can fight back by taking a whiff of your favorite smell every day for a few months. This forces your body to create new scent receptors.

▌ Search Out New Experiences

Look for interesting, rich and complex foods. Look for new and different tastes. Look for fresh, colorful foods. Look for spicy foods. Look for subtle and simple foods. Food is an adventure and you are an explorer. Go forth and eat well. The *20 Tastes to Try Before You Die* strategy suggests different foods to experience. You may find a few of them interesting.

This doesn't contradict the idea of *You Don't Always have to Try New Things*. Both principles work if you use them well.

▌ Plan Your Journey

The first time you experience a food may be the strongest experience you will have with it.

To re-create the first-time experience, you may want to leave time between eating the same kind of food. "Absence makes the heart grow fonder" applies to food as well. If, for example, you have dozens of strawberries every day it may be difficult to find the joy in each new strawberry. If you wait a week between strawberry tastings, you give your body a chance to forget about strawberries. Then the next strawberry will be a bolder experience.

If you plan your entire diet with this in mind, you can keep yourself at a continual peak of the eating experience. Certainly, there is also great delight in coming to know something completely. So mix it up. Keep your mind and taste buds off balance by combining short periods of new flavors with longer periods of focus on a single family of flavors.

Think of your eating life as a journey. The key to a lifetime of eating pleasure is to avoid most of the ruts in the road, continually travel to new places, while still managing to visit and stay with old friends along the way. You must consciously manage your journey otherwise you'll build up a series of habits and fears that will lock you into one boring path.

Planning your journey applies at many different points in time. You may pick different contrasting dishes within a meal. You may select different restaurant styles on a daily, weekly, or monthly basis. You may concentrate on wine from a particular region for a month. You may try cooking from different cuisines at home. You may fast for a day. You may go out to eat with different groups of friends. The possibilities are infinite.

. . . .

 ## Strategy 20. Refine Your Palate

Develop your sense of taste so you can better appreciate food.

Palate is a fancy word for your sense of taste, but it means more than just a sense of taste. When someone says you have a "fine palate" it means you are someone who knows good food. You can tell the difference between tastes. You have a feel for which flavors will taste good together and which flavors won't.

Most of us haven't spent five minutes considering the taste of food or refining our palate. But your palate can be developed. One way to do this is through an exercise Gordon Ramsay, a world famous chef, used on his *Hell's Kitchen* TV show.

Chef Ramsay prepared a group of foods and had blindfolded contestants identify each item they tasted. Whoever identified the most correctly won a prize. I don't have any prizes for you, but it's a fun way to start to pay more attention to food and develop your palate.

Here's a list of foods you might try tasting:

❖ Hot dog	❖ Short rib
❖ Oregano	❖ Swiss cheese
❖ Scallop	❖ Scrambled egg
❖ Chocolate	❖ Kiwi fruit
❖ Cucumber	❖ Seaweed
❖ Tuna	❖ Potato
❖ Chicken cubes each cooked with a different spice from your spice drawer. Cook as many as you can.	

It would be best to have the cook not take part in the test, but that doesn't really matter. With a small group of friends try tasting the different foods blindfolded and see who can identify the most items correctly. Each serving should be small, served with a toothpick. You'll need as many servings for each type of food as you have in the taste test.

Strategy 21. Twenty Tastes to Try Before You Die

Search for new peak taste experiences and dazzle your taste buds on these exciting food possibilities.

Part of the great fun of Joyful Eating is exploring and discovering new and interesting foods to eat. Using Joyful Eating as your magnifying glass you will gain endless hours of pleasure searching the world of food for new peak taste experiences.

On which foods should you apply your dazzling new tasting techniques? You will of course have your own favorite foods, but you will find many foods you might want try in this strategy.

This is a crucial strategy because by trying a large number of excellent foods, you start building up your unconscious database of foods and tastes. It is this internal database that helps you learn and experience more from all the food you eat. Nobody can tell you what is good or bad. You must explore for yourself what tastes and textures you like.

Becoming an accomplished taster is all about building memories of a lifetime of different taste experiences for comparison. Deriving pleasure from tasting food is a skill that is developed over years and years of practice and experience. So start now!

▌ So Why All the High Calorie Foods?

At first this strategy may seem out of place with the rest of the book. We will be talking about a lot of rich and fattening foods. The title of this book has "diet" in it, so how can I then turn around and encourage you to eat fattening foods?

It's not that kind of diet. It's not about telling you all the foods you can't ever have for about the rest of your life. Joyful Eating is about finding a way for you to have the foods you love in a way that brings pleasure to your life, while avoiding the harm of out of control eating.

Food is not a poison. Food is a joy. Food is a path to happiness. Food is an adventure you should have for the rest of your life. I can't and won't tell you not to eat a food just because it can be abused.

If you haven't tasted these dishes before, then get to it! It would be fun to make an event of it with friends. Try Joyfully Eating a new taste a week. It will be fun. And if you have tasted these dishes before, don't you think it's time to try them again?

Taste 1: Storm Wine

When the weather turns stormy, start by building a crackling fire. Pour a glass of your favorite beverage. Sit by the fire, slowly sip your drink, and experience the storm.

Taste 2: Hot Fudge Sundae Made with Mint-chocolate Chip Ice Cream

Together they are a spine-tingling pairing of tastes and textures: the hot of the fudge against the cold of the ice cream; the liquid flow of fudge against the solidness of the ice cream; the spike of mint against the constant deep flavor of the fudge. Perfect.

Taste 3: Icy Cold Water When You are Desperately Thirsty

Circumstance has a lot to do with how you experience food. To get a peak taste experience, you may want to consider creating a particular environment around eating. Hunger is the best spice. A meal always tastes better when you are really, really hungry. Even the plainest meal can seem like a feast in the right situation.

I have been on a few multi-week river rafting trips. After a long day on the river, you have to unpack the boats, put up your camp, and then fix dinner. When you get off the water you are starving, yet you still have to wait a long time for dinner to be ready. When dinner is finally ready you almost can't help yourself from tearing into it. These have been some of the best meals I have ever had.

Plain old simple water can be a world class taste experience too, even though water has no taste. Try this. When you are desperately thirsty, I mean so thirsty you feel like you will shrivel up and blow away without a sip, chug down an ice-cold glass of water. This may be one of the finest taste experiences of your life. There's something primal and eternal about drinking water. We take water for granted, but in the right circumstance drinking water can be heaven.

Taste 4: Oven-Baked Apples Sprinkled with Cinnamon

On a chilly night, cover a few apples with cinnamon and bake them in the oven. Almost immediately your house fills with the enchanting smell of apples and cinnamon. For hours this comforting feeling wraps around you like a warm coat. And when the apples are done, serve them in a bowl and top with fresh cream. Delicious.

Taste 5: Fresh Hot Bread and Butter

I vividly remember to this day a field trip we took in grade school to a bakery. The smell of baking bread was everywhere. We saw all the glistening automated machinery, but the highlight of the trip was eating hot fresh baked bread just out of the oven. Oh my, it was good!

Taste 6: Fresh Ripe Peach

Seek out a fresh peach that is just to the point of ripeness where when you bite in, the juice runs down your chin.

Fruits are under-appreciated miracles of taste. Don't forget to experience them when they're in season. Try fresh strawberries, cold watermelon, fresh nectarines, fresh blueberries, and fresh pineapple in Hawaii.

Taste 7: Warm Chocolate Chip Cookies Dipped in Cold Milk

Take a deep whiff of the warm chocolate chip cookie. Then dip the cookie slowly into a glass of cold whole milk. It's an awesome combination of flavors and textures.

Taste 8: A McIntosh Red Apple Just Picked Off the Tree

The McIntosh Red is a medium-crisp, tart-sweet apple that has a bright red skin that is sometimes tinged with green. You want to eat an apple fresh off the tree, partly because fresh picked apples taste better, but mostly because apple trees are so beautiful. The experience of eating an apple in the middle of an orchard can never be forgotten.

Taste 9: Vine Ripened Tomatoes Topped with Fresh Basil, Fresh Mozzarella, and Aged Balsamic Vinegar

The combination of flavors is truly surprising. A wonderful appetizer or snack.

Taste 10: Sit at a Sidewalk Cafe Sipping Cafe au Lait While Munching a Fresh French Butter Croissant

Make the Cafe au lait with French milk. French milk has more fat in it than US whole milk so the Cafe au lait seems sweet without adding sugar. Absolutely scrumptious.

Taste 11: Fresh Squeezed Orange Juice in a Long Stem Glass
Drink your glass of liquid sunshine while overlooking a garden in full bloom. The beauty of light tinkling through orange tinted glass cannot be matched.

Taste 12: Warm Homemade Chips and Chunky Salsa
Store bought chips cannot compare to homemade chips. I first discovered homemade chips at a block party. One our neighbors made homemade chips and I could not believe how good they were.

Taste 13: Orange Cut In Half Sprinkled with Chili Powder and Salt
A unique combination of tastes presented for your consideration.

Taste 14: S'mores Made Over a Campfire
Toast the marshmallows until golden, the insides should be soft. Make the fire big and the night cool.

Taste 15: Fresh Guinness in Ireland
Guinness is thought by many to be the finest beer in the world. It is also said that the finest Guinness can be tasted at James Gate Guinness Brewery in Dublin, Ireland. A dream vacation would be to go on a pilgrimage to Dublin and take a tour of the brewery. After the tour you are able to sample fresh Guinness! Reports from dazzled tasters find the beer so creamy it is out of this world good!

Taste 16: Roquefort Cheese with a Dry White Bordeaux Wine
A fabulous food and wine experience is Roquefort cheese with a dry Bordeaux wine. Roquefort is a blue cheese from the south of France. It has a complex, creamy and soft taste. White Bordeaux wines are also made in France. Dry white Bordeaux are usually brilliant in color, crisp, fruity, and have a delightful, fresh finish. Together they are like a dream French vacation without leaving your house.

Taste 17: Sweet and Spicy Hot Chipotle Cherry Pie
This is a pie with punch. It brings together heat and sweet into one happy cross-cultural marriage. First make your normal cherry pie recipe then add to

the pie chipotle (smoked jalapeño) that has been ground into a powder. The zing of the chipotle and the sweet of the cherry are a stunning complement to each other.

Taste 18: Thinly Sliced Prosciutto with Fresh Figs

Prosciutto is a salt-cured, air-dried raw Italian ham. Curls of prosciutto served with fresh fruit are a classic summertime appetizer. One of the tastiest pairing with prosciutto is figs. Figs are a soft and deliciously sweet fruit. Thin-sliced prosciutto adds a wonderful contrast to fresh figs.

Taste 19: Sweet and Sparkling Ice Kacang

A tasty Malaysian cooler. Perfect for a hot day, it's made of sweetened dried beans, strips of jelly and little droplets of starch in bright colors, small dried fruit, preserved sugar palm fruit and seeds, and long slivers of grass jelly are mixed with shaved ice, sugar syrup and sometimes evaporated milk. Wonderful.

Taste 20: Outdoor Barbecue on a Gorgeous Summer Day

The secret of a good barbecue may be smoke and time, but no matter how you cook it, there is no better way to spend a summer's day than having a big family picnic and barbecue. Load up the family, load up the dog, and find the perfect park. While your favorite meats slowly cook over an open fire, work up an appetite by swimming and playing baseball. Or maybe you would rather take a nap under a shade tree. The sensational aroma of barbecue will follow you wherever you go. That's a good day.

We'll always be adding more peak taste experiences at our website *http:// YourDesignerDiet.com.* Please drop by to find new taste experiences and to share your own discoveries.

Chapter 15

Put the Brake on Automatic Eating
Strategies 22–27

Have you ever opened up a bag of potato chips, ate the first chip, and then hundreds of hundreds of calories later realized you ate the whole bag? You probably don't even remember eating after the third bite. What happened?

That's automatic eating. It's eating when you don't even realize you're eating. It is eating mechanically, without thinking, one bite after another. It's the exact opposite of Joyful Eating.

Who hasn't had this experience in some form or another? It doesn't have to be potato chips. It could be cookies or candy or anything.

Imagine if day after day most of your eating habits were on automatic pilot. You would eat automatically and without thought. You would eat more than you wanted to, things you didn't want to, and when you didn't want to. You wouldn't stop eating when you should and would barely remember eating at all. You would gain weight year after year.

Sound familiar?

Creating Safe Zones, which we'll talk about in other strategies, helps minimize the risk of automatic eating, but they can't remove the risk completely. To control your weight, at some point you need to learn how to deal directly with automatic eating. And that's exactly what you'll learn in this chapter.

Strategy 22. Manage Your Triggers

A trigger is any event, feeling, or situation in which you are tempted to eat automatically.

If you can recognize what triggers your automatic eating, you can put yourself in a good position to stop the triggers.

▌ When Do You Eat Automatically?

The first step in recognizing your triggers is to think about the times when you eat automatically. Some common automatic eating triggers are:

- ❖ **Trigger Feelings:** stressed, anxious, lonely, sad, depressed, hungry, happy, bored, tired, angry, hopeless, a lack of control in your life, unappreciated.
- ❖ **Trigger Events:** party, sport, vacation, concert, funeral.
- ❖ **Trigger Situations:** stressful, embarrassing, alone, watching TV, going to the movies, talking on the phone, doing homework, sitting at the computer, reading, visiting a relative, driving in your car.
- ❖ **Trigger Foods:** candy, chocolate, ice cream, potato chips, pasta, fries.

Basically, it's almost anywhere or anytime. ☺

A visit from parents is an automatic eating trigger situation for some people. If it is for you, then you know that when your parents are visiting, you are in a trigger situation and you need to be more vigilant.

Some people find breakfast a trigger situation. Mornings are hectic and the brain isn't fully awake, and without thinking they will just grab a donut.

Other examples are buying a big bag of popcorn when you go to a movie, eating junk food while lying on the couch watching TV, eating candy while reading or studying, going to a party with lots of food begging to be wolfed down, worrying about an upcoming test or seeing a box of cookies on a table.

Sometimes you may not realize you have eaten automatically until after you've finished. In these situations, trace back through your day to figure out what the trigger was. You can start to deal with your triggers once you know them.

How can you deal with your triggers? There are a few ways:

- ❖ **Avoid Trigger Situations.** Discretion is often the better part of valor. Sometimes the best way to avoid automatic eating situations is to run away and save yourself. Don't feel you have to be macho and tackle every trigger situation head-on. It's up to you to figure out how extreme you need to be.

❖ **Dump Trigger Foods.** Dump all the foods you know tempt you to eat automatically. If it isn't available, you can't eat it. In a trigger situation, you're one short mindless moment away from tearing open a bag of cookies or popping the lid off a big container of ice cream. Just get rid of all these items. For support, ask a friend to help you dump all your trigger foods. This idea dovetails nicely with creating your *Home and Family Safe Zone.*

❖ **Make a Special Effort to Eat Joyfully.** You often feel compelled to eat in a trigger situation. In difficult situations, really focus on eating your food joyfully. Sometimes reconnecting to the physical feelings in your body can kick yourself out of automatic eating.

These suggestions can help with many of your triggers, but not of all them. Sometimes you can't avoid a trigger situation, sometimes trigger food surrounds you and you can't help it and sometimes even eating joyfully won't help. For those extra difficult situations, consider turning to the *Lifeguarding* strategy.

Strategy 23. Lifeguarding
Save yourself from slip-ups by becoming your own lifeguard.

Your brain is absolutely amazing, but that doesn't mean it is optimal or perfect in design. It can have flaws, **like feeling unwanted urges to eat.** Thoughts of eating just show up in your mind and chances are you will eat because your brain is telling you "I'm hungry."

See a luscious ad for a fine dessert and all of a sudden your brain throws up thoughts of hunger when a second ago you weren't hungry at all. Smell your favorite dinner cooking and your thoughts immediately turn to eating, when a moment before you may have been thinking about the twilight of a lovely sunset. Or perhaps your internal hunger control mechanisms are broken and you become hungry long before your time.

Whatever the reason, unwanted urges to eat can haunt you. You don't want them, yet they show up in your mind anyway. Because these are your thoughts, you think they are real and you should act on them. And that's the problem: you eat unnecessarily because of the unwanted thoughts. If you understand that these thoughts are often just brain noise, like static on TV, you can avoid eating just because you have thoughts of eating.

Not only thoughts about eating can be unwanted. In the middle of exercising, have you ever thought something like: you've done enough now, you are tired, and it's time to stop now. Where does that thought come from? In most cases it's not true, there's no reason to stop, but if you think your "stop exercising" thoughts are real, you'll probably stop. Yet in most cases your urge to stop exercising is no more real than your urge to eat.

In general, overcoming unwanted thoughts will help you do two things:

- **Stop doing** something you don't think you should be doing—like overeating.
- **Keep doing** something you think you should be doing—like exercising.

A lot of unwanted thoughts may flow through your mind. To control your weight, we'll be concerned mainly with the urges compelling you to eat and the ones demanding you stop exercising—in other words, thoughts that lead to slip-ups.

▌ Not All Your Thoughts Deserve Your Attention

At any time, a variety of thoughts fly through your mind, possibly like:

Eat the cookies...it doesn't matter anymore...I can have all the ice cream I want...nobody cares...if I have another candy bar I'll feel better...I am a big fat pig anyway...I am such a loser.

You may have had thoughts like these all your life.

There is a **big secret** about your thoughts you may not know: **just because you have a thought doesn't mean you have to pay attention to it.** A lot of thoughts are just unwanted messages from your brain that you can safely ignore. I call these **pop-thoughts** because they are thoughts that pop into your mind and will just as quickly disappear if you let them.

Cognitive scientists estimate that over 95% of your thinking is below the conscious level. That means less than 5% of your thoughts are made consciously and that most of your thoughts happen automatically.

A common example is what happens when driving a car on a long trip. When it's over, drivers often don't remember driving at all, yet they somehow completed a long complicated journey. Clearly driving requires a lot of thinking, but you are not always aware of it. If you can drive without thinking you can certainly eat without thinking!

▌ You are Not Your Thoughts

What this all means is **your thoughts are not you.** Thoughts just pop into your head for lots of reasons and not all of those reasons make sense.

Typically we think **all** of our thoughts are important and should be paid attention to because, well, we think our thoughts are us. Please consider that the voice in your head may sometimes be speaking rubbish that you can simply ignore. This is a pretty radical idea. We are not used to thinking that some of our thoughts may be unimportant; or even more radical, that many of our thoughts may be harmful.

Let's say you have a thought that you are hungry. Why did you get this thought? Where did it come from? Why did it show up just now? Why didn't you have this thought a little earlier or a little later?

Even after finishing a big meal, you can still think about eating more. You know you can't really be hungry. You just ate a giant meal! So where did this thought come from? Consider that it might just be an unwanted message from your brain. The key is to be able to recognize this thought as unwanted, so you know not to react to it. Imagine what would happen if you ate every time you thought you were hungry? Unfortunately, most of us don't have to imagine.

Here's a quote from the actor Willem Defoe about what his brain tells him:

> *Ever since puberty, whenever I cross a bridge I've felt a compulsion to jump off. I feel the same impulse with balconies.—Willem Dafoe*

Do you think he should pay attention to this message from his brain?

You don't need a death wish to get the same thought as Mr. Defoe. These kinds of thoughts may just pop into your head. Where do they come from? Why do you get them? Nobody really knows.

It's easy to say to just ignore these thoughts, but a lot of times they grab your attention with such strength and persistence they are hard to let go.

In Mr. Dafoe's case, he has ignored these thoughts because he doesn't want to die a painful death. In the same way, a lot of other messages from your brain should be ignored because they aren't any more real. They are just pop-thoughts.

Have you ever had thoughts like *you are stupid, you are ugly, you'll never amount to anything?* Where do these horrible little thoughts come from? In your better moments you know they aren't true, but they can still hurt. A lot.

They really are just **unwanted messages from your brain** and you don't have to pay attention to them. Let these thoughts pass through you. They are just mental events. They don't reflect reality. They come and they go. They only have a life if you give them attention. It's your mental attention that strengthens unwanted thoughts. Don't pay attention to them and they will go away.

The idea that you can consciously choose which thoughts to pay attention to is a radical and powerful idea, one of the most powerful ideas you may ever hear. We'll see how to apply the power of conscious choice in a few more sections.

▌ Just What are You Thinking? Keep a Thought Log

Do this exercise. As you go about your day, write down all your thoughts for a half hour. Be sure to write down all your thoughts. Don't only write down your big thoughts like *I have to go grocery shopping*. Write down all the quick automatic thoughts you may have, but do not always realize you are having because they seem so natural. When you see someone walking toward you for example, you may immediately think *What an ugly shirt*. Write down all of those kinds of thoughts too.

Afterward, take a look at all the thoughts you have written down. What do you think of your thoughts? Some are probably untrue, trivial, mean, or bizarre. Some may be wise, kind, and insightful. And other thoughts may not seem like you at all. You may be surprised to find your thoughts are all over the map.

After looking at your thoughts: Do you think all your thoughts are equally true or equally important? Do you think all your thoughts should be given equal weight?

▌ Some Thoughts are Unwanted

It's likely you don't want some of your thoughts. You probably don't want, for example, that thought to eat an extra piece of cake when you've already had a piece.

When is a thought **unwanted**?

❖ **When it doesn't make sense to you.** It's a thought telling you to eat when you aren't hungry, a thought to stop exercising when you should keep on going, or a thought telling yourself to jump off a cliff when the jump would kill you.

❖   **When it doesn't conform to who you want to be.** You have an
       image of the person you want to be. You know how you want
       to act. You know how you want people to think about you. Any
       thought that doesn't agree with the person you want to be can be
       considered an unwanted message from your brain.

How can you deal with unwanted thoughts and urges? Through a process
I call **Lifeguarding.** A lifeguard saves lives by the same process you can use to
manage unwanted thoughts. Once you can manage your unwanted thoughts,
you can stop slip-ups and save your diet. Think about how lifeguards perform
their job:

1.   **Go on guard.** When lifeguards go on duty they immediately
       become sensitive to everything around them. Anyone could need
       their help at any time. In the same way, you can go on guard when
       you enter a potential slip-up situation. When you are near food or
       exercising, you need to go on guard. At any time, you could need
       your own help to stop eating or to keep exercising. Once you are
       on guard it's time to be on the lookout for trouble.

2.   **Scan for signs.** Lifeguards continually scan the environment
       looking for potential problems to enable a reaction before a situ-
       ation becomes an emergency. In the same way you can scan your
       thoughts, visual images, feelings, and surroundings for signs
       of trouble. When you find something wrong, it's time to fix the
       problem.

3.   **Respond skillfully.** When lifeguards detected a problem the job
       is not done. Lifeguards must skillfully respond to any situation or
       lives will be lost. In the same way, when you detect a slip-up situa-
       tion, you must respond skillfully to save yourself from the slip-up.

You don't have to be a victim of your own random thoughts. Realize that
thoughts happen to you despite your intentions, not because of them. You
can learn to retrain your brain to stop the unwanted thoughts and we'll use
Lifeguarding as part of the retraining.

▌ Retraining Your Brain to Stop Unwanted Thoughts

You can retrain your brain to stop sending you unwanted messages
because of something called **neuroplasticity.**

Neuroplasticity is the ability of the brain to change itself. Once thought
impossible, we now know as Michael Merzenich tells us in the Scientific

American, "The brain was constructed to change." And from Dr. Jeffrey Schwartz in his groundbreaking book *The Mind and The Brain*, we learn, "The willful directing of attention can act on the brain to alter its subsequent patterns of activity."

What this means is that your brain is not hard-wired into its current behavior. Your brain can be retrained to reverse the years of bad weight-gaining habits.

One way to look at some of your current thinking processes is that they are like an old two lane highway that needs to be replaced by a new high-speed freeway. For years, when you've needed to go from A to B you've only been able to go on the old highway. There's only been one road and you've never had a choice to go any other way. You just got on the road and went. You knew the road so well that you didn't have to think during the entire trip.

By following the steps to avoid automatic eating you will be tearing down the old road and creating a whole new freeway, taking you exactly where you want to go.

▌ Rethink Yourself a New Brain

You can rethink yourself a new brain. The key is changing your behavior. **Changing your behavior changes your brain.** Why? Because it quiets activity in one part of your brain and shifts it to a new part. If you can consistently shift your attention away from the thoughts and behaviors you don't want, you can change the physical structure of your brain. You are building a new highway and tearing down the old.

Focusing your attention on a replacement behavior causes new synapses to fire, which strengthens those connections in your brain. After a while the old connections in your brain associated with the old thoughts and behaviors will weaken. More and more you'll turn to the new way of thinking and behaving because those pathways in your brain are stronger.

You might think this is all just mumbo jumbo. But it isn't. Dr. Schwartz has convincingly documented this amazing capability of your brain. Your brain can change and how you direct your attention is the force that makes the change. The **choices you make now matter** because they will influence the choices you'll make in the future. If you are willing to put in the work, you can literally retrain your brain away from old habits you no longer want into new habits that better represent who you want to become.

▌ The Three Steps to Retraining Your Brain

You can retrain you brain away from old behaviors using a series of steps I adapted from Dr. Jeffrey Schwartz's book, *Brain Lock*.

The Designer Diet steps to retraining your brain are:

1. **Become aware of your own thoughts.** When you notice an unwanted thought, go to step 2.
2. **Tell Yourself: It's Not Me; It's Just an Unwanted Message from My Brain!** Saying this statement to yourself identifies the thought as an unwanted thought, a thought you shouldn't take seriously or pay attention to.
3. **Immediately switch behaviors.** Changing your behavior changes how your brain is wired.

The idea of these steps is to focus your mind on solutions rather than problems. If you can shift your attention from problems to solutions frequently enough, your brain will reconnect itself to support your new solution-solving behaviors.

▌ Step 1: Become Aware of Your own Thoughts

The first step in the retraining process is to become aware of your own thoughts. This combines the *go on guard* and *scan for signs* Lifeguarding steps. Once you are aware of your thoughts, you can make a conscious decision about which thoughts are unwanted and which thoughts you should pay attention to.

You can become aware of your thoughts through a process called **mental note taking.** Mental note taking is similar to what you did when you wrote down your thought log. When a thought happens, you name or label it. Your goal is to observe your thoughts as they arise.

For mental note taking to really work, you need to stand outside yourself as an observer. You need to be able to observe your thoughts as they happen. This skill, also called "mindful awareness" or "bare attention," is described as calmly viewing your experience as an outsider.

Mental note taking is so different and strange from normal everyday thinking that you may find it difficult to do. That's OK. It's a skill you get better at with practice. Normally you just think and act without a lot of thinking about what you are thinking. You are being asked to do something totally different. Be patient. The payoff is worth it.

Mental Note Taking Example: Walking

We'll use walking as our first example of mental note taking. Walking is a fun example, because it's so simple and automatic we don't realize how complicated it actually is. Also, it's slightly easier to take mental notes of a physical activity like walking than it is of pure thinking. We'll move on to mental note taking for thoughts in our next example.

Let's say you are sitting down and you need to stand up to walk. What might your mental notes look like? In our examples, mental notes are marked with the phrase "note as."

Getting up from sitting requires a decision, which can be noted. On the decision to walk, note it as *wanting to walk*. The note is a thought about your thought. You generate the note by watching your thoughts as they happen.

When rising from your sitting position, note as *rising*. When standing, note as *standing*. When looking from here to your intended destination, note as *looking, seeing*.

At first, when you are walking, note as *right step, left step*. After you practice *right step, left step* for a while, you can break down each step into smaller components. For each step try noting it as *raising, dropping*. After you practice that for a while, you can become even more detailed. For reach step, note it as *raising, pushing forward, dropping*.

After you have walked enough and you decide to sit down again, note as *wanting to sit down*.

That's it. You're done with the example. Keep trying this exercise until it feels natural. When you try it for the first time, you will probably feel completely awkward and a bit silly. You may not even be able to note simple actions like *right step*. There won't be enough time. The step will happen, you won't have noted it, and you won't believe how you couldn't note such a simple thing.

After you try it for a while, you'll notice that you can make mental comments about many of your actions without tripping. Then you'll notice you can make mental comments about most of your actions. And eventually you'll be able to notice more and more of your actions with ever finer levels of detail.

That's the point of this exercise: **learning how to mentally comment on what you are doing and thinking.** Once you can do that, it gives you a little bit of time to see if a thought is unwanted. And once you know a thought is unwanted you can deal with it by moving immediately to the next step.

▌ Step 2: Tell Yourself: It's Not Me; It's Just an Unwanted Message from My Brain!

Using *mental note taking,* as you have a thought think about it and see if it is unwanted. If the thought doesn't make sense, or doesn't conform to who you want to be, then say to yourself:

> ***It's Not Me; It's Just an Unwanted Message from My Brain!***

When you notice an unwanted message from your brain, saying this statement to yourself identifies the thought for what it really is and interrupts your thought process so you can move to the *Immediately Switch Behaviors* step. In the beginning, it can help to say the phrase out loud. This is part of the *respond skillfully* Lifeguarding step.

Each phrase in *It's Not Me; It's Just an Unwanted Message from My Brain!* has a purpose.

The *It's Not Me* part is to remind yourself that you can't help which thoughts pop into your mind. You are not your thoughts. You don't consciously control your thoughts. Blaming yourself for your thoughts would be like blaming yourself for an itch you feel on your arm. You wouldn't think of blaming yourself for an itch. Don't blame yourself for your thoughts either.

The *It's Just an Unwanted Message from My Brain!* part is to remind yourself that this is a pop-thought. It's simply a thought that popped into your mind. Thoughts are not under your direct control, so don't worry about the thoughts.

Expect that you will have these thoughts. You will have these thoughts every day of your life. Understanding that will help you recognize and respond to them sooner.

And that's what is important to keep in mind. You are learning to be aware of your thoughts and then consciously deciding how to respond to them. If you decide that a thought is unwanted, then apply the next step: *Immediately Switch Behaviors.*

▌ Step 3: Immediately Switch Behaviors

After becoming aware of an unwanted thought and having said to yourself *It's Not Me; It's Just an Unwanted Message from My Brain!,* immediately **replace** your current behavior with a better activity.

The replacement activity can be **anything you enjoy doing.** Your goal is to focus your attention on your new activity. Ideally, your replacement behavior should be **active, useful, constructive,** and **require concentration** and **strategy.** Involving other people is a good idea. Biking alone, for example, is not as effective as biking with another person because it is less likely to refocus your attention on the new replacement activity. And passive activities don't work very well. You need to be active or your attention may drift back to your unwanted thoughts.

There are two different types of replacement activities: **Active Replacement** and **Drop the Thought.**

Active Replacement

Your goal is to immediately do something to interrupt the unwanted thought and replace it with an alternate, more desirable activity.

Some possible replacement activities are:

❖ Go for a walk or a bike ride.
❖ Work in your garden.
❖ Yoga.
❖ Play with your kids or your dog.
❖ Meditate.
❖ Talk to a friend.
❖ Play team basketball.
❖ Breathe deeply if you are in an awkward situation where you can't free yourself.

Can you think of other replacement activities based on your life and interests?

Switch for 15 Minutes

Have a goal of engaging in your replacement behavior for a minimum of 15 minutes. Dr. Schwartz found this to be about the length of time needed for urges to be noticeably reduced.

Drop the Thought

Ignoring an unwanted thought may be your only option when you are in a situation where you can't make an active response. Thought dropping is not as effective as an active response, but sometimes it's the best you can do and it's a lot better than obsessing on an unwanted thought.

To drop a thought just breathe, relax into your body, and let the unwanted thought drift through and out of your mind. A thought stays alive when you keep thinking about it. Do not think about it at all. Just let the thought pass through you like a gentle breeze. You may be tempted to analyze the thought, dissect it, figure out where it came from and what you should do about it. Don't. It's an unwanted message. You don't owe it anything. Don't let it own you. Ignore it.

Slowly Changing Your Brain

Over time the three step brain retraining process retrains your brain away from your unwanted thoughts and activities. Your brain actually changes to a new a set of behaviors.

It's not enough to tell yourself not to eat. That's why self-talk isn't as effective a strategy. You already know you shouldn't do something, yet you will still feel compelled to do it anyway. Unless you switch to another behavior, you won't be making the physical changes in your brain that will help prevent the unwanted thoughts in the future.

Making Up for Poor Executive Brain Function

There is a part of your brain called the frontal cortex that is thought to guide complex behavior over time. It is involved in planning, abstract thinking, learning rules, responding to events, and inhibiting inappropriate actions. Collectively these capabilities are called your **executive functions.**

Looking at the list you might be able to imagine what would happen if your executive functions were damaged. You would lose control of a lot of what we consider adult behaviors. And in fact, this is the last part of your brain to mature. Teenagers don't have a fully developed executive function, which explains why they behave like, well, teenagers.

A Kent State University study, and a few others, found evidence showing overweight and obese people have **impaired executive function** when compared to those of normal weight. Older adults also show a decline in their executive functions.

It's easy to see how maintaining a normal weight could rely on a strong executive function. What stops you from giving in to your impulses? Your executive function. What keeps your goals on track? Your executive function. What helps you respond to new situations? Your executive function.

With impaired executive function, it's going to be harder for you to control your weight. I think Lifeguarding may help make up for at least some of these problems because with Lifeguarding you aren't responding automatically to situations. You are consciously directing your behaviors. That should help make up for at least some of what your executive functions would have done for you automatically.

▌ Lifeguarding Example: Strolling the Food Court

Let's run through an example of Lifeguarding while walking into a food court at your local mall.

As you walk in you know you are entering a danger zone where slip-ups are as likely as browsing a 2 for 1 sale at your favorite store. Entering a danger zone means it's time to **go on guard** by starting to observe your thoughts using mental note taking. A true master is always on guard, but that's a skill developed over time. For now, it's a great start to notice when you are in a danger zone and then to go on guard.

What thoughts might go through your mind as you walk the food court?

That cinnamon roll looks incredible. Note as **seeing** food.

Oh, the smell is heavenly. Fresh baked dough…sweet icing…thick with cinnamon. Note as **smelling** food.

Maybe I should get one? Note as **wanting to eat.**

Oh, I am wanting to eat because I smelled the cinnamon roll. Let's see if this is an unwanted thought. Yes, it is. I can't have a cinnamon roll right now. It would blow my calorie budget and I would rather have a nice dinner tonight.

So: It's Not Me; It's Just an Unwanted Message from My Brain!

Now, what behavior will I switch to? I don't have a lot of options in the mall. I'll breathe deeply and drop the thought. I'll turn my thoughts to what I am looking for here and walk away from the tempting sights and smells.

And that's it. Once you're out of the danger zone you can go off guard again. It's not a complex process. What makes it possible is your ability to pay attention to your thoughts, think about what they mean, and then decide what to do based on your evaluation of the thought. For those prone to obesity, this is the **highest possible form** of weight control.

Previously you might have just smelled the cinnamon roll, bought it, ate it, and then afterward wondered how you could have possibly let yourself eat 1,000 calories on a single dessert. Oh the torment of hindsight!

Lifeguarding gives you a tool you can use to interrupt that automatic cycle of behavior and return control back to where it belongs—you.

Lifeguarding expands far beyond helping with automatic eating. If you have any negative thoughts about yourself, Lifeguarding can help with those too. Lifeguarding really can apply to every part of your life. *Go on guard* can apply to any potential slip-up situation. *Scan for signs* can be any way you notice that you are entering a danger zone. And *respond skillfully* can make use of any strategy in this book or any strategy you create.

Lifeguarding is potentially one of the most powerful and life-transforming strategies in this entire book. It's not for everyone as it takes discipline. But if you can master Lifeguarding, you'll have a skill nobody can take away and you'll have it for the rest of your life.

To Learn More

❖ *Mindfulness-Based Cognitive Therapy for Depression* by Zindel Segal, J. Mark G. Williams, and John Teasdale is a wonderful book for learning meditation and other useful Lifeguarding skills.

❖ *Brain Lock* by Jeffrey M. Schwartz, MD goes into fascinating and loving detail on how to retrain your brain.

....

Strategy 24. Visualize Your Own Automatic Eating Scenarios

Visualize each of your automatic eating trigger situations and imagine how you would handle them.

There's an old saying: luck favors the prepared mind. You can improve your success of dealing with automatic eating by visualizing how you want to handle these situations before they even happen.

▌ Don't Skip Visualization! It works.

When most people see a section on visualization, they skip it and move on to something seemingly more important. That might be a mistake. Visualization trains your brain almost as well as doing the real thing and without all the physical effort. And because you can visualize a scenario far more times than you can perform it, visualization is an incredibly cheap and efficient way of changing your brain. That's why world class athletes are taught visualization as part of their training. Please give it a try.

There are three steps to visualizing your automatic eating scenarios:
1.   List Your Triggers
2.   List Your Replacement Activities
3.   Visualize How You'll Handle Each Scenario

▌ Step 1: List Your Triggers

Earlier we listed a number of possible eating triggers. Now it's time to create a list of your own triggers so you can visualize how you will handle them.

Ask yourself: when are you likely to eat automatically? Take some time with this one. Think back to when you've done so. What have you eaten when you didn't want to? What were the situations? Where were you? Who was with you? Why do you think you ended up eating? Please write down your answers.

Hopefully you can handle many situations by removing your trigger foods and avoiding trigger situations, as we talked about in the *Managing Your Triggers* strategy, but unfortunately, not all scenarios are so easily solved.

▌ Step 2: List Your Replacement Activities

Next, create your personal list of possible activities you can switch to when responding to an automatic eating trigger. We listed several in the Lifeguarding strategy, but you'll also need to think of some of your own that fit your life and personality.

By creating your replacement activity list ahead of time, you won't have to think when you need to switch activities. You can just do it.

Keep in mind that you can **drop any unwanted thought.** You can just ignore the thought and let it pass right through you and out of your mind.

▌ Step 3: Visualize How You'll Handle Each Scenario

Now that you've created your list of triggers and possible replacement activities, it's time to visualize each of your trigger situations and imagine how you would react to them.

Think about a trigger. Think about what you are going to say and do when you encounter it. Keep going through all the trigger situations you've identified until you are confident that the next time you will know what to do when they happen. When a trigger does come up, you should be in an excellent position to counter it because you will have already practiced handling it. Your brain will have already started making changes toward the new behaviors.

When you find a new trigger, run through this same process again. Find an appropriate replacement activity and visualize how you will handle it when it happens.

Here are a few triggers we'll use as examples:

- Food Advertisement Comes on While Watching TV
- Hungry in a Meeting
- Urge to Stop Halfway through an Exercise Routine
- I am Stupid or Fat or Ugly or a Failure

You will certainly be able to come up with many more of your own.

▌ Scenario: Food Advertisement Comes on While Watching TV

Lusciously shot commercials of cookies and candy bars can immediately excite your mind with cravings that if left unchecked may turn directly into overeating. What can you do?

Watching less TV is a good answer, but what else can you do? Go through the Lifeguarding steps.

On seeing a food advertisement, *go on guard* immediately and start *scanning for signs* of cravings thoughts using *mental note taking*. Then *respond skillfully* to the advertisement.

One possible skillful response is to skip past the commercial if you are watching from a recording. For live TV watchers, consider changing the channel so you won't be affected by the commercial.

If neither if these responses work and your thought scans reveal a buildup of unwanted binge provoking cravings, it's time to move to step number two of *Retraining Your Brain*.

Say to yourself: *It's Not Me; It's Just an Unwanted Message from My Brain!* Then *immediately switch behaviors*.

Maybe you can leave the room (stay away from the kitchen!). Try breathing deeply and dropping the thought. Or try something else from your replacement activities list.

Using Lifeguarding, you don't have to let commercials compel you to eat. You can do something about it. You have the power.

▌ Scenario: Hungry in a Meeting

You are in an important meeting with ten other people and it happens: you suddenly get ravenously hungry. Oh no! Making an active response to the thought is impossible because you must stay in the meeting.

In this situation **start deep breathing, drop the thought,** and **bring your goal picture to mind** (see the *Bring Your Goal Picture to Mind* strategy). You don't have to react to the thought of being hungry. You don't have to pay it any attention. It's just a thought. Let the thought flow through you. The more you think about it the more energy is pumped into the thought and the bigger it gets. When it gets big enough you'll be forced to act on the thought. Shrink the thought. Ignore it and it will shrink to nothing and go away.

▌ Scenario: Urge to Stop Halfway through an Exercise Routine

You are about halfway through your exercise routine and all of sudden you're starting to get thoughts like these:

> *You've done enough already and you are tired, it's time to stop now...Hey, you can stop now...Oh, you can go eat that piece of leftover birthday cake, after all you deserve it, you exercised so hard today.*

I get thoughts like these all the time. What can you do about them? Lifeguarding to the rescue.

When you start exercising, *go on guard.* It's quite likely that almost every exercise routine will at one time or another prompt your brain to tell you to stop before you're done.

While exercising *scan for signs* of thoughts about stopping using *mental note taking.*

If you become aware of an impulse to stop, first determine if it's an unwanted thought. Sometimes you may really be hurt or drained enough that stopping is exactly what you should do. But most of the time, quitting in the middle of exercising isn't who you want to be, so it's an unwanted thought.

It's time to *respond skillfully.* What are some possible responses to thoughts demanding you stop exercising before you are ready? *Drop the thought* is one possible response, but you may prefer a stronger, more active response, something positive that will help pump you up and motivate you.

There are three pump-up-the-volume type strategies: *Repeat Your Power Phrase* (available on the website), *Bring Your Goal Picture to Mind, Play Big Goal Little Goal.* Take a look and see if any of these might work for you.

You don't have to pick just one strategy, but can use them all. And I'm sure you have strategies of your own. Lifeguarding helps you **realize when it's time to use a strategy.** A lot of the time you might just accept a thought to quit exercising and stop. Using Lifeguarding you will realize when a thought is unwanted and then you'll be able to implement your plan to deal with it.

Some people may be tempted to use a negative strategy like repeating something horrible to themselves like "I'm so fat I have to keep exercising." Avoid this. Always keep it positive. Negative motivation never lasts for long and it does a lot of damage along the way.

▌ Scenario: I am Stupid or Fat or Ugly or a Failure

This scenario is to let you know that Lifeguarding helps you deal with much more than automatic eating. You can respond to these unwanted thoughts using the same techniques. You don't have to let your brain put you down. Fight back. Retrain these thoughts out of your brain so you can have a better, more positive life. You deserve it.

Strategy 25. Bring Your Goal Picture to Mind

Power through adversity by thinking a mental picture of exactly how you wish to look, feel, eat, act and think.

Your *Goal Picture* is a mental picture of exactly how you wish to look, feel, eat, act and think. It is a **complete picture of who you want to be.** It may contain many overlapping images, feelings, and thoughts. It may even be a series of pictures, like a movie.

There will be times when you feel weak and unmotivated. You will want to quit. At these times, bring your goal picture to mind and it will help you remember what you are trying to accomplish and why. Sometimes that's all you need to outlast temptation.

The Goal Picture also works at the subconscious level to change the subconscious image you have of yourself. We often resist change because we see ourselves only a certain way. Our old image locks us into position. Your Goal Picture allows you to become the person you want to be.

▌ Steps to Creating Your Goal Picture

Here are the steps to building your goal picture:
1.   Think about who and what you want to be.

2.   Be honest with your goals. Don't set yourself up for failure.
3.   Think about how you wish to look, feel, eat, act and think.
4.   If you have a hard time coming up with a picture, think about people you admire and what you like about them.
5.   Picture your existing body then picture the new body you want.
6.   Picture exactly how you wish to look down to the smallest detail.
7.   Picture exactly how you wish to feel.
8.   Picture what you wish to eat and in what quantities.
9.   Picture exactly how you wish to act in specific situations.
10. Picture exactly how you wish to think in specific situations.
11. Make the changes real in your imagination. Begin to experience yourself as you want to be. Experience the changes you have made.
12. Make as many pictures as you need.

Keep building your Goal Picture in your mind until you can quickly call it up without too much effort.

You don't have to follow every step. Some of the steps may not make sense to you. Feel free to include only what you think will motivate you when you need to be motivated.

Pack your Goal Picture with vibrant symbols overflowing with personal meaning. When you look at or think about your Goal Picture, you want its meaning instantly clear to you. Don't worry what other people will think. If your motivation to exercise is best symbolized by an old pair of track shoes you wore in high school, then pick that as your symbol for exercise. All the motivation and health you felt at that time will be accessible via the track shoes symbol. Picking a different, more conventional symbol would drain it of all its power. That's the idea for all your Goal Picture symbols: make them deeply meaningful to you.

My Goal Picture is quite simple because I am not a very good visualizer:

> *I picture Superman looking up at a blazing sun and a full moon set against a green background. Green means good health to me because it symbolizes the vibrancy of nature. Superman symbolizes strength and goodness. The sun symbolizes vast power and endless energy. The moon symbolizes the loved ones and relationships I'll lose if I don't succeed. And the long distance between Superman and the sun reminds me of how far I have to go and that I want to live a long time. When I need more strength,*

I transform the sun into a roaring bear standing tall on its hind legs, claws extended. I imagine myself infused with the same power and energy a bear must feel in full roar.

In my mind these are the images that motivate me. They may seem laughably silly to you, but that's OK. You need to come up with images that are personally meaningful to you. It doesn't matter what they are.

Let your Goal Picture change as your life changes. A Goal Picture is never complete. Change it as you find new issues that need handling. Let your Goal Picture vary in your mind. Don't force it to be static.

▌ Create a Goal Picture Collage

If you aren't the kind of person who visualizes pictures easily, you may want to create a collage of your Goal Picture. Cut pictures out from magazines that represent all symbols in your Goal Picture and paste them into a collage. As you search for pictures, take some time and think about what they represent and what they mean to you.

This is a fun project and makes visualizing your Goal Picture a lot easier. Think about hanging up your collage in your workout area for extra motivation.

▌ How to Apply Your Goal Picture

Bring your Goal Picture to mind whenever you feel like you need support and motivation. This could be when you are eating too much, when you want to quit on your exercise, or for any other reason.

Mentally visit each symbol in the picture. Think about what each symbol means to you. Let your thoughts and feelings fill you with renewed strength and purpose. Sometimes your spirit just runs out of gumption and you need to get a refill. That's what your Goal Picture does for you. Visualizing your Goal Picture pumps you up when you need help the most.

▌ Experiencing the Goal Picture Meditation

Your Goal Picture can be used as part of an interesting experience called the *Goal Picture Meditation*. This is a 15 minute guided meditation that helps you make your Goal Picture more real to you. The meditation progressively relaxes your whole mind and body.

After you're completely relaxed, you're taken on a trip through your Goal Picture. This trip helps you experience and connect to your Goal Picture, which makes it more real and meaningful.

This is a wonderful experience. You'll need about 15 minutes and before you start, you should be in a comfortable space, wearing comfortable clothes.

The meditation is available as an audio file on our website at *http:// YourDesignerDiet.com.*

....

Strategy 26. Play Big Goal Little Goal

Set short term goals until you reach your long term goal.

This is a game you can play when your brain tells you to stop. Let's say you have a big goal, completing 35 minutes on the treadmill. But after a while you want to stop. A way to motivate yourself is to set a smaller goal you can reach quickly.

People do much better when they make regular progress toward a visible, well defined goal. For example, if you ask people to hold up their arm as long as they can they'll hold it up for a much shorter time than when they are asked to hold their arm up for 10 minutes. There's something about not having a specific goal that allows people to give up earlier.

So make little goals. Instead of thinking about your big goal, make a pact with yourself to reach a little goal, like just one more minute, or just reaching one more blinking dot on the treadmill display. Whatever works for you.

To reach the little goal, you can use the *Repeat Your Power Phrase* (available on the website) or *Bring Your Goal Picture to Mind* strategies. When you get there, set another little goal. And just keep setting little goals until you reach your big goal. Before you know it, you'll have reached your big goal without giving in to your unwanted thoughts to quit.

You can change each little goal too. You can say I'll do this little goal at a sprint or a higher treadmill elevation. Change up anything to make it interesting and different.

I use this strategy all the time. One of my favorite examples is a hike I take up this scary steep hill. Walking it is like inching up a flag pole. But it's not straight up. It undulates like a rock-armored snake. Each rise up the snake's back is about 100 yards. At the end of each rise is an arch, which levels off for a few yards. It repeats this pattern all the way to the top. Going up the hill is a constant cycle of hiking up the long rise, resting a little in the flats, tackling the next long rise and praying for the next flat to finally come again.

To get through the hike I make it a game of *Big Goal Little Goal.* The big goal is to get to the top. But five minutes into the hike I am breathing hard and

I don't care about the big goal anymore. So I make a little goal of hitting the next flat. About half way up a rise I get so tired I quit caring about getting to the next flat part of the trail. Remember, this is a steep hill! So I make an even littler goal of just taking the next step. I eventually get to the top one step, one rise, and one flat at a time. It's not heroic, but it works.

Strategy 27. Solving Emotional Eating with The Solution®

In The Solution program, you learn how to set limits and how to take care of yourself emotionally, to heal your sadness and anger rather than eating your way out of problems.

Hunger driven by emotion is just as real as any other source of hunger. If you suspect most or even some of your weight control problems are caused by emotional eating, then take a look at a program called *The Solution* created by Laurel Mellin. Here's how The Solution is described on their website:

> The Solution Method gives us the skills we missed in childhood. Based in the most up-to-date neuroscience, it teaches us how to rewire our feeling brain and turn off those cravings and those urges for sugar, fat, nicotine, alcohol—and other common life excesses, such as overworking, thinking too much and people-pleasing.

The Solution is based on solid research and has worked for many people. It's worth taking a look at and could become a very valuable strategy for you.

To Learn More

❖ The website for *The Solution* is at *http://www.thepathway.org/*.

Chapter 16

Weight-Proof Your Life

On my diet I feel deprived, I run to the kitchen, I eat. For a while
I am strong, I have the power, then I lose it and I gain 10 pounds
again! I do this over and over. I feel so stupid! Now I have the
power again... —Anonymous

Most of us understand exactly where Anonymous is coming from in this quote. For me staying on a diet used to feel like being a car with a very small gas tank. I would fill the tank up with willpower and my diet would run fine for a while. Then the tank would empty and I'd be off my diet. With such a small tank I couldn't go for long. I think that is what Anonymous is saying with "Now I have the power again."

But the power doesn't last. You won't stay motivated to eat less and exercise more. You can't rely on your environment anymore to help you maintain a healthy weight. This is why you are among the first generation of people completely responsible for their own weight loss.

Your willpower tank empties one slip-up at a time. A **slip-up** is when the threats cause you to eat more or exercise less than you intend. All it takes is one slip-up a week for you to gain weight. What can you do if you can't rely on willpower or your environment?

You create your own environment to minimize your chances of slipping up. These environments are called **Safe Zones.** A Safe Zone is a protected area you create—using strategies—in which you naturally achieve your goals without relying on willpower every minute of every day.

There are Safe Zones for many important parts of your life: Personal, Home and Family, Activity, Portion Control, Car, Shopping, Work, School, and Community. Each of these life areas can be changed to make it less likely you'll slip-up. And the less you slip-up the more control you have over your weight. We'll talk about how to create each type of Safe Zone in later chapters. You are by no means limited to these Safe Zones. Create Safe Zones wherever they make sense in your life.

The process of creating Safe Zones is called **Weight-Proofing.** Weight-Proofing **protects you from diet slip-ups by turning diet danger zones into Safe Zones.** Using Weight-Proofing strategies, you systematically **remove diet slip-ups from your life** by creating ever widening circles of Safe Zones around you and your loved ones.

Safe Zones are created by continually thinking of strategies that put you in the best position to succeed at four goals:

- ❖ Eating to your diet
- ❖ Burning more calories
- ❖ Finding more joy
- ❖ Avoiding slip-ups

The Designer Way and Weight-Proofing are perfect partners. Safe Zones are created by making little changes over a long period and that's exactly how the Designer Way works. Over time this creates an environment in which you don't have to rely on motivation to control your weight.

▌ Weight-Proofing is Like Baby-Proofing your Home

A good way of thinking about Weight-Proofing is that it's like baby proofing a home. The goal of baby-proofing is to remove any threat that could hurt a baby. The goal of Weight-Proofing is to remove any threat that could cause you to fall off your diet.

When baby proofing a home, you try to think like a baby and remove every possible way a baby might hurt itself. When Weight-Proofing your life, you **try to think like the threats** and remove every possible way they might cause you to slip-up and fall off your diet.

Think about how you go about baby proofing. You don't put up post-it notes asking your baby to please not touch the power outlets. You don't have a heart-to-heart talk to tell your baby not to go near the stairs. Why? Because babies don't understand. In the same way your body doesn't understand that it is no longer 25,000 years ago and not every food commercial means it's time to eat and you aren't going to starve if you don't eat for a few hours.

Weight-Proofing in real life looks a lot like the same process. When baby proofing a home you walk through the entire house looking for any possible threat to the baby and then implementing a strategy to counter the threat. You know what is dangerous because you have a good idea what might harm a baby. Let's say you walk into a kitchen and you notice a door leading down a flight of stairs. Stairs are definitely dangerous for babies so you buy a gate for the door. You look around the kitchen some more and you notice the cupboard drawers are easy to open, so you buy child proof locks. You repeat this process until all the threats to the baby have been neutralized.

When Weight-Proofing a home, you walk into the kitchen too. Only, this time you open the refrigerator because you know possible threats to your diet lurk there. Tucked in a side pocket are a few of your favorite candy bars. Half the candy bars are gone and you bought them two days ago. You know one of the threats says the easy availability of food leads to overeating. You also know you need to be extreme with candy bars because you find yourself automatically eating them during the day. There's a strategy we'll talk about later of removing all tempting foods from your house. So, you toss the candy bars and as a result you are much safer from the threat of temptation. Repeat this process anywhere and everywhere that could pose a threat to your diet. I call this process of finding all potential threats in a Safe Zone "making a **slip-up survey.**"

Weight-Proofing is: paying attention to your life, knowing what might be dangerous to you, and then removing the danger. Perform a slip-up survey in every Safe Zone we talk about in the following chapters. Look for any forces that might cause you to slip-up and do the best job you can at neutralizing them with counter strategies.

You can't change your genes or the world in which you live, but you can use the same incredible human qualities that made the modern world—your ability to think, learn, grow, and adapt—to create Safe Zones in which you have no choice but to succeed.

Chapter 17

Weight-Proof Your Personal Safe Zone

Strategies 28–37

Your Personal Safe Zone is a set of basic principles and ideas that will help you create, use, and manage all your Safe Zones.

· ·

Strategy 28. Forgive Yourself—Prevent a Lapse from Becoming a Collapse

Forgive yourself for slip-ups as you would a friend. Don't let a lapse turn into a collapse.

Controlling your weight is a daily struggle. It's a struggle you will sometimes lose. You've read about all the threats and you know how hard it is for a person in our modern, toxic environment to stay on a diet. You will slip-up. It's human nature to make mistakes. It's an inevitable part of life. What matters is what you *do* about a mistake.

What should you do about a mistake? **Forgive yourself.** Don't let a mistake throw you off your diet and into an eating binge. Don't let a lapse become a collapse. Forgive yourself like you would forgive a friend. We are often hardest on ourselves. We show ourselves less love and understanding than we would to our worst enemy. You may end up giving up if you can't see it in your heart to forgive yourself.

Forgiving yourself is called **self-compassion.** Self-compassion is the ability to treat yourself with kindness when things go badly. It's the secret of

291

why some people successfully roll with life's punches, face failure with grace, and eventually overcome their problems. Without self-compassion you end up dwelling on failures, making your problems bigger than they really are, and criticizing yourself into a downward a spiral of self-loathing. Life is tough enough without fueling the fire of your own anger and depression.

Self-compassion has three parts: self-kindness, common humanity, and mindful acceptance. Self-kindness is being kind and understanding toward yourself rather than taking the easy road of being self-critical. Common humanity is seeing your negative experiences as a normal part of life. Stuff happens and it sometimes happens to you. You can deal with it. Humans are incredibly tough. Mindful acceptance is being able to let things go rather than dwelling on them. If, like most of us, you need help on this one, please take a look at the Lifeguarding strategy.

Your emotions won't burn out of control when you practice self-compassion. You'll react more appropriately to events in your life. You'll be able to accept responsibility for your actions without feeling horrible for a long time. And your image of yourself will become less about the bad things or even the good things in your life. All of these changes help you control your weight because **your weight is much more likely to spin out of control when you are out of control.**

Think of every problem as a learning opportunity and not just another piece of evidence of how screwed up you are. If all you do is get down on yourself then you are missing an opportunity to improve your life. Use your problems as inputs into The Designer Way so you can help yourself avoid the same problems in the future.

All that matters is that you are continually learning and getting better. Time will take care of the rest.

. . . .

Strategy 29. Create Your Safe Zones Now, Using Your Logical Brain

Use your willpower when it's the strongest to create Safe Zones that will work all the time, even when your willpower runs out.

Like a lot of people, I contribute to my savings account by having money automatically deducted from my paycheck. If the process wasn't automatic I don't think I would save nearly as much money.

Think what I would have to do if money wasn't deducted automatically. I would get my paycheck and then rather than spend it I would have to write another check and deposit it into my savings account. How many times would I think of excellent ways to spend the money rather than saving it? Too many.

Now think back to *The Two Brain Threat* where we learned how short-term emotional thinking can overpower long-term logical thinking. Under the influence of dreaming about buying a shiny new toy (short-term thinking) I might make the decision to spend the money instead of saving it (long-term thinking).

How do I get around this problem? My logical mind knows I need to save for retirement. So at a time when I am at my most logical, that is, when I don't have a check in my hot little hands ready to spend, I set up an automatic deduction so I have no choice but to save money. It just works.

By setting up the automatic deduction once, the rewards are reaped every month with no effort at all. That's how the logical mind overcomes the emotional mind. **You plan and create your Safe Zones when you are at your most logical, so that you will naturally and easily attain your goals.**

Your logical mind knows you need help to stay on your diet. Setting up Safe Zones *is* that help. Setting up Safe Zones is like setting up an automatic deduction from your paycheck. If you have to rely on constant motivation not to eat, to always exercise, to always do the right thing, then you probably won't succeed. Few people can make that many right decisions under the continual bullying of their emotional brain.

By setting up Safe Zones when you are using your long term logical thinking, you are giving yourself the best chance to succeed when temptation comes knocking and you want to open the door. By creating Safe Zones, you guarantee success over the long run.

I have fond memories of applying this strategy on what I have come to call my Purge the Urge day. One of the Safe Zone strategies is to toss tempting foods out of your house so you won't eat them when hunger drives you to forage around your house looking for food to eat. This is "purging the urge." For me, ice cream is the temptress.

I did the deed from a position of strength. I had just eaten so I wasn't hungry. I was thinking about creating a Safe Zone so I was committed to throwing away the ice cream even though I had already paid for it and I knew I would really want to eat it later.

Tossing a perfectly good gallon of ice cream into the trash was really hard! But it paid off. Later that night, when I was looking for a snack and I would have normally made a big bowl of ice cream, the ice cream wasn't there so I didn't eat it.

You might be asking why I didn't keep the ice cream and use Joyful Eating to joyfully eat just one or two bites? Excellent question. That just doesn't work for me with ice cream. I know I can't control my ice cream eating so I know I have to **be extreme** and keep it out of the house.

From time to time I think I'm over my ice cream problem and I buy some, thinking I'll control myself. But I don't. I eat way too much of it. So I go extreme on this strategy and just don't have ice cream around. I really wish I could handle it differently, but I can't. It's not worth the risk.

Strategy 30. Out of Sight, Out of Mind

Create Safe Zones by looking at your life and determining where you can slip-up. Figure out a way to remove whatever is tempting from your direct attention.

The **single most important principle** when creating your Safe Zones is *Out of Sight, Out of Mind*. You may notice as you read the strategies how this idea cuts across a lot of them.

This strategy makes use of two powerful ideas:

1.   The harder something is to do the less likely you are to do it.
2.   If something is out of sight then you can't pay attention to it.

The first idea is pretty self explanatory. Moving a goody to an out of the way location, say on top of your roof, means you are much more likely to stay on your couch when the goody urge hits. It's too much effort.

The second idea is a little more interesting. Moving food out of sight means you won't pay attention to it which means you are less likely to eat it. A big part of creating your Safe Zones is being creative about how to focus your attention. You want to **focus your attention** on what is important and away from what's unimportant.

You may say to yourself, "I am stronger than that. I can be around anything and not be tempted." And that is surprisingly true. But remember our discussion on how little slip-ups add up. You don't have to slip-up often to make a big difference in your weight. If you have a bag of candy bars in your house and you only have one extra candy bar a week, that's about 4 extra pounds a year just by that one simple slip-up.

Look around your life and determine what threatens your goals and figure out a way to remove it. Get it out of your sight. Get it out of your mind. Create a world in which you do the right thing naturally.

Strategy 31. Be Less Inactive

Make a goal to be less inactive. The rest will take care of itself.

The **second most important principle** when creating your Safe Zones is to discover ways of being less inactive. The idea is you should be less idle and less sedentary because it means moving more and moving more burns calories. Seems obvious, doesn't it?

So why not say exercise more instead? Because, interestingly, it doesn't work as well as saying be less inactive. If you say exercise more, people feel you are ordering them around so they naturally resist. People like to have a choice. Once you give people a choice of how not to be inactive, they will naturally find other things to do and a lot of those things will be physical activity.

The research of Dr. Leonard Epstein, Professor of Pediatrics and Psychology at the University of Buffalo, has found that kids who reduced their inactive behavior lost weight, improved fitness, and maintained their weight loss. In his research **they did not tell the kids what to do.** They didn't say go play basketball or go for a run.

Instead, **they encouraged kids not to be idle** and let the kids figure out what to do for themselves. A lot of what the kids did instead was be physically active so the end result was better health. When kids were told to exercise the results weren't as good. Kids like a choice. So do adults.

One idea to try is to restrict the amount of TV and other media (games, music, etc.) kids can consume, to no more than a couple of hours a day. Then let the kids decide how to spend the rest of their time. They will naturally spend a lot of the time being active.

Do you see how this works? You aren't telling the kids to exercise. You just aren't letting them be inactive by watching TV. They'll be naturally more active on their own when they no longer have the option of being inactive. It's a twisted yet cool idea.

Other activities need to be available for this strategy to work. You can't tell kids not to watch TV when there's nothing else to do. Here we see how all the strategies work together. If your community is safe, then kids can go outside and play. If there are parks then they can go play. If there are sidewalks then they can walk and visit each other. All the strategies reinforce each other.

Another key is that if parents sit around watching TV all day and munching snacks, then so will the kids. It's critical parents act how they want their kids to. The whole family needs to be involved. All this may seem a little idealistic, but kids are now at a huge risk of dying earlier than their parents. You may want to be extreme on this strategy.

To Learn More

❖   The *Planet Health* website at *http://www.hsph.harvard.edu/prc/proj_planet.html* talks about how to improve the well-being of students.

Strategy 32. Get a Life—Making Your Life Interesting Helps Drive Out the Appeal of Food

Making an interesting life for yourself focuses your attention away from food.

We have lots of open ground where we live and a huge weed problem. Some years it seems we are growing a weed garden instead of a real garden. We weed and weed yet we can't keep up.

Then we discovered something interesting. Some of our plants were able to keep the weeds out all on their own. These plants are self-seeding, which means they spread and grow by themselves, so they crowd out the pesky weeds and don't give them any place to grow. We are growing more of these miracle plants in the hope that over the long run the weeds will never again be able to establish themselves in our garden.

It turns out that our relationship with food is similar to the plants that grow so well they crowd out the weeds. Dr. Nora Volkow, director of the National Institute on Drug Abuse, thinks you are less likely to need the artificial boost of food and drugs if you create meaningful connections to the world. The more naturally excited about your life you are, the less you need other substitutes. Dr. Volkow says:

> *If you don't get excited by everyday things in life, if things look gray, and the drug makes things look extraordinary, that puts you at risk. But if you get great excitement out of a great multiplicity of things, and intensely enjoy these things—seeing a movie, or climbing a mountain—and then you try a drug, you'll think: What's the big deal?*

Dr. Volkow bases her recipe for happiness on exciting new research on how our body decides what to pay attention to. Food isn't as potent as drugs, but it can still demand our attention when there aren't other interests to crowd out the thoughts of food. Food won't seem so important if we can give ourselves something else to pay attention to.

She is asking of us something we all want for ourselves, but is still hard to do: for us to have **interesting lives.**

The "Rat Park" experiments conducted in the 1970s by Dr. Bruce Alexander prove the wisdom of Dr. Volkow's often difficult-to-follow advice. Dr. Alexander and his research team thought rats became addicted to drugs in experiments because the rats had **awful lives.** They lived lonely lives in isolated wire cages.

To prove their idea, they created Rat Park, 200-square-feet of rat heaven featuring bright balls, tin cans to play with, painted creeks and trees and plenty of space for mating and socializing. The rats were given access to sweet morphine laced drinks. Another group of cage bound rats were also given access to sweet morphine laced drinks.

What the researchers found was surprising, especially if you, like I did, thought all the rats would become equally addicted to the morphine drink. After all, it's morphine, wouldn't any rat be attracted to the constant stream of morphine-induced pleasure? Curiously, the answer is no.

Rats living in Rat Park had so much fun they barely touched their sweet morphine cocktail. In contrast, rats stuck in isolated cages eagerly drank more than a dozen times the amount of morphine solution as the rats in the park.

The implication is clear: living unhappy and disconnected lives encourages addiction. A sunflower turns toward the bright sun as it grows. If you don't have something bright in your life, you may end up turning toward the darkness.

Strategy 33. Create Your Support Group—Long Term Support Systems Work

A support system can make you more than twice as likely to maintain your weight loss.

One of the reasons I like to see movies is because they remind me of thoughts and feelings that get lost in the repetition of daily life. I get busy and my attention narrows down to just the stuff I need to do to get through the day.

Seeing a good comedy reminds me to laugh. Seeing a good drama reminds me to find the deeper meaning in life. Movies reconnect me with parts of life that are easily lost without a little reminder.

A support system is like seeing a movie for your diet. A support system keeps your mind focused on your diet. Otherwise you are likely to just forget about your diet and drift back into old habits that never worked in the first place. Doing something, almost anything, about your diet on a consistent basis will help keep you on target.

Keeping you involved may be the secret of why support systems work so well. Studies show **a support system can make you more than twice as likely to maintain your weight loss.** That's a powerful force to have working on your side. And that's why you should think seriously about making a support system part of your Safe Zones.

Internet based support systems can be as effective as structured group or one-on-one in-person support programs. Pick whatever form of support you think will work best for you. Weight Watchers, for example, has excellent in-person support groups. And there are a bunch of support communities on-line for you to choose from.

When looking for a support system, think about what kind of support has worked for you in the past. Do want to bounce ideas off people? Do want people to share with? Do you want encouragement? Are you looking for great recipes? Do you need help with goal setting? Are you looking for role models? Are you looking for a positive environment? Do want education and mentoring? Do you want daily email reminders? Would on-line food, calorie, and exercise tracking help you?

Figure out what will help to keep you on target the best.

To Learn More

❖   At *http://YourDesignerDiet.com* we maintain a list of support systems that might work for you.

Strategy 34. Look Good Now—Don't Wait to Buy Nice Clothes

Looking your best at all times helps to transform you both inside and out.

Many people wait to buy new clothes until they've reached their goal weight. While this is understandable, don't wait. Buy clothes that fit you now. Look your best at all times. That includes both during the weight loss process and when you are gaining weight.

If you are squeezing into your old clothes, you will just end up feeling sad and bad. If you are wearing your old baggy clothes while losing weight, then you are keeping your old self around instead of building up your new self.

Clothes can make an amazing difference in how you feel about yourself. Your chances of staying on a diet are a lot higher if you feel good about yourself and the direction you are heading.

What Not to Wear Shows the Power of Clothes

The immense power of this strategy was brought home to me by watching the TV show *What Not to Wear* on BBC. In *What Not to Wear,* hosts Trinny and Susannah, a pair of brutally honest fashion writers, select a woman (and sometimes a man) who has been nominated by her friends and family as needing a complete style makeover.

The contestant is given about $4,000 to buy a complete new wardrobe. All her old clothes are thrown away. It's a fresh start.

The hosts don't just give her money and tell her to go shopping. They give her a set of rules about what clothes will look best on her and why. The rules teach her how to look the best she possibly can given her strengths and weaknesses. For the rest of her, life she'll know how to buy clothes that make her look her best.

You might think this show is mainly about fashion and clothes, and it is about those too, but what it's really about is the **inner transformation** these women must undergo before they will accept that they can be attractive, vibrant women again.

The women usually resist any change. They have reached a comfort zone with their clothes and their lives and they don't want to change, even though it's obvious to everyone around them that they could look so much better. And at the end of the show they usually **look astonishingly better.**

The before and after shots are dramatic. Selecting clothes that hide what needs hiding and emphasizes the strengths of each woman makes a stunning difference. What's clear from watching the show is that these women were never really as bland as their before picture. They had just given up and needed Trinny and Susannah's tough love and excellent advice to get going again.

We hide behind our clothes. We become invisible because we don't think we deserve any better. We lack confidence. We think looking better is impossible for us. *What Not to Wear* shows that's not true.

At the end of each episode, it's not the change of clothes we notice, but the change in the women. We see them smiling and happy, strong and confident, amazed at how much better they look. We see them with hope.

That's the transformation proper fitting and well styled clothes can help to make in you.

This was a very hard strategy for me. I've never paid much attention to clothes. I never liked clothes and I hated shopping for them. But *What Not to Wear* made a big impact on me. Seeing these women bloom motivated me to give dressing better a try.

And I do try now. I've upgrade my wardrobe and I feel a difference inside. I feel more confident in myself. I still hate shopping though.

▌ Clothes Help Prevent Kids from Being Teased

Clothes are important for kids too. For kids, looking "fashionable" with clothes that fit is especially important because it will help reduce teasing and bullying. Being overweight with comical clothes is like putting a big "tease me" sign on a kid's back. Look good, don't look dumpy and the other kids will move on to another target.

. . . .

Strategy 35. Manage Your Stress

Reduce your constant desire to eat more fat and sugar by managing stress.

Humans love the right amount of stress. Stress energizes, stimulates and excites. That's why you go on wild rides at the amusement park, watch horror movies, crank up the music or go a little too fast on the freeway. The goal is not to have a stress-free life. A little bit of stress is fun.

And that's what you are built to handle: a little bit of stress at a time.

Historically, stress did come in short bursts. Let's say it's late at night and suddenly you see someone possibly lurking outside your window. To respond to the threat, you body immediately mobilizes all its resources and shuts down everything nonessential. You release energy so you can either fight or flee. Your heart rate goes up. You start to sweat. Your pupils dilate. Your body turns off growth, digestion, reproduction, and your immune system so you save energy. There's no reason to worry about reproduction in a crisis. You need to worry about surviving. Now!

All these physical responses turn on when you think something threatening is happening. The threat doesn't have to be real. You just have to think it is. If the stranger turns out to be a burglar, you are prepared. But let's say the scary stranger is really your roommate. Then your thinking immediately changes. You sigh with relief and all the physical stress responses reverse and you go back to normal again.

That's exactly how your stress response is supposed to work. Stress stays low normally, a crisis happens and your stress response ramps up, and once the crisis is over you return back to normal.

▌ Chronic Stress Decreases Your Life Expectancy

The problem is that in the modern world you can experience stress all the time. You may experience stress in traffic, waiting in line at the grocery store, or worrying about your mortgage. The number of stressors in modern life is potentially infinite.

All these are psychological stresses. They **come from your belief** that something threatening is happening. You think yourself into feeling stressed. The good news is that you can learn to manage these stresses.

Psychological stresses, like worrying about being fired from your job, can be chronic, which means they happen all the time. The problem is that your stress response is not meant to be on all the time.

When you suffer chronic stress, all those wonderful fight or flight responses start causing damage and you get sick. You can suffer from hypertension, impotency, osteoporosis, exhaustion, muscle wasting, ulcers, heart disease, and loss of memory. And we've seen the strong link between weight gain and stress in the *Stress Threat*. Chronic stress is not good for you.

▌ What can you do about chronic stress?

Dealing with stress is a lot like dealing with weight problems. Stress management isn't something you can fit into a five minute break between meetings or just do on the weekends. It's something you have to do all the time, which is exactly like staying on a diet and is why managing stress and staying on a diet are both so hard.

Some common stress management techniques are:

- ❖ **Relaxation Exercises**—You learn to relax muscle groups through-out your body. When a stressful event happens, you can use this skill to reduce tension.
- ❖ **Breathing Exercises**—You learn to breathe deeply when you become stressed, like you do when you are calm, so you can control your fight-flight response.

❖ **Meditation**—Meditation is a skill that has been shown to be very calming and improves your ability to handle stress.

❖ **Visual Imagery**—You learn to take time during the day to imagine you are in a pleasant and calming place.

❖ **Physical Exercise**—Exercise helps to relieve stress and improves your physical, emotional, and mental health.

❖ **Positive Self-talk**—Talk to yourself with positive calming phrases like "I am calm, I can stay relaxed," "Breathe deeply and slowly, let the tension go," or "I can handle this." Too often the way we talk to ourselves inside our own heads just makes things worse.

❖ **Balanced, Healthy Lifestyle**—Eat a balanced diet, get enough sleep, don't work too much, have fun, develop meaningful relationships, and put some effort into spiritual growth.

❖ **Avoid Alcohol and Drugs to Cope With Stress**—You only create more stress by using drugs and alcohol.

All these techniques can work well for you. But in the end these are all just rules. What is hard is consistently applying them. Overcoming temptation is always the challenge.

To go beyond techniques, you have to look at attitudes. Why does one person get stressed in a traffic jam and another person sing along with the radio, apparently unaffected by the traffic disaster around them? What makes the same exact event psychologically stressful for one person and not another? Why does one person see the glass as half-full and another person see the glass as half-empty? It stands to reason that if you can be more like the people who handle stress better then you can avoid the bad effects of chronic stress.

▌ The Long-Lived Nuns

A really interesting study called the Nun Study shows how certain personality traits help some people handle stress better and that handling stress better leads to much better health as you age.

Data has been collected for over thirty years from the School Sisters of Notre Dame. Nuns are a good group to study because they live in very similar environments over long periods of time.

Researchers noticed that the nuns who had the most positive attitude at a very young age were twice as likely to be alive late in life when compared to sisters who were more negative at a young age. That's a dramatic difference.

The nuns who aged well showed a sense of humor and the ability to adapt to new challenges. It's not that these nuns didn't experience psychological stress. They did. But because of their positive attitude, it's thought they **shut down their stress response sooner** and quickly returned to normal. They didn't experience chronic stress.

So the obvious next question is: how do you get a better attitude?

▌ Develop a Better Stress-Handling Attitude

Robert M. Sapolsky, a top stress researcher, has come up with a few characteristics of better stress handlers:

1. **Can you tell the difference between a big thing and a little thing?** A lion attacking you is a big thing. Is a traffic jam really a big thing or is more likely a little thing? Better stress handlers know what is a real threat to them.

2. **If it's a big thing, do you try to get a little control?** Do you take control by acting or do you just sit around and mope? Better stress handlers don't sit passively by and let events happen to them. They try to get some control of a situation by acting.

3. **Can you tell if the outcome is good or bad?** Can you tell when your life is improving? Can you tell when you've won or lost? Or do you get just as stressed over a good outcome as a bad outcome? Better stress handlers can tell when they've won and there's no reason to be stressed anymore.

4. **If the outcome is bad, do you at least have an outlet for dealing with the stress?** Do you take your frustration out in other ways or do you just bottle it up? Better stress handlers find a way to let out their pent up emotions rather than keeping it all inside.

Approaching events in your life with these steps in mind will help you become a better stress handler.

▌ Develop a Supportive Social Network

Unfortunately, it won't be enough to manage stress using only the stress management techniques we talked about earlier. Neither is developing a better stress handling attitude. There's a much bigger source of stress in your life that we have yet to talk about: **isolation.**

Sapolsky says you are much more likely to have high stress levels if you are socially isolated. There is a **threefold difference in mortality rates** for people who are socially isolated.

Being alone is a major source of stress. This is especially true as you age. As you get older, the people in your life may get sick, grow apart or die. Many older people find themselves all alone and this is a major health risk for them.

We are social animals. A big part of our well-being seems to come from connections to other people. It's crucial to keep and develop relationships with family and friends, especially as you age.

To Learn More

❖   *Why Zebras Don't Get Ulcers* by Robert M. Sapolsky. A truly excellent and witty book on every aspect of stress.

Strategy 36. Daily Reminders—Keeping Your Diet In-Sight-and-In-Mind

If you don't think about staying on your diet regularly, then you probably won't.

It takes only a couple of days for me to slide out of my good habits and back into the bad ones. How long does it take for you? Not very long either?

A recent study showed that people who got daily diet reminder emails had a BMI lower than those who didn't. That helps to validate the idea that you need to be continually involved with staying on your diet or you'll fall off.

How can you build into your life the mindfulness needed to control your weight?

1.   **Keep a Journal.** People who regularly keep a journal have been found to better maintain their weight loss.
2.   **Sign Up for Mindful Email.** A mindful email service sends you a daily email with a helpful suggestion on how to control your weight. It's not really the suggestion that helps, though it may; it's more the reminder that keeps you aware of your need control your weight. Researchers at the University of Alberta in Edmonton have shown that emails promoting healthier eating and increased physical activity are effective at lowering people's weight.
3.   **Participate in On-line Groups.** Talking with other people in on-line groups keeps you involved in your diet.
4.   **Join a Challenge.** Challenges kick in your competitive spirit to help you lose weight. You may, for example, choose to participate in a "pedometer challenge", where you and a group of like-minded

adventurers come up with your daily step goal and track the number of steps you take each day. You might like a "vegetable challenge", where you are asked to creatively include more vegetables in your daily meals. The most common challenge is the "weight loss challenge" where you challenge yourself to lose a certain amount of weight in a certain amount of time. You might even compete against other people to see who can hit their weight loss target. What makes challenges fun is your built-in support community. Challenge participants get together and talk about different ideas and generally help each other. More and more challenges are being created all the time.

We maintain lists of all these different services at *http://YourDesigner Diet.com*.

Strategy 37. Create Your Own Strategies—Use the General Concepts and be Creative

Use your own creativity to think of more strategies. It's a never ending process.

Always ask yourself how you can build new strategies into your life. That's the idea behind Safe Zones. Building strategies into your Safe Zones makes it **harder to slip-up because you aren't relying on willpower.**

The number of strategies you can apply to your own life is limited only by your imagination. We have covered many of the major principles in this chapter. You will read many more strategies in this book. Now use your own creativity to think of more.

You can work with new ideas from any source. If a new book comes out and it has a good idea, then snatch it up and make it a strategy. If you watch a talk show and something makes sense to you, then make it one of your strategies. Creating new strategies is a never ending process. Always be on the prowl for more ways to Weight-Proof your life.

For inspiration or to share the ideas you have created please visit *http:// YourDesignerDiet.com*.

Chapter 18

Weight-Proof Your Exercise Safe Zone
Strategies 38–52

The goal of creating your *Exercise Safe Zone* is to get you to burn more calories by naturally incorporating **more physical activity** into your daily life.

You may be thinking "physical activity" is really just a code word for exercise and that I want to avoid the word "exercise" because people don't like to exercise. And you are right, sort of.

I think of exercise as a more intense form of physical activity, done just for the sake of exercising. We'll talk about exercise, but what I mean by physical activity is calories burned from your normal everyday activities.

Going for a run is exercise. Running requires a special effort. Walking more by parking farther away from the store entrance is an example of getting more physical activity. Both exercise and physical activity play vital roles in creating your Exercise Safe Zone.

Before you say that trying to burn more calories from these small increases in physical activity is a waste of time, please take another a look at Threat 5, *The Power of Rest Threat*. This threat shows that some people naturally burn up to 350 calories a day through unconscious fidgeting. That's a lot of calories a day. In fact, that's 35 pounds a year's worth of calories that people with high NEAT levels naturally and easily burn off. Yet other people are not natural fidgeters and don't burn any extra NEAT-related calories.

Increasing your physical activity levels by small amounts everywhere in your life is like trying to create a higher NEAT level for yourself. With relatively little extra effort, you can dramatically increase the number of calories you burn each day by taking advantage of every opportunity to increase your physical activity levels.

When considered alone, each weight loss move will have a small effect. But if you keep making move after move, the results will change your life. **Small changes over time make for big results.** This is especially true for all the strategies that increase physical activity.

You may think I am saying you shouldn't exercise. That's not what I mean. What I am saying is you don't have to rely on exercise alone. Besides, you already know you should exercise more. Study after study shows exercise is good for you. Every New Year you probably resolve to exercise more. And you may exercise more for a little while, but most of us will exercise less and less until one day we just stop. This is a shame because the people who have been found to keep their weight off the longest are those who can manage to exercise consistently.

Here are a few reasons why exercise is good for you:
- Increased life span.
- Better sex life.
- Reduced chance of cardiovascular disease.
- Reduction in osteoporosis.
- Reduced insulin resistance.
- Reduced LDL.
- Increased HDL.
- Reduced triglycerides.
- Improved control of osteoarthritis.
- Improved blood pressure.
- Improved lung function.
- Reduced chance of retinopathy.
- Increased endorphins.
- Increased number of dopamine receptors.

Why is it so hard to exercise regularly when exercise is obviously so good for us? From *The Power of Rest Threat* we learned that exercise is not a drive for humans. In our past we had to exercise to survive so an instinct to exercise wasn't needed.

If we exercise, it's because we **consciously make it happen.** It's hard for us to do anything consistently, especially when more interesting distractions pile up and drive our attention elsewhere.

If you are one of the many people who find regular exercise difficult, then you need to use your long-term thinking brain to figure out a way to make more physical activity a natural part of your Exercise Safe Zone. When you work physical activity into your Safe Zone then it will happen, even if you don't intend it to.

Not all the physical activity related strategies are in this chapter. Physical activity is a broad topic so you'll find related strategies throughout the rest of the book too.

I know many of these physical activity strategies aren't original. But I hope you see the bigger picture here. What's important is not the type of activity, but the idea that every little extra bit of activity adds up. Find any way you can to increase your activity levels.

If you love exercise, then great. Whatever works. But most people don't like exercising and they need to be clever about weaving more activity seamlessly into their daily lives. And that's exactly what we'll be talking about in the rest of this chapter.

· ·

Strategy 38. Leverage Your Metabolism—Your Muscles Help You Lose Weight 24 Hours a Day

Muscles continuously burn calories so you can eat more and still lose weight.

The difference between losing and gaining weight can be just a few hundred calories a day. If you could change something about your body to burn a few hundred more calories a day, would you?

Excellent. You can burn more calories by building muscle through weight lifting. You knew there had to be a catch, didn't you?

Adding muscle increases your resting metabolism. This is the calories you burn when you are doing nothing, when you are absolutely at rest. Your brain, for example, is only about 2% of your weight, but consumes about 20% of your total energy! Your body must burn calories to run your brain, even when you aren't doing anything. And it's the same for every other part of your body. Running your body takes a lot of calories.

If you have a faster metabolism, you burn more calories and store less fat. If you have a slower metabolism you burn calories less efficiently and therefore store more calories as fat. You want your metabolism always working for you by burning more calories and keeping you out of starvation mode.

Your resting metabolism is responsible for 50–75% of the calories you burn each day. Digestion accounts for about 10%, and physical activity for 15–40%.

What is the single biggest calorie burner in your resting metabolism? Your muscles. **Simply by building muscle and becoming more active, you can increase your resting metabolic rate by 15% or more.**

This is why many men can seemingly eat all they want when they are younger and not gain weight. Men tend to have more muscle mass than women, so the extra food is burned up. But old age makes the sexes equal. As we age we lose muscles, which is one of the reasons we gain weight as we grow older.

▌ Replace Fat with Muscle to Lose Weight

How do you get a faster metabolism? By **replacing fat with muscle.** One pound of fat burns about 4 calories a day. One pound of muscle burns a whopping 50 calories a day. So the more muscle you add, the more calories you burn.

The exciting benefit of burning calories by adding muscle is that you are burning these calories 24 hours a day without any extra effort on your part. Muscle is like interest on your bank account balance. You get interest on your money and you don't have to do anything but let the money sit in your bank account. Muscle works the same way.

The more muscle you add, the more calories you burn and the easier it is for you to lose weight. Another benefit of adding muscle is that when you get to your target weight, you can afford to eat more food because of all the extra calories your muscles are burning. You'll also feel stronger, be happier, have more energy, and look better in clothes. What a deal! A free wonder drug. How can you not take it?

▌ Creating Your Resistance Training Program

You've learned about many of the wonderful benefits of muscles, so how do you build them? With resistance or weight training! The key point is it's not as hard as you may think. We always hear about those hard charging folks who spend hours in the gym. Fortunately, you can lift twice a week for about 20 minutes each day, and see significant results.

Skeptical? Here's a 15 minute workout routine created by Jesse Cannone, a certified personal trainer:

1.   Jumping Jacks—1 minute.

2. Bodyweight squat—15–20 reps.
3. Push-ups—as many reps as possible.
4. Kick butts (jog in place and kick your rear with each heel)—
    1 minute.
5. Hamstring floor bridge—15–20 reps.
6. Superman (lying on stomach with arms out to side, lift legs and
    chest off floor)—15–20 reps.
7. High knees (jog in place lifting knees as high as possible)—
    1 minute.
8. Stationary lunge—15–20 reps.
9. Torso rotations/twists—20 reps each direction.
10. Side bends/reaches—20 reps each direction.
11. Mountain climbers—1 minute (if you can).
12. Wall sit—as long as you can hold it.
13. Dips (use chair/bench/stairs)—as many reps as possible.

This short, intense workout delivers excellent results and you can do it anywhere with no special equipment. I do a variation of this routine when I am on the road or in the office. Of course, this is just one example to show how little time you need to spend on a workout. Please figure out what works best for you. The larger point is everyone is pressed for time. Fortunately, you don't really need a lot of time to get a good workout.

You'll see some strong benefits if you can work weight lifting into your life.

To Learn More

❖ *Strong Women Stay Slim* by Miriam E. Nelson, PhD. This is a wonderful all around guide to get you started. Despite the title, it's a good book for men too.

❖ *Burn the Fat Feed the Muscle* by Tom Venuto. This is more of a hard core body building book, yet is still very usable by beginners.

Strategy 39. Move to a Place Where You Will Naturally Be More Active

Move to a location where you will naturally walk more and drive less.

Imagine that you are thinking of moving and you are considering two different locations: Sit City and Active Town.

You like Sit City because you can buy a great house for a good price. But there are a few problems with Sit City. There are no sidewalks in the suburb you would be moving to, and you're concerned it would be hard to walk safely on the roads. There aren't any parks or schools close by so you couldn't walk there either. Your house is miles and miles away from a real town center and all you have close to you are strip malls. Strip malls mean most of your eating options are fast food restaurants and you'll have to drive everywhere. And strip mall living means you won't have stores close by offering quality fresh fruits and vegetables at reasonable prices.

You can see what your life will be like in Sit City. You will eat bad food, drive everywhere, and sit inside your house all the time watching TV. Year after year, you can just see the pounds being packed on.

You like really like Active Town, but it is more expensive and the house is smaller. It's one of those new communities organized like older small town centers. Near your house is a mix of parks, shops, bike paths, golf courses, offices, and stores with fresh fruits and vegetables. You can walk everywhere and you hardly need to drive at all.

You can see what your life will be like in Active Town. You won't have the giant house you always dreamed of. That hurts a little. But your life will be better in most ways that matter, kind of like how small-town living used to be. There's a main street where you can shop for fresh food and room to get outside and play. And you'll have a better chance of meeting people too.

Which place should you pick to live? In making your decision, you may want to consider the impact on your weight. You may not have thought about where you live as having a lot to do with your weight, but it does.

People who live in a community where they can walk to shop, work, eat and socialize have been found to be thinner. The reason is simple: they walk more and drive less. A University of Maryland study found people who live in the most sprawling counties are the most likely to be overweight.

The best predictor of not being obese is, amazingly, having shops and services near where you live. The environment in which you live is the driving force for how much physical activity you'll naturally get in your daily life. Your environment also has a lot to do with the quality and cost of the food available to you. In Sit City you'll naturally get far less exercise and worse food than you would in Active Town.

If you currently live in a Sit City **you may want to think about moving** to a place like Active Town. Moving may seem extreme, but it may be the easiest way for you to create a situation in which you will naturally walk more. Creating situations where you naturally walk more is the core of creating your *Exercise Safe Zone.*

Just give moving some thought. You may find this to be one of the most effective strategies you could ever implement.

▌ Active Towns are Being Built

Active Town is not a fictional place, well the name is fictional. Verrado, near Phoenix, Arizona, is one impressive example of an Active Town development. Their vision of the future is to re-create a modern version of the classic American small town instead of sprawling suburbs connected by overcrowded roads.

You'll find a small-town feel in Verrado. Many houses have front porches. There's a core downtown with a main street lined with shops, cafes, and restaurants. Open spaces are scattered throughout the development and are an easy walk from homes. Neighborhoods are walkable and schools are close and accessible.

This is the kind of place where you'll want to walk and that could make all the difference in staying on your diet. Verrado is not alone. Many communities like Verrado are now being built.

. . . .

Strategy 40. Take it Easy

You can't exercise if you get injured or sick, and you won't be able to control your weight.

A study supported by the National Heart, Lung, and Blood Institute shows that women trying to lose weight can benefit as much from moderate physical activity as from an intense workout. **It's more important for you to exercise regularly than to force hard exercise.**

For you hard chargers out there, this should be news you can use. You don't need to kill yourself, especially as you grow older.

How many times have you pushed and injured yourself? It can take months to come back from a pulled muscle. Tendonitis, a classic overuse injury, can take years to clear up. Ignoring a cold can add weeks and weeks to the time you're sick.

So use your judgment. It's much more important that you keep exercising over time than it is for you to give it all you have one week and then nurse an injury for the next few months.

This is a very hard lesson to learn for competitive people. You've spent your entire life pushing and pushing and pushing some more. And there comes a time your body starts pushing back. This time comes for everyone, even you.

If you are in doubt, wait it out. Avoid injuries. Nothing stops an exercise program faster than getting hurt. You can't exercise if you are injured, so be careful out there.

....

 ## Strategy 41. Walk the Walk—Add 2,000 Extra Steps a Day

You can find more steps to take almost anywhere, anytime. Every additional step adds up to more calories burned.

Walking is the king of all exercise because it is free, available and good for your health. Walking requires no equipment, can be done almost anywhere, lowers blood pressure, shapes and tones your body, burns calories, strengthens back muscles, reduces the risk of heart disease and diabetes, and reduces stress.

I've read that if walking were a drug it would be the most prescribed drug on earth. We humans are world class walkers. Our ancestors walked miles each day to hunt and gather food. You have this incredible innate ability to walk a lot longer and farther than you think.

America on the Move is an organization dedicated to helping you exploit your walking genius for weight loss. Their initiative is to improve health and prevent obesity with a goal for each person to move more and eat less by making 2 small daily changes.

1.   Add an extra 2,000 steps (or activity equivalent) to your day. Two thousand steps is about one mile.
2.   Choose one smart way to eat 100 fewer calories each day. One hundred calories is about one tablespoon of butter.

If you can implement both of these steps, you will prevent the current average American weight gain of 1–2 pounds a year.

The long term goal of *America on the Move* is for **everyone to take a total of 10,000 steps a day,** which is approximately 5 miles. That's about how far our hunter-gatherer ancestors walked each day. Even an inactive person takes 1,000 to 3,000 steps a day.

Every little bit helps. Start with a few extra steps and then add more as you can. We'll be covering a number of strategies on how to add more walking to your *Exercise Safe Zone*.

The America on the Move program has you use a pedometer to count the number of steps you take each day. A step counter is a simple device you attach to your waist band or belt. It counts the number of steps you take as you walk. Pedometers can be bought at any sports store.

You start by using the step counter to get an idea how many steps you take in a day on average. Then you make a goal of walking 2,000 more steps a day. If you can manage to do that you are getting more exercise and burning more calories. After you reach your 2,000 steps you can make an even higher goal.

At first I thought this program was, well, silly. The idea of counting your steps rather than going running or something more substantial didn't seem useful to me. But I've totally changed my tune.

Now I seek extra steps everywhere. Thinking about adding a few extra steps wherever you can is a very powerful idea. And the extra steps really add up. How much do all the extra steps add up to? That's why the step counter is useful. It's excellent feedback on how you're doing and having a good source of feedback is critical for keeping any strategy on target.

▌ Measuring Activity Using Steps is Better than Using Time

Using a pedometer and having a **goal of walking a certain number of steps** a day may be more effective than setting a goal of exercising a certain amount of time. One study found the actual physical activity recorded was significantly lower for women whose goal was to exercise 30 minutes a day when compared to women who had a goal of reaching 10,000 steps a day.

The reason was that the women who had a 10,000 step a day goal **would still come close to their goal,** even if they didn't quite reach it. Women who had a goal of exercising 30 minutes may have had an all-or-nothing attitude that caused them to give up when they couldn't fit in their 30 minutes of exercise.

This study is an exciting confirmation of my own experience. When your goal is to get more steps each day, you can seize any opportunity to add more steps to your total. If your goal is to exercise 30 minutes, it's all too easy just to skip it.

For some reason, when I had a goal of adding an extra 2,000 steps a day, I started looking for all sorts of ways to add additional steps. Just having a goal makes a difference. Goals get your mind unconsciously plotting on your behalf.

Now I find more steps almost everywhere. I can take a longer path through the grocery store. I can get up from my desk at work and take a short walk. I can park farther away from entrances. I can take the stairs instead of an elevator. I can get up during TV commercials and take a little walk. Once you start looking, steps are everywhere for the taking.

▌ Get Your Home, Work, School, and Community on the Move

America on the Move has a ready-made program you can use to set up their program for yourself, for work, for school, for your community, or for any group you belong to. Their website gives a complete set of materials for starting a realistic weight loss program. It's a great way of getting people started.

To Learn More

❖   The *America on the Move* website is at *http://www.americaonthe move.org*. On this site you'll find their complete program offerings.

. . . .

 Strategy 42. Ration TV

Rationing TV time can increase your kid's physical activity by 65%.

We watch TV like we eat goodies. We get big heaping servings and eat until it's all gone. The problem is TV is on 24 hours a day. It never ends. Kids watch an average of 4 hours of TV a day and now spend more time watching TV than in school.

What can you do? One study suggests rationing your kids' TV viewing.

In the study, for every hour of physical activity the kids participated, in they got a token that would allow them to watch on hour of TV or play an hour of video games.

The results of this simple-sounding scheme were very impressive:

1.   Kids increased their physical activity by 65%.
2.   Their daily TV watching time went down dramatically, from almost three hours a night to only forty-five minutes a night.
3.   TV-related snacking went way down because they weren't watching as much TV.

This study shows a clever way of implementing the *Be Less Inactive* strategy. Remember that the idea was not to tell kids to go exercise more, but to get them to be less inactive and they would figure out how to exercise on their own. Rationing TV is a way of getting the kids to be less inactive.

One cool bit of technology this study had that you won't have is a TV operated by tokens. The tokens the kids received for exercise operated the TV, like a video game. Although you don't have a token operated TV, you can still probably figure out a way of making this strategy work for your family.

Is this strategy just for kids? I don't think so. I think you can use it for yourself too. Of course you can always cheat, but you can always cheat on anything. The process of awarding yourself tokens redeemable for TV viewing time may be **just the amount of structure** you need to help lower your TV viewing time.

▌ Or Just Yank the TV

Researchers found kids with a TV in the bedroom had a higher BMI and were significantly more likely to be overweight compared to kids without a TV in their bedroom. So consider yanking the TV out of your kid's bedroom.

Electronic gadgets of all kinds (computers, phones, TVs, etc.) are linked with children sleeping fewer hours at night than they used to. Since not getting enough sleep is strongly associated with obesity, you just might want to pitch all the **electronics out of their rooms.** The gadgets may seem harmless on the surface, but they could be a significant cause of your child's weight problems.

To Learn More

❖   TV Allowance is a device connecting your TV to the power outlet. It allows you to control the amount of time the television is allowed to be on. Their website is at *http://www.tvallowance.com.*

Strategy 43. Park Far Away from an Entrance

Don't park as close as you can to an entrance, park far away. You will naturally walk more.

Long ago I heard the suggestion to park far away from entrances and I rolled my eyes at it. How much of a difference could it really make? As I was thinking of how to create my *Exercise Safe Zone,* I decided to try parking far away from entrances. It really works! Now it's one of my favorite strategies because it's so simple, easy, effective, and there are so many opportunities to use it. Think of all the times you park your car and enter a building. That's a lot of opportunities.

Let's run some numbers on this strategy. When I park at work, for example, I park far enough away that I add a total of 400 additional steps (200 steps each way) to my daily total. Now, let's say I park at five different places during the day and each time I find 400 additional steps. Over a day that's 2,000 extra steps! That's an extra mile of walking from just this one simple strategy.

Strategy 44. Take the Stairs Instead of the Elevator

Lose over 3 pounds a year by climbing up and down 5 flights of stairs a day.

An easy way to add a few more steps to your day is to take the stairs. Over a year you can easily lose 3 pounds using this one simple strategy. You don't think it can be that much? Let's run some numbers.

You burn about 10 calories per minute going up a flight of stairs and 7 calories per minute going down. It takes about 2.5 minutes to climb 5 flights of stairs. It takes about 1 minute to descend them. When you add all that up, you burn 32 calories ascending and descending 5 flights of stairs.

If you can make this one simple change a day—ascending and descending 5 flights of stairs—you can burn off over 3 pounds a year! That's a lot of weight. It could be all you need to keep from becoming obese.

Most people don't take the stairs. Researchers found that only 6–9% of people chose to use the stairs instead of elevators or escalators. If they were aware how many calories they could burn, maybe they might change their minds.

For a while I worked on the fourth floor of an office building. I noticed that people who worked on the second floor used the stairs a lot of the time. Once you worked on the third floor or above forget it, you used the elevator.

When I first started working there, I was excited I would be able to use this strategy. I could see the calories just dropping off as I happily climbed stairs everyday. It didn't turn out exactly as I expected.

I was going up and down stairs 10 times a day! That's a lot of stairs to go up. I was getting tired and sweaty and neither is a good way to get ahead on your job. So I decided to modify my strategy.

I decided I would aim to go up the stairs once or twice a day, depending on how I felt, and I would always go down the stairs. Most days I was able to go up the stairs twice and down the stairs 10 or so times. That's still a lot of extra calories burned for one simple change.

Strategy 45. Exercise in the Morning

Ninety percent of people who exercise consistently exercise in the morning.

The longer you put off exercise the less chance that you'll do it. You'll be tired, or something will come up.

Morning exercise has other benefits too. When you exercise in the morning, you'll feel energized for the day. Many people find they are less hungry after morning exercise. And many people think morning exercise puts them in a healthier mindset and that helps them make better food choices throughout the day.

Strategy 46. Work with a Personal Trainer

A personal trainer can help keep you on a schedule and force you to exercise, even when you don't want to.

Many people work better when they are working with other people in accomplishing a goal. Going it alone can be hard. That's where working with a good personal trainer comes in.

Working with a personal trainer sets up a system of **accountability.** It's just natural to not want to disappoint your personal trainer so you are more likely to work harder and keep with the program.

A personal trainer also serves as a **mentor.** You'll learn a lot about being healthy. You'll learn about exercise, nutrition, and what it takes to succeed.

When you are busy with life and everything is saying you don't have time to exercise, your personal trainer will be the one person **motivating** you and creating a positive environment in which you can succeed. Sometimes you just need an ally who supports your goals.

Even if you have never considered using a personal trainer, you may want to give one a chance. If you are shy or the cost of a trainer is a bit high, then maybe you and a few of your friends can share a personal trainer.

By hiring a personal trainer now, when you have the willpower, you are making it more likely you will exercise later, even when you don't feel like exercising. And that puts you in the best position to succeed.

Strategy 47. Take Streaming Video Exercise Classes on Your Computer

Exercise classes over your home computer may be a good option for you.

Let's say you don't like the gym, or perhaps the inconvenience of commuting to the gym is keeping you away, or maybe you are just bored by your exercise videos at home. You can now find services that will stream exercise classes over the Internet for you to follow on your home computer. You can find all sorts of classes including weight lifting, aerobics and yoga.

The advantage of this setup is that you can work out where and when you want, even if you are traveling. And you may already have a nice, but underutilized workout room in your house just waiting to be used. Another advantage is you may find it less embarrassing to try something new like yoga or Tai Chi.

To Learn More

❖   We keep a list of web-based classes at *http://YourDesignerDiet.com.*

Strategy 48. Increase Your NEAT

Sit rather than lie down, stand rather than sit, and walk rather than stand. Find ways to move even a little bit more during the day.

We learned in *The Power of Rest Threat* how obese people naturally sit more than lean people. Fidgeters can burn 300–800 calories a day not from exercising, but from everyday activities. Think about this: running 8 miles burns about 800 calories. By fidgeting you could burn as many calories as running 8 miles!

How fidgety you are is called your NEAT (non-exercise activity thermogenesis) quotient. Even those of us not blessed with a high NEAT can consciously learn how to change our daily activity levels.

Your goal is to figure out little ways through which you can increase your NEAT. In the past you may have felt, like I did, that those little bits of activity didn't count, but it turns out they may be what counts most of all.

The increased calorie burn from fidgeting is amazing. Fidgeters, for example, burn 40–60 more calories per hour when seated than people who sit motionless. Standing fidgeters burn 70–100 calories more per hour than people who stand still. Those are big differences.

Here are some suggestions on how to become NEATer:

❖ Get up and out of your seat. Stand up instead of sitting down.

❖ You could lose one pound a year simply by sending one less email each hour. Instead, walk down the hall to talk to the person you would have sent the email to. That short walk burns off one pound a year.

❖ Laughing for 10 or 15 minutes burns about 50 calories. Laugh that much every day and you've lost 5 pounds in a year.

❖ Walking around instead of sitting while on the cell phone burns up to 50 calories in 10 minutes.

❖ Put a portable pedal exerciser in front of your TV and pedal slowly while you watch. You can do the same while reading.

❖ Put a treadmill in front of your computer at work. Every hour on the treadmill at 1 mph is about 100 calories.

❖ Pick a time each hour when you get up and take a little walk. Maybe go look out a window. Take a turn around your building. Go to the bathroom.

❖ Tap your feet. Wiggle your fingers.

❖ Performing sit ups during commercials while watching TV burns up to 65 calories an hour.

❖ Dance while you cook.

❖ Watching TV while sitting down burns about 72 calories an hour. Do light housework while watching TV and you bump the calorie burn up to 216 calories per hour.

❖ Take walking meetings.

❖ Hold meetings while standing.

❖ Don't use your remote control.

❖ Walk to the mail box instead of driving.

These are just a few ideas. Take a look and see where you can add even a little more activity. The general rule, even if you aren't a natural fidgeter, is: sit rather than lie down, stand rather than sit, and walk rather than stand.

 Strategy 49. The Integrative Workout

You can easily burn 500 calories a day through normal everyday activities.

Lee Labrada, a former Mr. Universe, has written a book titled *The Lean Body Promise,* in which he advocates burning more calories through the activities you already do each day. To make this work, you need to get a feel for how many calories you burn in your daily activities:

❖ **Activities That Burn About 4 Calories per Minute:** calisthenics, slow cycling, light gardening, social golf, general housework, line dancing, table-tennis, doubles tennis and slow walking.

❖ **Activities That Burn About 7 Calories per Minute:** aerobics, basketball, baseball, moderate cycling, active dancing, football, racquetball, skiing, swimming, singles tennis, and brisk walking.

❖ **Activities That Burn About 10 Calories per Minute:** competitive basketball, fast cycling, strenuous dancing, competitive football, jogging, kick-boxing, running, cross country skiing, jumping rope, vigorous swimming, vigorous walking, heavy weight training.

These calorie burn numbers are just estimates. Your mileage may vary depending on how much you weigh, your metabolism, and how intensely you perform an activity. A good general rule is to figure your **normal everyday activities to burn about 7 calories a minute.** If you aren't sure if the physical activity you are performing is 4, 7, or 10 calories a minute, then run your calorie burn calculations using 7 calories per minute.

You can use this information to create your own integrative workout. **Your goal is to find between 1 to 1.5 hours of physical activity and integrate it into your daily routine.** Here's an example of an integrative workout routine from Mr. Labrada:

❖ **Monday:** to burn 500 calories: carry your child, vacuum, do other housecleaning chores, carry and put the groceries away, run up and down stairs, squat and lunge.

❖ **Tuesday:** to burn 600 calories: run up and down stairs, walk to the store, clean windows, play with the kids.

❖ **Wednesday:** to burn 750 calories: walk the dog, play with kids, sweep the driveway, carry baby, run up and down stairs, squat and lunge.

❖ **Thursday:** to burn 700 calories: push stroller through the park, play with kids, vacuum, mop floors, carry laundry up and down the stairs, run to the mailbox and back.

❖ **Friday:** to burn 800 calories: run errands on foot, walk your dog, carry baby, do lunges and squats, carry and unpack purchases, play with kids.

❖ **Saturday:** to burn 500 calories: wash car, walk to the store and buy the paper, play with kids on the playground, work in garden.

❖ **Sunday:** to burn 675 calories total: walk through park, swim and play with the kids.

What are the results? Let's add up the calories. It looks like you'll burn 4,525 calories a week on this plan, which is a weight loss of over one pound a week. That's a remarkable result from everyday activities you may not have thought about as burning a lot of calories.

Of course, you may not have a child to carry, but the general idea is sound. You just need to figure out replacement activities that fit your life. For example, if you spend two hours in the mall searching for that perfect shirt, you'll have burned about 500 calories. A half hour of shoveling snow off your sidewalk burns about 350 calories. An hour of raking leaves burns about 200 calories. Walking around your neighborhood looking at Christmas lights burns off a lot of calories too. When you are on the phone, walk around instead of sitting. Carry in groceries one bag at a time.

With a little creativity, you can find more exercise almost everywhere. And as we have seen, the calorie burn numbers are not trivial at all. Searching out and finding more physical activity in your daily life is a very rewarding weight loss move.

To Learn More

❖ Lee Labrada's website is *http://www.labrada.com.*

· ·

Strategy 50. The Playground Workout

You can get a good workout from playing with your kids in the park.

Getting a workout, while playing with your kids, is fun and effective. This integrative workout idea is from Lee Labrada's book *The Lean Body Promise.* You burn calories, work your muscles, and have a good time. Doesn't that sound better than exercising? Plus, you are spending quality time with your kids.

Here are some of the possible playground exercises:

❖ **Swings.** Pushing someone on a swing is like a mini chest press. It works your triceps, chest, and upper back. You burn about 50 calories in 10 minutes.

❖ **Slide.** Helping your child on the slide works your calves and back. You burn about 50 calories in 10 minutes. Don't be shy, go down the slide yourself too!

- ❖ **Merry-go-round.** This dizzying delight works your legs, butt and back as you push your kids around in circles. You burn about 75 calories in 10 minutes.
- ❖ **Monkey-bars.** Hanging and climbing on the monkey bars works your abdominals, biceps, and upper back. You burn about 75 calories in 12 minutes.
- ❖ **Throw and catch.** Playing catch works your arms, shoulder, and lower back. You burn about 50 calories in 5 minutes.

The important idea here is that you can integrate exercise into your daily life if you look for opportunities. Before researching the Playground Workout, I wouldn't have thought about this venue for increasing fitness.

Thinking about play as exercise can sometimes give you that extra push you need to go out and have fun. We get so wrapped in life that taking time out for play, even with our children, may seem a frivolous waste of time. Now, in the back of your mind, you can think that you aren't just having fun, but you are burning calories and building muscles at the same time. Maybe just that little bit of motivation is all you need to get moving.

Strategy 51. Just Don't Sit, Sit Actively

You can burn up to 350 calories a day by changing how you sit.

Office workers face a real problem getting more physical activity into their daily lives. They spend hour after hour sitting at a desk. What if you could turn sitting into exercise that could burn up to 350 calories a day?

Sounds good, doesn't it? Sitting can be made to burn calories by using an **exercise ball** as your desk chair instead of a more traditional chair. In fact, as I am writing this sentence, I am sitting on an exercise ball instead of a regular chair.

The reason why using an exercise ball burns calories gets back to *The NEAT Threat,* which showed us how the little bits of unconscious fidgeting we do all day adds up to big calorie burns.

Sitting on an exercise ball burns calories because it is an **unstable surface.** The ball is round and mushy so you sink into it a little. You can't stay in one place without constantly using your muscles to keep balanced on top of the ball. That's why sitting on an exercise ball is called **active sitting.** You are actively engaging your abdominal and back muscles to keep balanced.

Contrast active sitting to a traditional chair where you sit passively. The chair completely supports you and you need very little effort to sit. With active sitting you aren't even aware you are burning calories, it's just a side effect of trying to stay balanced on the ball.

Exercise balls aren't for everyone. They take a bit of getting used to at first. They can also be tiring because you use a lot of muscle power to stabilize the ball. Start using your exercise ball as a chair in short chunks of time, slowly building up to using it all day.

Don't think exercise balls are just for work. You can use them everywhere. We have used exercise balls as chairs on our deck and for chairs at our dinner table. You could even have a house rule saying you can only watch TV while sitting on an exercise ball. Such a policy transforms passive TV viewing into a calorie burning exercise!

To Learn More

❖ *FitterFirst* at *http://www.fitter1.com* is a quality supplier of exercise balls and other balance equipment.

Strategy 52. Go On the Dog Diet

Your dog needs walking and so do you. A perfect match.

Every morning our two dogs, Annie and Stout, get restless. They want to go for their walk. Every time I go in the direction of the front door, Annie races ahead of me thinking it's walk time. And when I don't open the door, I can see the excitement whoosh right out of her.

Later in the day, Annie will get more and more direct. She'll just come up in front of me, sit down, and stare. I know what she wants. She knows I know what she wants. The question is: will I go for a walk?

Even if I wasn't planning on it, the dogs can encourage and cajole me into going because they are just so darn cute and excited. Their energy is contagious and it makes me want to go even when I feel a little down. No, that's not quite it. The dogs help me walk especially when I am in one of those "I don't want to do anything" moods. It takes a hard person to ignore their "go on a walk dance" day after day.

So, you may want to consider getting a dog. Of course, you should only do so if you can commit to taking care of a dog, but if you can, a dog will help keep you active.

This strategy isn't all just fanciful tales of puppy dog tails. There's real science behind it too. A University of Missouri-Columbia study found **walking a dog can help you lose more weight in a year than most diet plans.** Dog walkers in the study averaged a weight loss of 14 pounds a year. If you can't see yourself getting a dog, maybe you can become a dog walker or volunteer at a dog shelter.

And dogs don't just help you get more exercise. They will be more than happy to help control your portion sizes by eating your leftovers!

Chapter 19

Weight-Proof Your Portion Control Safe Zone
Strategies 53–66

Maybe you've had a morning that runs something like this: You overslept, you are in a hurry, and you are hungry. You pop two pieces of bread in the toaster and you think cereal. Cereal is fast and yummy and almost healthy too. You grab a box of cereal from your many options. It's one of the sweeter choices, but it tastes awesome and you deserve it on such a horrible morning. Next, you pull down any old bowl off your shelf and completely fill the bowl with cereal. Then you take milk from the fridge and pour it to the brim. Ah, the toast is done. You slather on some butter. To make breakfast complete and healthy, you top it off with fruit.

This scene is replayed every morning across America. The details may change a bit, but the end is the same: overeating. What's wrong with this breakfast, you may ask. It's just cereal, toast, and fruit. That's good, isn't it?

Let's run the numbers. How many calories do you think are in our example breakfast? A few hundred? What if I said it's closer to 1,000 calories? Would you be shocked? How can it be so many calories? Because your portions are much bigger than you think. Let's see why.

The bowl you are using is probably a big salad bowl which, surprisingly, is for salad, not cereal. You want to eat a lot of salad so it's a fine bowl for salad, but not for cereal or ice cream or spaghetti or most anything else you eat from a bowl.

You will almost always fill the bowl to the top and eat the whole bowl, which is probably 2 cups of cereal. The box says one serving only has a pleasant sounding 120 calories, but a serving is only ¾ of a cup. You are eating a lot more than one serving. For two cups of cereal you are eating 300 calories!

Next the milk. Covering the cereal probably takes one cup of milk. A cup of 2% milk is 122 calories. A cup of whole milk has 146 calories but let's say you are using 2% milk. So now your breakfast total is 422 calories.

Two pieces of toast has about 200 calories. Your breakfast now comes in at a total of 622 calories.

A tablespoon sized pat of butter has about 100 calories. So that's 200 calories worth of butter for two pieces of toast. Breakfast now weighs in at a hefty 822 calories. But wait, there's more.

Let's say you have about 1½ cups of fruit. That's 150 calories.

Your grand total for this very common and normal sounding breakfast is 972 calories!

For a woman that means you've unwittingly consumed nearly half your calories for the entire day at breakfast! Let's assume snacks, lunch, and dinner follow a similar pattern and you eat more than you expect at those meals too. What's the result? Overeating and weight gain.

What can you do? **Practice perfect portions:** stay within your calorie budget by eating the right amount of food at every meal.

Let's look at breakfast again using more perfect portion sizes. Let's switch to a lower calorie cereal choice that has 120 calories per one cup serving. It's still tasty, but it's a bit healthier than the other cereal. Two cups is a lot of cereal; eating one cup of cereal is a more appropriate serving size. That means you are only spending 120 calorie on cereal.

Less cereal means less milk, about ½ cup of 2% milk is 61 calories. A lower calorie move would be to use non-fat milk for only 42 calories.

Two pieces of toast with butter is a lot. Instead, try eating ½ an English muffin at 63 calories topped with sugar free jam at 10 calories.

Half the fruit is still a nice portion. That's ¾ cup of fruit at 75 calories.

Your breakfast now totals a more reasonable 328 calories. Remember, the first breakfast came in at 972.

If your daily calorie budget is 2,000, you still have nearly 1,700 calories to eat for the rest of the day, which is more than enough for satisfying meals and snacks.

Let's take a look at how much weight you'll gain by eating bad breakfast number one. The difference between the two breakfasts is 644 calories. You'll gain over an extra pound a week just by eating the more caloric breakfast!

What's going on? **You probably have almost no idea how many calories you are eating each day.** The reasons are simple, as we read in the threats. People are horrible at estimating how many calories are in a meal, even experts are horrible at it. And our plates and bowls make it all too easy to eat too much food. You will naturally fill a bowl to the top with cereal and you will just as naturally eat the whole bowl. The sizes involved almost don't matter. And because you've probably come to think of larger portion sizes as natural, you may not think twice about eating larger portions.

What's really interesting, as we learned in the threats, you won't feel any fuller from eating the larger, more caloric breakfast. **You would feel just as satisfied eating the smaller, less caloric breakfast.** Does practicing perfect portions seem like a useful skill to learn now?

▌ Can't you always just eat more food?

Perhaps you've been convinced that all that stands between you and diet heaven is portion control. And that's partly right. Portion control battles with exercise for the top title of the best way to successfully lose weight and maintain weight loss. Some studies show portion control as the most important factor, others show exercise as the most important. Let's just say both are important.

Portion control is probably the most difficult strategy to learn, because your body doesn't want to control your portions. It wants you to eat as much good tasting food as you can. Overcoming that diet-busting instinct takes some work.

Some people question the effort at portion control altogether. The common response to portion control is: can't I always just eat more food? I don't have to stop at a given portion size.

Yes, you can always eat more. Nothing ever stops you from eating more. Nothing. If you want to hijack a candy truck and eat 10,000 candy bars a day for a week—you can.

But that's not how you create your perfect diet. Your perfect diet can't assume that strategies always work because nothing always works. Instead, we are trying to get the probabilities to line up in your favor. We anticipate what will most likely happen and how we can get what is most likely to happen to **go our way** instead of against us. Right now portions go against you.

That can change. Portions can work for you and become one of your most powerful Safe Zones.

With portion control, this means ensuring that most of the time you eat an amount of food close to what you need. And if you should eat more, hopefully your exercise strategies will be enough to overcome the difference.

Over a lifetime, if you can shift the balance so your portions are in line with your calorie budget, you'll be able to lose weight. I think you can do that much, if not more, with the portion control strategies presented in this chapter.

▌ How do you learn to practice perfect portions?

The goal is to always serve yourself the right amount of food. How do you know how much that is?

1. **Figure out how many calories you need each day.** You've already done this in the *How Many Calories Can You Eat Each Day?* strategy. As you eat, keep a **mental ticker** in the back of your mind about how many calories you have eaten. Your mental ticker tells you when you are crossing over into weight gain territory and then you can do something about it. If keeping a mental ticker doesn't work for you, then keep a food diary of what you eat. This will allow you to calculate how many calories you've eaten. And if keeping a food log is more than you want to do, then keep a general feeling for if you are eating too much, just enough, or not enough. This feeling, though not perfectly accurate, may be enough to create a bright red stop light in your mind, telling you if you should eat or not.

2. **Learn to figure out about how many calories you are eating.** The goal of this step is not to turn you into a calorie counting maniac. Few people can count calories every day over the long run. You just need to develop a good feeling for approximately how many calories are in the foods you are eating. *The Honest Calorie Estimation Method* strategy will show you how to estimate portion sizes and calorie counts.

3. **Decide on your perfect portion size.** A perfect portion has as many calories as you are willing to spend on whatever you are eating. Typically, the ideal portion is considered to be 3 ounces of meat. In contrast, I suggest that you have as much meat as you want as long is matches your calorie and nutritional goals. How

do you know how many calories you have to spend on a portion of food? From steps 1 and 2. In step 1, you track how many calories you have eaten so you know how many calories you have left to spend. And in step 2, you learn how to judge the calorie content of a meal, so you can decide how much to eat based on the number of calories you have available and the number of meals you have left to eat. If you want to eat 6 ounces of meat and it fits within your goals, then that is a perfect portion.

4. **Learn different strategies for creating your *Portion Control Safe Zone.*** Once you know how much food you can eat, you'll need to learn the strategies to help you not slip-up and eat more than you think you should. You'll find many strategies for creating perfect portions in this chapter.

After practicing perfect portions for a while, you shouldn't have to count calories at all. Your portions will be close to the appropriate size, and you'll be able to control your weight without too much effort.

You don't have to be exact in all your portions. Small weight changes become obvious with the daily and weekly feedback mechanism you created in the Designer Way. When you start to gain weight, be more careful about your portion sizes, look for new portion control strategies, and get better at the strategies you are practicing. With this approach, you put yourself back in control of your weight.

▌ Example: Using the Portion Control Strategies

Let's run through an example of how you might apply the portion control strategies in your daily life. This example will be in the form of a conversation between Coach, our portion control expert, and Annie, someone worried about controlling her eating during a long road trip.

Annie: I don't know if I want to go on this trip.
Coach: What's wrong?
Annie: I gained so much weight while my family was over. It's amazing how fast it came back on.
Coach: You don't have to be afraid. Let's see how we can use a few strategies to help you control your weight.
Annie: I know, but I've failed so many times in the past. I don't think it will work.

Coach: That was before you knew **how** to control your weight. All you had before were a bunch of marketing slogans. People telling you to "eat less and exercise more" and "stop eating when you are full" isn't very helpful. With the strategies you can help make sure you won't overeat.

Annie: OK, let's give it a try. I think I'll have to run the spin more often while on the road so my weight doesn't get out of hand.

Coach: You have your daily weight feedback techniques like how your clothes fit, trying on a belt, how you look in the mirror. You don't necessarily need to run a spin more often. When any of these tell you that you're gaining weight, you can make some moves to tighten things up a bit.

Annie: OK, that makes sense.

Coach: Have you calculated your calorie budget?

Annie: Yes, it's 1,600 calories.

Coach: Did you decide how you were going to spend your calorie budget on meals? Are you going to eat many small meals during the day or eat three meals a day with snacks?

Annie: I'll like three meals a day with snacks.

Coach: How do you want to spend those calories on breakfast, lunch, dinner, and snacks?

Annie: I need about 800 calories for a good dinner. So that leaves about 300 for breakfast, 300 for lunch, and 200 for snacks during the day.

Coach: Sounds good. If that doesn't work out, you can always make adjustments later. How about we use breakfast as an example of applying the portion control strategies? Let's start with an important first question. Are you someone who does better eating breakfast or not?

Annie: I don't usually eat a big breakfast, but we'll be on the road and my husband likes a good one, so I'll probably eat with him.

Coach: What do you to have?

Annie: I usually have two eggs, toast, and hash browns.

Coach: How many calories is that?

Annie: I don't really know.

Coach: But if you eat a breakfast without knowing how many calories you are eating, how do you stick to your calorie budget? Why don't you try the using *The Honest Calorie Estimation Method* strategy to figure out how many calories you'll be eating?

Annie: Two eggs have about 160 calories plus the calories in the fat used to cook them. Two pieces of toast with butter has about 300 calories. The hash browns are harder to estimate. I'll guess about 200 calories plus calories for the fat used to cook the hash browns. Plus, I'll usually get an orange juice and that's about 100 calories for an 8 ounce glass. So my usual breakfast probably has more than 700 calories! Holy cow! That's almost half my calorie budget just for breakfast.

Coach: That's the power of estimating calories. You know when you are getting in trouble and you can do something about it before real damage is done. So, what do you think you can do to meet your calorie budget?

Annie: What are my options?

Coach: All the strategies in this book! But your basic options are: **select it, raise it, skip it, change it, doggy bag it,** or **share it.** "Select it" means select a correctly portioned meal from the start. "Raise it" means increase your calorie budget so you can afford a larger breakfast. "Change it" means change what you are planning to eat so it has fewer calories. "Skip it" means don't eat breakfast. "Doggy bag it" means you put the food you don't want to eat in a doggy bag. "Share it" means share a meal with a friend.

Annie: On the road, there's no way to know how much food I'll be served so selecting the right portions from the start won't work. And I don't want to increase my calorie budget for breakfast. And I don't want to skip breakfast. I'll have to figure out something else to do.

Coach: That's good. You are considering your options. With a little thought, you can still enjoy a fun, tasty breakfast without going off your diet. You don't have to give in and eat everything or nothing.

Annie: But if I've paid for the food I should eat all of it!

Coach: So, no matter how much food they serve you, you'll eat it all?

Annie: Well, I guess not. That could be a lot of calories.

Coach: Exactly. You can't ever control how much food you're served, but you can control how much you eat. What are some of your other options?

Annie: I could change my breakfast. I could eat poached eggs on toast. I like that and it'd get rid of the butter. Or maybe I could eat just one piece of toast and use sugar free jelly instead of butter. I could have fruit instead of hash browns. Or maybe I could have a few hash browns. I don't like any of these options. I'm paying good money for a breakfast I am not eating and that I don't want to save for later. And most of the changes I make don't bring down the calorie total by much. Yet I want to eat breakfast with my husband. Argh!

Coach: It's tough to have a satisfying breakfast for only 300 calories.

Annie: My husband and I could share breakfast. He doesn't need a full breakfast either because it has so many calories. Maybe I can just have some of his breakfast? We'll split the toast and hash browns, I can have some of his eggs, and I'll drink tea instead of orange juice. It might work.

Coach: Well done. You've managed to stay on your diet and meet all your goals.

Annie: But I am afraid it won't work. My husband may not get enough food, I may not get enough, and we'll have to agree on what to order.

Coach: That's true. It may not work. But at least try. If it doesn't work you can always try something else. Maybe you can share part of a breakfast and order a side of eggs?

Annie: That might work. We'll give it a shot. We'll find something that works. Thanks, Coach.

This scenario shows the give and take involved in creating a weight control
solution that balances all your goals and concerns. For the rest of this chapter,
I will talk about a variety of useful portion control strategies.

. . . .

Strategy 53. Servings vs. Portions

**You are probably eating many more calories than you think because
you aren't looking at serving sizes.**

In the chapter introduction, we discussed an example of how easy it was
to overeat by pouring too much cereal into a big bowl. When we calculated
how many calories are in the cereal you may have been surprised because the
label on the cereal box said 120 calories. But that 120 calories is **per serving.**
How much cereal you actually ate is called your **portion.**

A key to practicing perfect portions is to be aware of the difference
between serving sizes and portion sizes. The *serving* size is a standard measure selected by manufacturers for figuring out how many calories and other
nutrients you are eating. Your *portion* size is how much food you actually put
on your plate.

In the cereal example the serving size is ¾ cup, which has 120 calories.
In reality you ate 2 cups of cereal for 300 calories. I don't know if anyone has
ever served themselves ¾ cup of cereal without really trying to because ¾ cup
of cereal looks really small in a big bowl.

When you eat something out of a package, look at the serving size and
figure out how many calories you'll really be eating. If it turns out you'll be
eating too many calories for your calorie budget, then move to another food.
Or you need to accept the smaller portion sizes.

A trick manufacturers often play is to make serving sizes smaller than
you typically eat. You look at the nutrition label and see a calorie per serving
number that looks reasonable and then what do you do? You eat the whole
package of course! Remember the idea of unit bias; that we tend to see the
whole package as what we should eat. The end result is you eat a lot more
calories than you think. Don't fall for this trick.

We have become very used to large portion sizes in American culture.
The ¾ cup serving size for cereal is really the right amount. It's the larger

amount of cereal you normally eat that isn't right. And remember from the threats we learned that you don't need to eat larger portions, you'll still feel satisfied from the smaller portion sizes. You just need to make sure you use the right portion sizes to begin with.

How do you practice perfect portions when eating from packages? Here are a few steps to consider:

1. **Decide how many calories you have in your calorie budget to spend on eating this food.** You can decide not to stick to your budget, but you should at least make a conscious decision when you ignore it. Keep a background ticker going in your brain for estimating how many calories you are eating. You can use one of the web calorie counting services to help you get a more accurate calorie count.

2. **Look at the number of servings on the label.** Look at the size of the package compared to the number of servings. Packages often advertise themselves as single serving sizes, but really have several servings per package. You can easily make the mistake of eating a package of food and hugely underestimate the amount of calories you are eating.

3. **Multiply or divide according to how much you plan to eat.** If you plan on eating the entire package, then multiply the number of calories per serving by the number of servings per package to get your calorie total. Something to keep in the back of your mind is that not all labels are accurate. Even though you are doing everything right, you may still gain weight because the labels can be wrong.

I love using spaghetti as an example because it's stunning how many calories you eat when you eat as much spaghetti as you really want.

My box of spaghetti says there are 8 servings in the box. Each serving is 2 ounces and has 190 calories.

Let's say I've already eaten about 500 calories for breakfast, 900 calories for lunch, and 300 calories in snacks, which leaves me about 1,000 calories for dinner. I plan to spend about 500 calories on spaghetti. My remaining calories will be spent on chocolate, vegetables, cheese and some other dishes.

I don't know my calorie counts exactly. I just keep a mental ticker in the back of my mind that tracks about how many calories I am eating. If I start gaining weight within a spin of the Designer Way, I'll suspect I am not counting very well and I'll try harder to be more accurate in my future estimates and portion sizes.

For the purposes of this example, I first take as much spaghetti as I would normally serve myself without considering the serving size. It turns out that this amounts to about 5 servings of spaghetti for a total of about 1,000 calories. That's 500 calories above my target!

Now I want to figure out how much spaghetti I should eat. First I need to know how much is 2 ounces of spaghetti. I have no idea, so I weigh it out on a scale. Two ounces of spaghetti is about a ½ inch circle. That's not much. I only need about 2½ servings, not the 5 servings I would have dished out for myself. So considering serving sizes when eating really works. I prevented myself from eating 500 extra calories in just this one meal.

Imagine how many calories you'll save yourself from over a whole lifetime.

▌ Using Servings of Food Groups Instead of Calories

The Portion Teller, by Lisa Young, PhD, RD, recommends against using calories to keep track of how much you can eat. Instead, she recommends eating a certain number of servings of vegetables; fruits; grains, and starchy vegetables; dairy; fats; fish, poultry, meat, and meat alternatives; treats and sweets.

So instead of a calorie budget you would have a serving budget for each food group. Let's say your budget is 3 servings of vegetables where each serving is ½ cup. Instead of a calorie ticker counting in the back of your mind you keep a servings ticker for each food group.

The reason for this approach is a good one: it helps you select a good mix of food groups in your diet and you never have to worry about calorie counting.

Personally, I eat a variety of foods so I am never worried about getting a wide enough mix of foods in my diet. And I don't recommend what you should eat, so I couldn't possibly recommend how many servings of each food group you should have.

Yet the servings approach is very sensible. I thought you should know about it, so you can decide if it would work better for you than the calorie approach.

Strategy 54. The Honest Calorie Estimation Method

Figure out how many calories you are eating by comparing portions to parts of your hand and by estimating each item on a plate separately.

How many times do you look at what you are eating and think: how many calories is this? Or maybe you think about it, but you have no idea how to calculate the calorie content of a meal. And why should you know how? Calorie estimation is not a skill you learn in school or summer camp. But the good news is you can learn to estimate how many calories you are eating and once you do, you'll never look at a plate of food in the same way again.

You've learned one calorie estimation method already in the *Servings vs. Portions* strategy. When eating food from a package, it's relatively simple to figure out how many calories you are eating.

But what if you are at a restaurant that doesn't tell you how many calories are in its meals? What if you are at a buffet? What if you are at home serving food from huge casserole dishes? How can you tell how many calories you are eating then?

It's hard to estimate, because you don't know how much food is being served, nor do you know how it was prepared. But we aren't trying to get a perfect calorie count. We merely need a good enough guess that you'll be able to stay within your calorie budget. Just one restaurant meal can throw off your whole calorie budget for that day and cause you to gain weight.

Two skills will help you master calorie estimation:

1. **Handy estimation.** If you can visualize how many servings you are eating in every meal, you will always be able to make a good guestimate of how many calories you are eating. One fun and practical method for visually sizing-up how many calories are in the foods you're eating is called the Handy method: you compare food portions to parts of your hand. For example, your index finger equals about 1 ounce of cheese which equals about 100 calories.

2. **Piecemeal estimation.** Using the Handy method alone isn't good enough because the larger a meal is the more likely you are to underestimate the calories. To get around this problem, don't worry about the meal as a whole, but **use the Handy method to estimate the number of calories of each individual food item in the meal.** Estimating each item individually can make your estimates up to 30% more accurate.

▌ Handy Estimation

The Handy method of calorie estimation uses your hand as a reference for figuring out the approximate calories in various foods. Perhaps you've heard some people say one serving of chicken is about the size of the palm of your hand or a deck of cards. Both your palm and the card deck are ways of visualizing food serving sizes. The advantage of using your hand instead of other items like card decks is that your hand is always with you. Handy, isn't it?

Some people may object to the hand method because everyone's hand is different. That's true, but larger people tend to have larger hands and also need more calories, so it all works out in the end.

The calorie counts in the table are useful only for creating a very approximate estimate of whatever you're eating. For really accurate counts you'll need to use a calorie counting computer program. But when you don't have a label telling you how many calories are in what you are eating, these are good numbers to use as a start.

To use the table on the following pages to estimate calories:

1. Look at the food on your plate and match it to the most similar food item under the food column in the table.
2. Visualize how many of the hand portions of food you are eating.
3. Multiply the number of calories for the hand portion size from step 1 times the number of hand portions you estimated in step 2. This gives you the total number of calories

The visualization step may be difficult because few of us are skilled at guessing how many of one thing fits inside another. It's hard, but don't worry about it. You are just aiming for a good enough approximation so you can decide how much to eat. The main step is just to think about how much you are eating. The rest is low fat gravy.

▌ Piecemeal Estimation

People prone to being overweight tend to eat larger meals. Because of the difficulty of estimating the number of calories in larger meals, overweight people **underestimate** how many calories they are eating. That's why it's perfectly reasonable for an overweight person to think they are eating fewer calories than they are. Now, if you could better estimate the calories, don't you think you could make better eating decisions? I think so and that's the point behind this strategy.

Unfortunately, people think they are pretty good calorie estimators, but they aren't. People are way off. You were not born with a calorie estimator in your brain. Your average person estimating the number of calories in a large plate of food will underestimate them by over 30%. Even dietitians underestimate large plates of food by nearly 9%. **The larger the meal, the less accurate your estimations.**

Why would you have an instinct to estimate calories? When food is scarce the rule is to eat whenever possible. Maybe someday they'll develop magic glasses that automatically see everything you eat and track calories. Until then, calorie counting is a skill you'll need to develop.

The smaller a meal, the more accurate your calorie estimates. And that's the main idea behind Piecemeal estimation: **mentally break up your meal into small parts** and estimate how many calories are in each part using either the Handy method of estimation or package-supplied serving information. Researchers have shown that your calorie estimates can be much more accurate using the Piecemeal approach.

▌ Fajitas Calorie Estimation Using Handy and Piecemeal Skills

Let's run through an example of how to use the Handy and Piecemeal calorie estimation techniques to estimate one of my favorite meals, sizzling steak fajitas from Chevy's. If you've never seen one, it's a giant plate of tortillas, beans, steak, sour cream, guacamole, tamalito, onions, and peppers. All the parts of the meal are probably familiar except for perhaps the tamalito, which is a delicious concoction made from sweet corn.

The first time I ordered this meal, I had to estimate its calorie content, so I could determine how much of it I should eat. At the time, my calorie budget for the meal was 700. Just from looking at the giant, gorgeous, multilevel fajitas plate I was pretty sure it had more than that. I would have to either not eat some of the meal or put some of it in a doggy bag. The question was, how much? How do we figure out how much to eat? By using the Handy and Piecemeal calorie estimation techniques together.

With so many small portions of different foods, this meal is a nightmare for the calorie estimator. What makes the job easier is that all the food items are separate. Each item being separate makes them easier to visualize with the Handy method. Calorie estimation becomes really difficult when food has a sauce or is all mixed together in a casserole.

Let's give it a try. Just so you know my first estimate for the meal was 1,375 calories. It turned out the meal was really 1,513 calories. I was off by about 140 calories, which isn't too bad. It's close enough to make realistic food choices.

Handy Estimation Table

	Fist = 1 Cup	Leafy Veggies	20 calories
		Carrots	50 calories
		Popcorn (movie)	85 calories
		Potato	115 calories
		Beans	225 calories
		Soups	
		Broth Based	160 calories
		Cream Based	230 calories
		Soft Drink	100 calories
		Whole Milk	150 calories
	Cupped Hand = ½ Cup	Grains	
		Cooked Rice	100 calories
		Cooked Pasta	180 calories
		Spanish Rice	180 calories
		Fruit	
		Bananas	70 calories
		Strawberries	35 calories
		Sweets	250 calories
	Flattened Hand = 1 Slice	Bread	
		Thin Slice	70 calories
		Thick Slice	120 calories
	Palm = 3 Ounces	Meat	150 calories
		Nuts	200 calories
	Finger = 1 Ounce	Cheese	100 calories
	Finger Tip = ½ Teaspoon	Butter	35 calories
		Olive Oil	20 calories

I am basing the real calorie counts of the meal on a nutritional information sheet from Chevy's website. Some of the calorie counts aren't directly available from their site, so my estimations could be a bit off.

The meal comes with a pack of 3 tortillas. Using the food table, a slice of bread has about 70 calories and the tortillas were about the same size so I guessed about 70 calories for each tortilla. Looking up the calories on the web I found their tortillas are 80 calories each, so not a bad guess. My estimate was 30 calories too low.

I thought there was one handful of cooked onions and peppers, which is about 10 calories. I don't know the actual calorie count because they include these ingredients with the steak calorie count.

A palm sized piece of steak has about 150 calories and I estimated, by visualizing all the steak pieces against my palm, that I had three palms worth of steak for 450 calories. The actual calorie count was 546 calories, which includes the cooked peppers and onions.

The Spanish rice looked to be about one handful for about 180 calories. The actual calorie count is 176.

The black beans looked to be a little more than ½ a fist for about 125 calories. The actual count is 175 calories. I am guessing that the difference may be additional fats included in the dish.

There's no sour cream entry in the estimator table, I'll use cheese as a close approximation. I know sour cream has fewer calories than cheese so I'll use half the calorie value for cheese as a better guess. There looks to be about 3 fingers worth of sour cream for 150 calories. The actual calorie count is 121 calories.

There's no guacamole entry in the table either. And like for the sour cream, I'll use half the calories of cheese as an approximation. There looks to be about 2 fingers worth of guacamole for 100 calories. The actual calorie count is 79 calories.

I have no idea how many calories are in tamalito. Since it's like a dessert, I am going to use the sweets entry in the table as a close approximation. There's about ½ a handful of tamalito for a guess of 125 calories. The actual calorie count is 144 calories.

There's salsa, which I didn't estimate at all because it has so few calories. The actual count is 4 calories.

There's a little bit of cheese. I thought there was about a ¼ finger of cheese for 25 calories. The actual calorie count is 28.

Using the Handy method combined with the Piecemeal approach is pretty accurate. My total calorie estimate for the meal is 1,375 calories. The actual calorie count is 1,513. So I am off by about 140. Some of my estimates were a little high, some were a little low, but they balanced out. If I were to just look at the entire plate of food and make a guess I wouldn't be even close. I would have underestimated the number of calories in the meal by a lot.

If you ate all the tortillas in this meal, you would be at almost your daily calorie total without even realizing it. This is one important way you gain weight: **unknowingly eating large portions.** Is this Chevy's fault? Not at all. They are serving you a great meal. It's up to you what you do with it.

We just went through a calorie counting exercise that gave you enough information to make good eating decisions. If you hadn't estimated the calorie count, you probably would have eaten the whole meal. But since you did an estimate, you can ensure you won't overeat by taking action. What can you do?

One option is to immediately divide the meal in half, ask for a doggy bag, and eat half of the meal saving the rest for later. Using this approach I would be close to my 700 calorie budget, eat a wonderful meal, and have lunch tomorrow.

This whole process goes a lot faster in real life. The calorie estimates become second nature after a while. Scanning your plate and making size estimates isn't too difficult. What can be hard is remembering how many calories there are for each food type and serving size. A good solution is to copy the table and take it with you.

In this example, we've tackled estimating a difficult and complex meal. You can use the same process for any meal. And once you get in the habit of practicing perfect portions, your chances of overeating go way down and your chances of staying on your diet go way up.

To Learn More

❖ *The Portion Teller* by Lisa Young, PhD, RD. This excellent book gives a lot of great advice on how you can practice more perfect portions. The history of how portion sizes have increased over time is worth the price of the book by itself.

❖ *Picture Perfect Weight Loss* by Dr. Howard Shapir. Packed with beautiful pictures comparing different portion sizes, you'll learn a lot about how many calories are in the foods you eat.

Strategy 55. Decide Exactly How Much You'll Eat Before Taking the First Bite

Create situations in which you won't eat more than you should. You can't trust your body to tell you when to stop eating.

Has something like this happened to you? It's been a long day and you're excited to take a break and go see a new movie. At the movies you buy a giant bag of popcorn, a large soda, and a box of candy. Your usual. You could have bought the small popcorn, but the giant box was only a dollar more and it comes with free refills. Who can pass up that deal?

About halfway through the movie, you notice that all the popcorn is gone. How did that happen? You don't remember eating it all. Well, it happened one handful at a time. You think about how many calories you just ate and you are amazed. A large bag of movie popcorn has about 1,700 calories. A large soda has about 1,200. A large box of candy has about 900 calories. Oh boy. That's almost two days worth of calories in one sitting!

You may not have intended to eat everything. You may have intended to eat just part of the popcorn, or the candy, or the soda, but once you are in the middle of eating it's almost impossible to stop.

That's why the goal of this strategy is for you to **decide how much you'll eat before you start eating** and only have that amount of food in front of you. Follow this one rule and your chances of overeating nose-dive. It's hard to eat food that isn't there.

You can always choose to eat more. Sometimes we consciously make such a choice. No problem. We like the food. We want to have fun, but make the choice to overeat consciously. Don't let how much food happens to be served on your plate dictate how much you eat.

It's tempting to romanticize your body and think that if you could just learn to live in harmony with it then all would be well. You could become a "natural" eater and your weight would naturally stabilize at a nice slim and trim level. I have no doubt this works for some people. And these people may think it will work for everyone else. But it doesn't work for me. It may not work for you either.

I can eat a whole cake and my body is whispering "good job" the whole time. That's what "natural" means for me. My body is happy I found a good source of food and is all for eating as much as I can just in case I don't get to eat for a couple of days. If I ate what I "naturally" felt like, I would do nothing but gain weight.

Don't get me wrong, I would love to be a natural eater. And if the natural eating strategy works for you then go for it. Whatever works. But don't expect natural eating to work and if it doesn't, don't feel like you are broken. We are all different and not being a "natural" eater is just part of your uniqueness.

To implement this strategy, follow two steps:

1. **Decide how much to eat** using the calorie estimating techniques we've already talked about. Make your decision at the beginning of a meal, because that's when your long-term thinking is at its strongest.

2. **Get rid of the food** you don't want, using strategies we'll cover later in this chapter. The strongest strategy is to put all the food you don't want to eat in a doggy bag **before** you start eating.

 Strategy 56. Start with Soup or Salad

Have a salad or cup of soup to take the edge off of your hunger.

The idea behind this strategy is to fill up on tasty, high volume, low calorie food so you can enjoy smaller portions of great tasting main dishes while still feeling full.

When you start a meal with a large portion of a food that has a lot of bulk and few calories, like soup and salad, it makes you feel full so you end up eating less for the rest of your meal.

Researchers have found that people who ate a big salad before eating a main course ate fewer calories overall than those who didn't have a salad. One study found that eating a large low calorie salad reduced the overall calorie total for the entire meal by 107 calories. Eating a large high calorie salad had the opposite result: the total calories for the entire meal increased by 145 calories.

This strategy is surprisingly effective and easy. I use it almost every day now. Both soup (not cream based) and salad taste wonderful, so you aren't losing any quality from your meal. And by eating the salad, you feel full enough that you can eat a smaller portion of a food you really love and still feel full. It's a win-win.

We'll talk more about similar ideas in the *Pump Up the Volume* strategy.

Strategy 57. Ask for a Doggy Bag Immediately

You've decided how much you are going to eat before you take the first bite. Put the rest in a doggy bag *before* you start eating.

Restaurant portions are about twice the size they were 15 years ago. A full restaurant meal may supply most of your daily calories. **You can't change how much food a restaurant serves you, but you can change how much you eat.**

As you order, **immediately** ask your server for a doggy bag. Don't wait. Do it now.

When your food arrives, **immediately** divide it into your **correct portion size** as soon as it is brought to your table. Don't wait. Do it now.

Immediately put all the food you shouldn't eat in the doggy bag. Don't wait. Do it now.

Don't fool yourself that you'll stop eating later. You probably won't. Once you start eating the food will taste so good you simply won't stop.

By following this strategy, you are both cutting down on how much you are eating and you also have an excellent meal for the next day. Think of it as getting two meals for the price of one with the added bonus of staying on your diet!

Strategy 58. Split Meals with a Friend

Buy one meal and split it with a friend.

Gigantic restaurant meals make it realistic now to buy one meal and split it between two people. If you need a little extra food, then buy an appetizer or two. Most restaurants will give you an extra plate if you ask nicely.

Remember to leave a full tip for your server. They are still doing all the work. Leaving a tip based on the price of one meal wouldn't be fair.

Strategy 59. Use Meal Replacements

Meal replacements are convenient, portion controlled, relatively low calorie meals that fill you up.

A meal replacement is a drink or bar you eat instead of fixing a meal using "real" food. Your breakfast, for example, would be a meal replacement bar or shake instead of your normal cereal and toast or bacon and eggs.

Nobody was more skeptical about using meal replacements than I was. I was sure they were a scam created by food manufacturers to extract yet more money out of consumers.

However, when I looked into the research, there was a lot of evidence showing meal replacements work, even over many years of use. Using meal replacement, people are able to stay on their diets, lose up to 8% of their body weight, and keep the weight off.

Why do meal replacements seem to work so well?

1. **It's easy so you can do it every day.** Eating a bar or fixing a shake is easy so people can stick to it over the long term. It's not a strategy you easily get tired of.

2. **It protects you from slip-ups by reducing the number of decisions you have to make.** When fixing your own meals, there is always the chance of overeating. Using a meal replacement guarantees you a fixed meal size and number of calories. It's an easy form of portion control.

3. **You feel full.** Meal replacements are formulated to help you feel full after eating them. This reduces your need to snack which reduces your total number of calories.

In short, meal replacements work because of portion control. You are eating a fixed size, relatively low calorie meal that fills you up. A breakfast, for example, may have three times the calories of a meal replacement. By eating meal replacements you are creating a Safe Zone in which your portions are controlled.

Usually, people replace only one meal a day, but it has been shown to be safe and effective to replace two daily meals. Just make sure you eat healthy snacks and dinner during the rest of the day.

▮ Which meal replacement should you use?

Through experiment and research I have created my own meal replacement shake, but if you look around you'll find plenty to choose from. There are all different kinds on the market for all different needs and ways of eating.

Experiment with different products to see which you like best. Do you prefer a bar or a shake? What mix of protein, carbs, and other nutrients are you looking for? Does it fill you up? What flavors do you like? How much does it cost?

There are so many products it may take a bit of research to find which one works for you. But if you have trouble with portion control, the meal replacement strategy may be an excellent choice for you.

Strategy 60. Try Pre-Prepared Meals Instead of Cooking

Using pre-prepared meals you can control your portion sizes while still eating good quality food.

The art of portion control is in figuring out ways to make yourself eat only the amount of food you intend to. For many of the same reasons we discussed in the *Use Meal Replacements* strategy, you might find pre-prepared meals an excellent strategy for enforcing portion control.

Pre-prepared meals are ready-to-eat or near-ready-to-eat, are quick and easy to make and have a known calorie count for a known portion size. With a little calculation and measuring, you can determine exactly how many calories you are eating. That's a big advantage over eating out or even fixing your own meals.

Pre-prepared meals have another portion control advantage because they are naturally limited in size. While you might go get another serving from your casserole dish, it's unlikely you'll make another pre-packaged meal.

Companies are now targeting the busy family market with pre-prepared meals, so you can expect to see even more products in the future.

One of the under-appreciated benefits of using pre-packaged foods is they **teach you what proper portion sizes look like.** We have become so used to large portion sizes we don't know what a proper sized piece of chicken or serving of pasta looks like anymore.

One way to teach yourself proper portion sizes is to use pre-prepared meals like those supplied by NutriSystem, South Beach, Lean Cuisine, and other vendors. You don't even need to eat their food for weight loss reasons. By eating their meals, you'll begin to learn and get a feel for how much food you should be eating. The small size of the portions will be quite shocking at first. Once you get used to them it will be easier for you to eat the right portion sizes in the future.

What are some of your pre-prepared meal options?

1. **Healthy Frozen Dinners.** Frozen dinners were horrible at one time. That's not as true anymore. Many good-quality, low-calorie frozen dinners are available now.

2. **Prepackaged Dinners.** Look in the refrigerator section of your store for complete prepackaged ready-to-cook meals for your family. New products are coming on to the market all the time.

3. **Fresh Preparation.** This is a service combining the benefits of meal preparation services and frozen dinners. They provide a menu of meals you can choose from, do all the shopping, and then perform some of the more time consuming meal preparation steps. You cook the meals in their facilities and take the finished masterpieces home with you to serve later. The advantage is that you get a wide variety of fresh food with known portion sizes. You also get to cook, which is a lot of fun, especially once you remove all the labor of shopping and chopping from the process!

4. **Personal Chef Service.** Meal preparation services have become a lot more popular lately. They can include personalized meal planning, grocery shopping and preparation of dinners. They do all the cooking for you. There is a wide variety of different options, depending on your budget and preferences. You can pick up pre-prepared meals each day, or you can take home a bunch of meals for later. The advantage of using a meal preparation service compared to frozen or prepackaged dinners is that the food should be fresher, higher quality, more nutritious, and better tasting.

5. **Full Time Personal Chef.** If you have the resources, a personal chef is a good hire. Your expert cook can make a wide variety of the foods you like while keeping your calorie budget in mind.

6. **Restaurant Pickup and Delivery.** Most restaurants aren't a good source for meals because they generally serve large portions of high calorie food. That's why we like them, I know, but it's not good portion control. I would like to see restaurants creating healthy, good tasting meals with known portion sizes and nutritional information. To me this seems a natural market for restaurants. They are often conveniently located and are already set up to cook fresh good quality food. They just need to take that extra step of helping people stay on their diet.

You can build an almost impenetrable Safe Zone around these ideas. You don't always have to make your own meals. You are minimizing your chances of slipping-up by limiting your portion sizes using pre-packaged meals. That's how you put yourself in the best position to succeed at controlling your weight.

You still have chances to cook if you want. You don't need to eat every dinner as a pre-prepared meal. You may want to cook on the weekends when you have time and use pre-prepared meals on the weekdays when time is short.

Even when using pre-packaged meals, you may need to fix a salad or other side dish, as most won't provide enough calories on their own. To go along with a frozen dinner, I usually fix a big salad, some fruit, and a dessert. Sometimes I'll even toss in a small appetizer. The salad helps fill me up and provides excellent nutrition. My fruit of choice is either a crisp apple or sliced strawberries spiked with cinnamon. For dessert I'll toss in a couple of squares of high quality chocolate.

Overall the meal is healthy, portion controlled, and there's very little opportunity for slipping-up. All fine attributes of a Safe Zone.

 Strategy 61. Use Smaller Plates and Bowls

Your plate size determines how much you will eat. Eat from smaller dinnerware and you'll naturally control your portion sizes.

We've learned how we unconsciously eat more from larger packages and in *The Dish Threat* we learned how much larger plates have become in recent years. That's a weight gaining combination if ever there was one.

A good counter-move is to right-size all your plates, bowls, glasses, cups, and spoons so that they fit your portion sizes. You may think this strategy is a bit silly, but it's **amazingly effective.**

Think about how you serve food. If you are filling a big a plate from a big serving bowl, you are very likely to fill the entire plate with food. Your plate size then determines how much you will eat.

Simply by using smaller dishes, you reduce the amount of food you serve yourself without even trying (or thinking about it).

One of my most successful strategies ever was **replacing a standard soup bowl** with a much smaller dessert bowl. Now I use a dessert bowl that is already the correct portion size for the amount of dessert I should eat. Using a dessert bowl for dessert, what a radical idea!

Dessert bowls always looked small to me. But they aren't. Carefully measure how much ice cream you put in a soup bowl. It could easily be over 1,000 calories. Do the same for a dessert bowl. The calorie numbers will be much more reasonable.

I also bought smaller plates. A big plate just demands to be filled up. The smaller plate is more like the portion size I should be eating so it is much easier to eat the right amount of food.

Where do you find smaller dishes and utensils? It's not easy. You have to look around. Dishes were smaller in the past so you can often find old sets of smaller dishes at garage sales. I hope in the future some manufacturers will step up and make attractive portion-controlled dishes.

I try never to rely on my ability to stop eating. I use every strategy I can to make sure I always eat the right amount of food so it's not possible for me to fail and eat more than I should.

Strategy 62. Break Up Food into Smaller Packages

Smaller packages ensure the proper serving size and give you a chance to stop eating after each serving.

After grocery shopping, repackage your food into the appropriate serving sizes. This strategy helps ensure you won't eat too much. Let's say you have cookies. How many cookies do you want to eat at one time? Let's say three. Now take the cookies out of the box and put three cookies each into separate plastic bags.

Breaking up the larger container into individual serving sizes accomplishes two goals:

1. **You don't have to think about the proper serving size.** It's built-in to your packaging. This means you won't accidentally overeat because the portion sizes will be correct.

2. **You give yourself a chance to stop eating after each serving.** When food is in a large package, there is no natural stopping point so you just keep eating. With smaller packages, you get a natural place to stop and think to yourself that you have had enough.

When I get home from shopping, I break out the zip-lock bags, the scale, and I repackage food into its proper portion sizes. It's not something I look forward to, but I find if I don't do it, I will eat too much.

The first time you measure and repackage your food, you may be shocked at how much you have been eating. I repackage the hamburger into ¼ pound patties for my wife and ½ pound patties for me. A ¼ pound is a lot smaller than I remember.

I was stunned by how much spaghetti I was eating before I started using pre-packaged quantities. A serving of spaghetti, for the kind I buy, is 2 ounces for 190 calories. The quantity I used to eat was easily 5 times that!

I have found several ways of making the packaging job easier:

1. **Use a good electric scale.** It makes measuring a lot faster.

2. **Buy a lot of zip-locked baggies.** You need something to put those smaller portions into.

3. **Buy right-sized pre-packaged food portions from the start.**
    Cheese, for example, comes packaged in slices. Even though the
    slices are more expensive, it's worth it to me. Cookies and crackers
    are now sold in one hundred calorie serving sizes. Carrots are now
    sold in single serving sizes. It's a trend I expect will continue.
4. **Don't repackage vegetables.** You want to eat more of them.
5. **Some foods aren't easily repackageable.** Nuts, for example, are
    difficult to repackage because there are so many of them and the
    serving size is so small. I know I should only eat 10 almonds at a
    time, so I just take 10 from the jar. I'll consider not buying some-
    thing if it's hard to repackage. Other foods are just hard, like salad
    dressing. It's not practical to repackage salad dressing, yet it has a
    lot of calories in a small amount, so I make sure I am careful when
    measuring out a serving.
6. **Be creative.** You can usually overcome any problems with a little
    thought and a firm understanding of the reason for repackaging
    food. The idea is to make it hard for you to slip-up and eat more
    than you should. Just apply the no slip-up idea whenever you can.

Repackaging is a strategy you should definitely revisit when your feedback
strategies show you are gaining weight. Over time it's so easy for portion sizes
to creep up. Repackaging food into smaller portion sizes helps create a Safe
Zone where portion creep isn't so creepy.

Strategy 63. The Goody Rules
Reduce the goodies and save your weight.

The Goody Rules are strategies for reducing the pressure goodies exert
on your brain to eat them. When goodies are around, and you know they're
around, your brain targets them like a laser pointer. To control your weight
you need to change your environment to reduce the goody threat. Here are a
few strategies for countering the power of the goody:

▌ Put Goodies in Cloudy Containers

Simply using a container you can't see into helps stop unintentional eating. One study found that people ate many fewer chocolates from an opaque
bowl, meaning they couldn't see the contents of the bowl. Out of sight, out
of mind.

▌ Place Goodies Far Away

We've learned how the closer food is to you the more food you will eat. So put the goodies out of the way.

Simply by placing food out of reach you will reduce the amount you eat from mountain to mole hill. If you didn't have a remote control how often would you change channels? The same strategy works for food.

Two Weight-Proofing ideas combine in this strategy: the harder something is to do, the less you will do it, and placing food far away gives you the natural pause you need to rethink your urge to snack. It's similar to the idea of repackaging foods into correct portion sizes instead of eating from a large container. The **distance you must travel** to eat your goody gives you time to rethink and stop what you are doing.

This strategy applies in every area you can think of: home, work, school, and in your car. Don't leave convenient jars of snacks in your office, on a counter or in your desk. Keep candy-filled vending machines far away.

Treat bad foods like vampires—never invite them in.

▌ Go Out for Goodies

If your environment contains goodies, you will hunt them down and eat them. The best way to put yourself in a position to succeed is to simply not have goodies in the house. If you want a treat, go out and get it. Pack up the family, zoom off and get a scoop of ice cream. The mere fact that you have to make a special effort prevents the majority of treat trips.

How extreme do you need to be in this strategy? As always, you have to decide for yourself and for your family.

I decided I had to be extreme. I found myself eating too many ice cream bars (even low calorie ones) when they were around, so I simply got rid of them. If I really want one I can go down to the store. If you look in our house there aren't any goodies.

Well, that's not completely true. I keep around bars of high quality dark chocolate. Dark chocolate is a wonderful dessert because I feel completely satisfied Joyfully Eating two squares. And get this…two squares of delicious dark chocolate only have 100 calories! And for some reason I don't pig out on the dark chocolate, which means I can keep it in the house without worrying I'll make an occasional slip-up.

▌ Use Tall Thin Drinking Glasses

People naturally pour up to 32% more of a drink into shorter and wider containers. That's a lot of extra calories! You can help prevent yourself from drinking too much simply by buying different shaped glasses. How's that for creating a Safe Zone!

Strategy 64. Don't Eat from a Container

Take the amount of food you want to eat out of its container and put it in a separate dish, especially for binge foods like potato chips and ice cream.

When you eat potato chips out of the bag, how often do you keep eating until you reach the bottom? Portion control is almost impossible when eating out of a container. Avoid the temptation entirely by not eating out of containers in the first place. Instead, serve yourself exactly how much you think you should eat into a separate appropriately sized dish and eat out of that dish, not the container.

This one is very difficult for me. After dinner I place the leftovers in a plastic container. The next day when I am hungry, the most natural thing in the world is to eat directly out of the container. Why dirty another dish? I always have to remember to take just my portion size out or I'll eat too much almost every time.

Strategy 65. Don't Bring Serving Dishes to the Table

Fill your plate with as much food as you are going to eat for the entire meal *before* sitting down to eat at the table.

At family style meals, it's traditional to bring big heaping serving dishes filled with food to the table. Individuals then serve themselves directly out of the huge serving dishes using gigantic serving spoons. Can you guess why this style of eating may be bad for your waistline?

1. The serving dishes and utensils are large, so chances are you'll spoon more food than you should onto your plate.
2. The serving dishes tease you by staying on the table while you are eating. Your chances of having seconds and even thirds go way up.
3. Eating with friends and family encourages you to linger over the meal, which increases your chances of eating more.

Who knew the family dinner table was such a minefield? To avoid temptation, serve each person's plate with their appropriate amount of food and put the rest of the food out of reach. To be really safe, put all the leftover food away before you eat.

....

 ## Strategy 66. Trick Yourself into Eating More Healthy Food

You can reverse a lot of the "do not" suggestions made in previous strategies to trick yourself into eating more healthy foods instead of just figuring out how to avoid bad foods.

Let's say you, for example, want to eat more baby carrots because they are filling and healthy. What do you do?

Put the carrots into a large clear container and put this close while working. You can also put the carrots within easy reach in the refrigerator. This combines a lot of the research from the threats section to get yourself to unintentionally eat more of a healthy food. You can use the same idea with salads, vegetable plates and anything else you want people to eat more of.

I am constantly amazed at the difference this approach makes. If I hide carrots in the vegetable drawer of the refrigerator, I won't think about them when a snack attack hits. But if they're plain view, I'll eat them first instead of settling for a worse choice.

We keep hard boiled eggs in our refrigerator as a filling snack. Eggs are healthy, fixed sized, and have a natural stopping point to discourage over-eating. A funny thing happens though. When only a few eggs are left in the bowl, we stop eating them. This is right out of the threats. When more eggs are in the bowl we eat more of them. We don't want to believe these threats are true, but they are.

So when the egg bowl goes low, I make sure to fill it up again. If we didn't, we'd probably switch to a less healthy snack. I've noticed the same situation happens with apples too.

If you want your family to eat more fruit, then have a big fruit basket displayed proudly on a kitchen counter, next to the refrigerator. Don't have junk food in the house. It has been found that even when healthier foods are available, people will still eat the junk food if it is around. **If you only have good food around then that's all you can eat.**

With a little thought and creativity, I am sure you can come up with a lot of ideas that will work for you and your family.

Chapter 20

Create Your Home and Family Safe Zone
Strategies 67–76

Your home and family environment is the number one danger zone for falling off your diet. It's a simple matter of time and opportunity. Your home bristles with food and exercise slip-up traps just waiting to be sprung. And because you spend so much time at home, your chance of giving in to temptation is almost certain.

What do I mean by slip-up traps? Cookies in the pantry. Ice cream in the freezer. Candy in the drawer. A TV that almost begs you to sit down instead of exercise. If not TV it could be video games or talking on the phone. Everywhere you look, another potential slip-up trap waits to make you fall off your diet.

That's why you have to take special care when creating your *Home and Family Safe Zone*. Scour your house for every possible slip-up opportunity and figure out a way to remove it. Transform your home into a Safe Zone and your chances of staying on your diet sky-rocket.

Strategy 67. Eat More Meals at Home with Your Family

Your Home and Family Safe Zone protects you from the threats of eating out.

People eat away from home more than ever these days. The temptation of eating at a restaurant combined with the huge portion sizes is a definite threat to your diet. Staying on a diet while eating out all the time is like running with a hundred pound rock on your back. You can probably do it, but it's really hard.

Try eating at home more often. Make use of the home Safe Zone you've created; it helps protect you from overeating. At home you can't eat off your diet because you've only purchased the foods you have purposefully decided to eat. Another advantage is you'll spend more time with your family.

Strategy 68. Learn to Cook

Until you can answer the "what's to eat" question, you are always vulnerable to slipping up and eating the wrong foods.

Is this you and your family?

Cook? Me? You must be kidding. I can't even boil water! We eat out a lot. Mostly pizza and fast foods. There are so many choices and the kids don't make a fuss. But, we keep sandwich fixin's around and stuff you can pop in the micro too. —Anonymous

As late as the 1960s, it may not have been possible to feed a family without cooking. The environment has changed. Now a family can eat out every day. Fast food is cheap, kids love it, and you'll never get bored because of the huge variety of available fast food restaurants.

The problem is, fast food is associated with poor nutrition and obesity. Yes, I know, you can make better choices, but most of the time people don't.

What's the easiest thing to do when you don't have a plan for a meal? Go out. Restaurant portions are huge and it is so very tempting to eat something you shouldn't. If you choose not to eat out, then the chances are you will go home and graze, eating lots of different things without much control over the quantity or quality of the food. A bag of chips may seem like the perfect answer when you are hungry.

How can you answer the "what's to eat" question? We've already talked about a few possibilities: meal replacements and pre-packaged foods. Another answer is: **learn how to cook.** Cooking takes control of your *Home and Family Safe Zone* and more importantly, the Safe Zone of your kids.

A family that eats together eats better says a recent study in the journal *Archives of Family Medicine.* The study showed children who report frequent family dinners have healthier diets than their peers who don't.

There are a lot of places to learn to cook. Hopefully someone in your family is a good cook and is willing to teach you. You can also consider books, magazines, school, community colleges, gourmet food stores, and formal cooking schools.

Try involving your children in the meal-making process from a young age. When they are preschoolers, teach them how to set the table. Take them grocery shopping and let them pick some treats, fruits, and vegetables. Have a family night and let the kids cook some of the meal. Giving children more and more supervised responsibility over time helps them become very capable and better able to make healthy decisions as they grow older.

The sheer joy of cooking is one of life's gifts many in the modern world have lost touch with. The ritual of preparing food and eating together is as ancient as humanity and it can reconnect us in a deep and satisfying way, if we let it.

....

 ## Strategy 69. Pump Up the Volume—Feeling Full from Fewer Calories

To feel fuller, eat foods that have the same weight with fewer calories.

There's a weight control strategy most people haven't heard of called *Volumetrics.* Volumetrics was created by Dr. Barbara Rolls, a well respected food-nutrition researcher at Pennsylvania State University. She found the "eat less" part of "eat less and exercise more" isn't true. You can eat less and gain a ton of weight. You can also eat a lot more and still lose weight.

This amazingly counterintuitive finding hinges on Dr. Rolls' research showing that people eat about the same weight of food each day, regardless of the food's calorie content. Your body doesn't seem to pay attention to the number of calories in food when deciding if you are full or not. This finding has big implications for your weight.

The idea behind *Volumetrics* is that if you eat food that has the same weight with fewer calories you can eat more and weigh less. The relationship between what a food weighs and the number of calories it has is called its **energy density.**

Cookies are an excellent example of a high energy dense food. Cookies have a lot calories in a little package because they are made from a lot of fat and sugar. Fat has the most energy, at 9 calories per gram. If your food is high in fat it is also high in calories.

Celery is a good example of a low energy dense food because it has a low number of calories for its weight. Celery has a lot of water and fiber, at almost no calories.

The difference between raisins and grapes is a good example of how eating a low calorie dense food can help you feel full for fewer calories. You may think you feel full faster on higher calorie food, but unfortunately that's not the way it works.

Let's say you are eating a small, high calorie food like raisins. You'll eat a lot of raisins before you start feeling full because each raisin is small. And because each raisin is high in calories, you end up eating a lot more calories than you probably intend. One-quarter cup of raisins is 100 calories. One and two-thirds cups of whole grapes is 100 calories.

For the same 100 calories, which do you think will fill you more: ¼ cup of raisins or the 1⅔ cups of grapes? The grapes! Grapes are a lower energy dense food than raisins. The grapes take up more space for the same number of calories. Grapes are a good deal then. You get to eat more grapes than raisins and feel fuller.

So the big idea of Volumetrics is to **lower the energy density** of the food you eat. This allows you to eat a lot more food for the same calories, just like you can eat more grapes than raisins for the same calories.

You can lower the energy density of a common dish like a casserole by **adding more vegetables** and **using less cheese** and low-fat milk. Using less cheese and a reduced fat milk means there are fewer calories because there is less fat. Vegetables are high in fiber and water while being low in calories. The overall result is a dish that has the **same weight but fewer calories** and you'll still feel full!

The same idea can be applied to hamburgers. Add vegetables to your hamburger and you lower its calorie density, yet it will still be filling, and it will taste just as good. Adding fruits and vegetables to most dishes reduces the number of calories in the dish while at the same time keeping you feeling full.

You may be asking, why you can't just drink water? Your stomach knows the difference between food and water. You have to eat real food to feel full. But you can make use of broths because the broth will contain food. It combines a lot of liquid and real food. This is why soup is so filling.

Volumetrics works. One study found that increasing the amount of fruits and vegetables in your diet means that you **eat 400 fewer calories a day.** And at the same time you don't feel hungry. It's not hard to understand why. It's the volume of food that makes you feel full. You can eat a large volume of water and fiber from fruits and vegetables without eating a lot of calories. The same volume of fatty foods would be an enormous number of calories. A series of Swedish studies found **simply adding carrots, spinach, and other high fiber vegetables to your meals** can significantly lengthen the time it takes you to feel hungry again.

Volumetrics isn't a fad diet. It's a well researched idea. The trick is getting fewer calories for the same weight of food.

To Learn More

❖   *The Volumetrics Eating Plan* website at *http://www.volumetrics eatingplan.com/* has more information.

....

 ## Strategy 70. Structure Your Meal Plans—Plan Exactly What You're Going to Eat and Why

People using meal plans lost 50% more weight than people not using meal plans and kept the weight off better over time.

A meal plan is an exact plan of what to eat every day, combined with a shopping list of which foods you need to buy to cook all the planned meals. Your meal plan tells you exactly which foods to buy, how much to buy, what meals you will make and when you will eat them.

Why is using a food plan such a strong strategy for losing weight and staying on your diet?

1.   Following your chosen diet becomes much simpler because **you've reduced the number of decisions** you have to make. It will be difficult to eat outside your meal plan because that's the only food you'll have easily available.

2. Your portions will be **correctly sized** because you planned them to be the right size. There's no guessing involved. And by having known portion sizes, you are also learning better calorie estimation skills. This also helps to stop overeating.
3. You will eat **better quality food.** You can pick better recipes that are more nutritious so you end up eating better.
4. You will **snack less and eat more regularly.** Eating breakfast, lunch, and dinner decreases the temptation to skip meals and snack.

The problem is, meal planning can be hard because it, well, requires planning! It's always easier not to plan.

How might you go about creating a meal plan?

1. **Realize that this isn't easy.** Meal planning is a skill you develop with practice.
2. **Pick a planning day.** When are you going to plan your meals? Sunday is a common day, but it can be any convenient day for you. A typical meal plan lasts a week because food can normally stay fresh for that long, but you can use any time period that works for you.
3. **Who will do the planning?** Consider rotating the task if someone doesn't take the job on permanently. Remember to involve kids in the process, so they can learn how to plan meals for when they grow up.
4. **Pick a shopping day.** When will you go shopping? Sunday is a common shopping day, but again, you can pick any day. You can also make several smaller trips during the week to pick up fresh foods like fruits and vegetables and anything else you might have forgotten.
5. **Know your way of eating.** What type of diet will your family eat? What's the target calorie budget for each person? Do any of your family members have special dietary needs? If so, how will you accommodate them?
6. **Have a backup plan if you're busy.** What happens when life gets in the way and you didn't get the meal planning done or didn't go shopping yet? Have a backup plan so your family can still eat a healthy meal.
7. **Find sources of meal plans.** Meal planning is a huge topic. You can find lots of advice in cookbooks at your local library. Ask your

family and friends too. A lot of people love to cook and will be full of great ideas. There are also many meal planning services available on the Internet. And you may already have a huge batch of cookbooks. Always be on the lookout for new sources of meal ideas.

8. **Recycle meal plans.** Find out what your family likes and keep making it. People don't really get bored with meals when they are served relatively far a part. Include new meals in your plans, but don't think you always have to be inventive. This puts too much stress on you and the more stress you feel the less likely you are to plan meals. Old favorites are old favorites for a reason: people like them.

9. **Use seasonal meal plans.** Vegetables and fruits are usually much cheaper and better tasting when they come into season.

Your risk of overeating is almost non-existent if you only buy what you plan on eating.

To Learn More

❖ We maintain a list of meal planning resources you may find helpful at *http://YourDesignerDiet.com.*

Strategy 71. Use a Shopping List—Buy Only the Foods in Your Meal Plan

A shopping list prompts you to plan meals, prevents you from buying foods you don't need, and encourages you to eat the portions and type of foods you desire.

Here's how I used to shop. I had no regular shopping day. When I was out of enough stuff, it was time to go shopping. I hate shopping so delaying to the last possible minute was the standard plan. I could go days without vegetables or any other good foods, because it just wasn't time to shop yet. Meals were made from whatever I could find or pick up on the way home.

When it finally was time to shop, I had no plan. I just went to the store and bought stuff that looked good. I didn't really know how to cook so I had no idea about making meals. I had no meal plan so a balanced diet hung on whatever moved me as I stalked the aisles. What did I pick to eat? Lots of spaghetti. Ice cream, of course. Cereal. Not many fruits or vegetables.

Oh the bad old days! What do the good new days look like? Make a meal plan, as we talked about in the *Structure Your Meal Plans* strategy, of what you are going to eat each week. Part of a meal plan is a shopping list of exactly which groceries you plan to buy. A lot of people stumble on the creating the shopping list step because it's hard. Fortunately, there's a secret to painless shopping list maintenance.

▌ Keep a Running Shopping List

The secret to easy pain-free shopping list creation is to **update your list as you run out of an item.** Keep a pad of paper in the kitchen. As soon as you run low on something, turn around and write it down on your shopping list. With this habit you'll never run out of what you need.

For an even smoother shopping experience, divide your shopping list into different sections based on where you need to go to shop for an item. For example, if you run out of dog food, then write it under the pet store section. If you run out of a spice then write it under a section for your spice store. And so on for all your items. Organizing your shopping trip is much simpler using this approach.

Shopping becomes less stressful because you already know most of what you need. You'll add more items when creating your meal plan, but most of what you'll need will already be written down.

This strategy helps to create your Safe Zone because you won't wander around the store wondering if you need this or that. You'll know exactly what you need to buy and you'll be confident of having what you need. Otherwise you'll buy food you don't need and you'll buy more food than you need, both of which encourage you to overeat.

▌ The List Should Specify Quantities

Your shopping list should list all the foods you need to buy along with the quantities of each. For example, don't just add "chicken" to the list. That doesn't help anyone. Say exactly what type and quantity of chicken to buy. Providing quantity information helps you make smarter decisions about where to shop and what cuts will be cheapest. You'll also reduce your chances of buying too much food.

▌ Only Buy What's on the List

This is a hard one: **only buy what's on your shopping list.** Learn to trust your list. It's probably right and your memory of what you have or need is probably wrong. If you update your list when you run out of items and you plan your meals, the chances of your list being wrong are small. And even if your list is wrong the world won't end. You'll be able to fix something from what you have on hand.

Why such a strong rule? Two reasons:

1. **The more food you buy the more you will eat.** So don't buy it. Disregarding your list encourages you to buy more food than you need.

2. **You will probably buy foods you shouldn't eat.** You are at your strongest when you make your shopping list. You are being thoughtful about what you should be eating and why. Sticking to your shopping list prevents you from buying the wrong foods.

The shopping list is life. Planning and creating a shopping list of only what you need creates an incredibly powerful Safe Zone for you and your family.

Strategy 72. Parents Rule—You Have More Influence Over Your Kids than You Think

Hold firm to your meal plan and your shopping list. Don't give in to your kids' food desires and demands.

Parents have the hardest job in the world. While shopping one day I watched as a mother and her twin boys rolled their cart down the cereal isle. The kids were nagging and nagging mom to buy a sweet cereal they see advertised on TV all the time. I am pretty sure I would have lost it after a while, but mom didn't. She calmly ignored their cries and said no, you can't have that cereal, you need to choose a healthy cereal. And one of the boys shot back, saying the box says the cereal is healthy! Ouch. But she didn't fold. Later I looked at the cereal he was talking about and it was about as healthy as a candy bar combined with a cheap vitamin pill. The kids eventually picked a better cereal. Score one for parent power.

This is what parents have to live with every day. How can a parent be strong all the time, especially when their kids are being marketed to all day, every day, in every part of their lives? I don't have an answer.

But as we learned in *The Pestering Kid Threat* the desires of the child, which aren't usually for nutritious foods, often drive the food choices for the whole family. And when this happens the whole family suffers.

I don't know how to do it, but as a parent try to hold firm to your meal plan and your shopping list. Don't give in to your kids. They won't starve.

Quite the opposite. You will be teaching them how to eat. Hopefully you are teaching them how to cook too. These are skills that will serve them well for their whole life.

One way to think about it is that you are the creator of the Safe Zones for your kids. If you put them in the best possible position to succeed, they will. If you give in to them they will fail, become obese, and die early. Sorry to be so blunt, but those are the stakes you are playing for.

To Learn More

❖   *Consuming Kids* by Susan Linn tells the troubling tale of how marketers directly encourage kids to nag their parents into making favorable purchasing decisions. Don't read this book at night. It's really scary.

Strategy 73. Eat Calories, Don't Drink Them

Don't drink sugary sodas or juices. Soft drinks are our largest single source of daily calories, providing more than 7%.

SODA HAS A LOT OF CALORIES! Sorry for shouting, but for some reason a lot of people don't realize that all the soda they pound down throughout the day has a lot of calories. Just because a soda is a liquid doesn't mean it's a free food. Soft drinks are our largest single source of daily calories, providing more than 7% of them. The 7-Eleven Double Gulp holds 64-ounces of soda and comes in at **800 calories.**

It's not just sodas that are the problem. Fruit juices have become popular, but they are equally high in calories while providing little nutrition. Children who drank more than 4 glasses of fruit juice on the day of a study were more than twice as a likely to be overweight or obese when compared with children who did not drink these drinks.

Here are some potential alternatives to drinking sugary sodas and fruit juices:

1   If you hate diet soda, then go heavy on the ice when filling up the glass. You'll save a lot calories by fooling yourself into thinking you're drinking a full glass of soda.

2.   Adding some lemon to diet soda may make it taste better to you.

3.   In general, liquid calories are far more fattening than filling. Eat your fruit rather than drinking fruit juice. For the calories in one

box of apple juice, you can enjoy an apple or orange. And whole foods fill you up better than liquids and they are more nutritious.

4.   Try drinking water in the morning instead of fruit juice. Fruit juice has a ton of calories. If you want the nutrition, then eat the fruit instead.

Switching to diet soda will save you hundreds of calories a day. For every 20 ounces of regular soda, you're consuming 250 calories. Drink several sodas a day and you can easily down 1,000 calories. That is most of your daily calorie budget spent for nothing!

Not drinking your calories also reduces your exposure to fructose, which as we read in *The Fructose Threat,* can trick you into thinking you are hungrier than you should be. That's a big win for your diet too.

 Strategy 74. Snack Smart

Always have healthy snacks available for when you are hungry. Otherwise you'll eat unhealthy snacks.

Snack time is danger time. You are the most likely to go off your diet when you are hunting and gathering food for a snack.

Here are a few ideas on how to deal with snacks:

1.   **Always have healthy snacks available for when you are hungry.** Try baby carrots, fruit, hard boiled eggs, some food that makes sense for you. If you don't have foods you can eat on demand, then you'll make poorer food choices.

2.   When you get the urge to splurge on a snack instead of sitting down to the entire bag of chips, **take only a handful** and put it in a separate dish. This will probably be enough to satisfy your craving.

3.   Eating chips with **fresh chunky salsa fills you up** and reduces the number of high-calorie chips you would eat.

4.   **Pay attention to hidden calories.** When you grab a candy bar at the check-out counter and then super-size dinner, you are adding a lot of calories you might not notice.

5.   **Try fat-free microwave popcorn** sprinkled with some Cajun seasoning or a packet of sweetener. Use an oil-free microwave popper to save on fats.

6.   **Cut out fried foods.** Healthier choices are grilling, baking, roasting, broiling or boiling.

You need to take steps now to make sure that you are prepared when a snack attack hits.

Strategy 75. Eat More Fruits and Vegetables to Eat Less Fat and Sugar

Eat more fruits and vegetables for lower weight and better health.

Let's assume you think eating more fruits and vegetables and less fat and sugar are important. What's the best way to eat more of the good stuff and less of the bad stuff?

▌ Focus on What You Should Eat, Not What You Shouldn't Eat

Interestingly, it has been found more effective to focus on what you should eat rather than what you shouldn't eat. Don't say, for example, eat less fat and sugar. Instead, concentrate on eating more fruits and vegetables. By eating more fruits and vegetables you may naturally eat less fat and sugar. It's very similar to the idea we discussed earlier about being less inactive as the way to get kids to exercise more.

Sometimes the indirect way is best.

▌ Kids Follow their Leader

It is more effective to get parents to eat more fruits and vegetables than it is to only concentrate on getting children to eat healthy. The family follows the parents.

This makes sense, doesn't it? If you have an overweight child, just trying to make the child eat healthier doesn't seem to work. What kid won't eat a bag of chips if they see their mother or father doing so?

What seems to work are parents leading by example, showing their children how and what to eat. Parents have a lot of power in this area, far more than they realize.

The problem is, of course, that parents are often overweight too so their family environment helps keep everyone overweight instead of on their diet. Ideally, parents need to educate themselves about the benefits of fruits and vegetables in their diet, then educate their children, and then translate what they have learned into changes in the food they buy and cook.

▌ So Why Eat Fruits and Vegetables Anyway?

You might think everyone just knows to eat more fruits and vegetables. We hear through public service announcements that we should do so, but we have all learned how to tune out advertisements by now.

Before I did the research for this strategy, I have to admit I didn't really know why I should eat more fruits and vegetables either. There are many reasons: they can help you lose weight, protect against heart disease, cancer, stroke and numerous other health problems. Now I really try to put more fruits and vegetables in my diet.

The recommendation is, we should eat 5 servings of fruits and vegetables every day, but they never say how much is in a serving! I eventually tracked down this information. A serving size may not be not as much as you think:

- ¾ cup (6 ounce) 100% fruit or vegetable juice
- 1 medium fruit (apple, orange, banana, pear)
- ½ cup cut-up fruit
- ½ cup raw or cooked vegetables
- ¼ cup dried fruit (raisins, apricots, mango)
- 1 cup raw, leafy vegetables
- ½ cup cooked or canned peas or beans

This is a pretty low requirement. There are so many obvious health and weight benefits to eating more fruits and vegetables that you may want to consider adding more to your diet.

For a few ideas on how to increase fruit and vegetable consumption in your household, take a look at strategies *Trick Yourself into Eating More Healthy Food, Pump Up the Volume, Snack Smart* and *Learn to Cook.*

. . . .

Strategy 76. Don't Skip Meals

Skipping meals seems like a good idea to lose weight, but it won't lead to healthy, permanent weight loss.

People who eat breakfast every day are **35–50%** *less* **likely to be obese** as those who seldom or never eat breakfast. That's an impressive statistic. Why might eating breakfast encourage a normal weight?

One possible reason is that people who eat breakfast may be less likely to snack during the day or binge at other meals. You may tend to snack if you don't eat a meal because **few people actually skip a meal.** You say you are skipping a meal, get hungry, and then go buy some junk food from the vending machine. Then you eat more in the next meal to make up for the food you didn't eat during the skipped meal! You end up eating more food overall, the food you eat is bad, and you feel worse because you're hungry.

If you do manage to skip a meal you may end up under-eating. Eating a lot less than your basic calorie requirements **slows** your metabolism down. Your body will enter **starvation mode** and you won't lose weight even though you are going hungry. Not a good deal. Plus, unless you are very careful, by skipping a meal you may not being getting all the nutrients you need.

Yet many people say breakfast is unnecessary and the big push to eat breakfast is based on shaky science.

What should you do? **Experiment.** And it's not just for breakfast either, the same idea applies to any strategy.

Skip breakfast for a few days and track your calories and how you feel. Do you end up eating more food when you skip breakfast? Are you starving during the day? How do you sleep at night?

On other days eat breakfast. Make sure the number of calories you eat matches your calorie budget. It's not fair to overeat. Track how many calories you eat during the day. Are you eating less overall? Do you feel less hungry? Are you sleeping better?

If you eat less total calories, feel good, and sleep well eating breakfast then maybe you are a breakfast person. Otherwise, maybe you aren't a breakfast person.

See what works best for you—always.

Chapter 21

Weight-Proof Your Car Safe Zone
Strategies 77–79

Calories in the car don't count! Haven't you said that to yourself? I have. But we know it's not true. This magic ability of being able to treat cars as an anything-goes-food-orgy-palace makes your car a danger zone.

All the threats and strategies apply while eating in your car. You still have to worry about portion sizes. You still have to worry about calories. You still have to worry about compulsive eating. This chapter will talk about car specific strategies too, but the major point is that calories eaten in your car count. You need to find ways of converting your car from an extreme red flag danger zone into a Safe Zone.

Strategy 77. Drive Away from Temptation
Change your driving route if it puts you in temptation's way.

Every day for years when going to work I drove by a donut shop that had the best donuts I've ever tasted. These were awesome donuts. And because I am an early-to-rise sort of person they were always hot and fresh. I can still taste them in my mind, though I haven't had a donut for many years now.

I didn't have a donut every day as you might expect. I would have a donut once a week. Then, later, I was able have a donut once every two weeks. But as we have seen, little slip-ups add up and that was enough for me to gain weight.

Part of my environment was a risk to me. Good willpower got me a long way, but I needed to be extreme and put myself in the best position to succeed. So I changed my route. I drove a different way to work so I wouldn't drive by the donut shop anymore. Out of sight, out of mind.

Strategy 78. Don't Eat in Your Car

How extreme do you need to be? Maybe you need to ban eating in your car.

It's so easy to overeat in a car. For many people, eating in their car is simply too dangerous. Perhaps you should consider making it a rule that you just won't eat in a car.

Strategy 79. Pack Your Own Food

Pack good food for the road rather than buy fast food on the run.

A lot of people live on the road. Salespeople, parents, commuters and vacationers are just some of the groups who spend a lot of time in their cars. When the hunger drive hits, the next stop is usually the drive through window of one of our many fine fast food restaurants and then it's back on the road again.

And while it's possible to eat healthy at a fast food restaurant, the chances are very much against it. So if you spend a lot of time in your car, how can you put yourself in the best position to succeed at controlling your weight?

Buy a small cooler and pack your own food to take along with you. You can pack healthy snacks and tasty meals. It can be even more convenient than fast food because you don't have to stop traveling to eat.

And there are advantages to packing your own food other than staying on your diet. You'll save money. You can reload food supplies from any grocery store. And you can decide to either eat in your car, or you can stop and picnic at any beautiful spot along the road. Fast food restaurants aren't known for their beautiful locations. Picnicking in a lovely park or beside a river transforms any meal into a feast.

Chapter 22

Weight-Proof Your Shopping Safe Zone
Strategies 80–83

Entering a store is entering temptation alley. The store's job is to sell merchandise and they use all kinds of tricks that lead you into overeating. That's why the topic of shopping gets its own Safe Zone. Every year, millions of dollars are spent on research whose only goal is to get you to spend money on things you didn't know you wanted until you got to the store.

Poor grocery shopping means you won't be able to make good meals and you will eat all the foods you know you shouldn't. Protect yourself by creating a *Shopping Safe Zone*. Learn how to buy only what you want to buy, when you want to buy it, for as much as you want to pay.

Strategy 80. Use the Hunt and Gather Method of Shopping

Eliminate temptation by taking each item on your list and going directly to that item in the store.

There are two main styles of shopping: visit every aisle, and hunt and gather.

In the **visit every aisle** approach, no matter what is on your shopping list you go up and down every aisle. The problem is, you end up buying stuff that's not on your list. You see a treat, imagine how good it will taste, and plop it in your cart. When shopping with kids this happens a lot.

The other approach, the strategy I recommend, is to **hunt and gather.** With hunt and gather you go directly to each item on your shopping list. This approach eliminates a lot of chances for temptation. If you are not shopping every aisle, you are far less likely to buy items you don't need. And once you remember the layout of your store, hunt and gather shopping is a lot speedier.

The key to hunt and gather shopping is to have a **complete shopping list.** We have already talked about meal planning and shopping list creation in the *Home and Family Safe Zone* chapter. Without a list that has everything on it that you need, you'll fall back to visiting every aisle which means you will buy stuff you don't need. One time we had three large bottles of ketchup because I kept thinking we needed more ketchup!

Strategy 81. Don't Stockpile Food—You'll Eat It If You Have It

Eliminate temptation by only buying as much food as you need.

Let's say the store had a great deal on cookies so you bought 5 bags of cookies. It was a great deal you couldn't pass up. Will you eat more cookies because you bought more?

Yes! Studies show **the more of a particular food you have on hand, the more of it you will eat.** It's an unconscious process. You don't know it's happening and it doesn't make logical sense, but it makes a sort of body sense. When food is available you eat it so having a larger supply of food may unconsciously encourage larger portion sizes. And of course buying treats in bulk and keeping a large cache of sweets around is like a beacon, broadcasting to your brain saying "come eat me."

How might you combat this threat? **Buy only as much food as you need and no more.** Buying food in bulk may seem like a deal from a money perspective, but the extra weight has its own cost too and may not be such a bargain when you consider the extra insurance and medical costs.

Strategy 82. Know the Quantity of Each Item You Want to Buy

Buy only the amount of each item you specify on your shopping list and no more.

Your shopping list must specify exactly how much of each item you need. For example, don't just write down spaghetti on your shopping list, write down how many packages or ounces of spaghetti you should buy.

Why is this so important? If you don't buy the exact quantity you need, you will be tempted by store signs suggesting how many you should buy. Research has shown a sign that says, "Soup, no limit per person," will cause you to buy more, even if there isn't a special on the soup. Just putting a number in the price tag, like saying 3 for 2 dollars, makes you think about buying 3 items instead of the one item you really needed.

Stores have many of these tricks. Putting items at the end of an aisle or candy at the checkout line makes you more likely to buy them. These tricks are so subtle and silent you won't even notice they are working on you.

That's why stores are such a major danger zone. You will be tricked into buying foods you weren't planning to and don't need. The end result is overeating.

Sticking exactly to your shopping list prevents all these problems from happening in the first place. If your list says you need so much of a food item, that's all you buy. You don't have to think about it. If there's a sale on candy bars and it's not on your list, you don't buy it. You don't have to think about it.

The list creates your Safe Zone by reducing the number of decision you have to make. You created the list at your strongest. When you are in a store, you're at your weakest because all the tricks are working on you and you are imaging what a deal you are getting, or you are imaging how good something will taste.

Just stick to your shopping list and you'll be safe.

Strategy 83. Ignore Promotions

Don't buy food because the store is having a promotion. As the song says, just walk on by.

Don't buy something because it promises you the chance of winning something. Store promotions are a powerful inducement to buy stuff you don't need. Ignore them.

Chapter 23

Weight-Proof Your Work Safe Zone
Strategies 84–90

Work can be a dangerous environment, continually challenging your diet. At work you find vending machines serving nothing but junk food. Kind people bring in delicious home baked cookies. Every Halloween candy parents don't want their kids to eat magically shows up on desks and counters. Leftover pizza sits in the lunch room. You go out to lunch with coworkers to all sorts of wonderful restaurants. Some particularly cruel people buy those giant jars of candy and set them on their desk. And the cherry on the sundae is that many of us sit all day so we don't get any exercise. All this adds up to make work a diet-busting environment you must live in every day.

Companies have a huge stake in encouraging people to lose weight and stay on their diets. One study showed a 77% increase in medication costs and a 36% increase in outpatient care costs for obese people when compared to people in the normal weight range.

If trends continue, overweight people may simply not be hired because of the increased insurance costs. And even if it doesn't go that far, the increased health costs related to the overweight might decrease the quality of health care for everyone

Companies can help Weight-Proof work and lower their health care costs. A work place program implemented by Colonial/Unum showed a $700 a year per person reduction in medical costs for those who participated. Motorola's wellness program led to a return on investment of $3.93 for every dollar spent. These are major savings other companies can replicate too.

There are two parts to creating a Work Safe Zone: what you can do for yourself on your own and what your company can do for everyone. Work with your company to help implement Weight-Proofing strategies. You can also reach out and get together with your coworkers on Weight-Proofing ideas. Most of your coworkers probably want to stay on their diets as much as you do. Regardless of what your company does or doesn't do, there is a still a lot you can do to create your own Safe Zone at work.

In the future, weight is sure to be a hot workplace topic for everyone.

Strategy 84. Take Walking Meetings and Breaks

Find extra steps in your day by holding meetings while walking, and walking during breaks. Every little walk adds extra steps.

▌ Walk During Meetings

Not all meetings have to be held sitting down at a table under artificial lights. If you are just talking, then take a stroll in the hallways, or better yet, outside. You'll probably be more creative as exercise pumps up your brain.

▌ Walk During Breaks

Get up every hour or so and take a short walk.

We weren't meant to stay in one place all day. By taking a short brisk walk, you increase the number of steps you are taking, you reduce the chance of getting repetitive strain injury (RSI), and you jump start your brain so you'll be sharper during the day.

Put your walk break in your calendar so you'll remember to take it. Get a few other people in the office to walk with you so all of you can help each other to remember. It may take some creativity to find a place to walk. You can walk the hallways if there is nowhere outside or the weather is uninviting.

Strategy 85. Pack a Healthy Lunch—It's Cheaper Too

Packing a healthy lunch makes it easier to stay on your diet.

Packing lunch makes it harder to fall off your diet at work. Part of your meal planning and shopping will be about what you should eat for lunch. This helps to create your Work Safe Zone because it's much harder to overeat when eating from a well planned lunch.

Going out to eat every day makes it so easy to go off your diet. Yet, a big part of building work relationships is going out to eat. You still should go out with the gang, but you don't have to go out all the time.

If you need to snack during the day, pack snacks as well. Don't graze from vending machines. They are dangerous. Baby carrots make a great snack. Carrots are filling, low in calories, nutritious, and have a very satisfying crunch when you eat them. When you eat carrots you feel like you are eating real food. Carrots can also easily be eaten in the car and aren't messy.

This strategy isn't just for work. It applies to your kids' school lunches too.

. . . .

 # Strategy 86. Stock Good Food in the Vending Machines

Put healthy food alternatives in the vending machine so people have a choice.

When hunger hit at work, I would walk to the vending machine and all there was to choose from was junk. I was hungry so I ate the junk. Fellow workers and I would often complain to each other how there was never anything good to eat in the machine. Then we would insert our quarters and buy the junk anyway.

We should have done something about it, but what? I had no idea so the easiest thing to do was to do nothing. Now I would go the extra step and do something. One extra candy bar a day at work packs on over 20 extra pounds a year. I would try and find out who is in charge of the vending machines and see if I could get them to include healthier alternatives. Even something as simple as switching to baked pretzels from fried chips could make a difference.

Companies interested in health care costs should put good food choices in their vending machines anyway. Unlike schools it's not possible to get rid of vending machines at work, but they can be made healthier. And healthier impacts the bottom line with lower health care costs.

. . . .

 # Strategy 87. Make Stairways Clean and Safe

Increase the number of steps you take in the day by skipping the elevator and take the stairs.

One of the big reasons people take the elevator and skip the stairs is they often look like the set of a horror movie.

To make it easy for people to take the stairs consider:

- ❖ **Displaying clear signage pointing to the stairway.** In a lot of buildings it's hard to even find the stairs.
- ❖ **Bring up using the stairs in company wide memos** so people know it's an option. It's all about marketing.
- ❖ **Make sure the stairway is clean, well lit, and safe.** A lot of stairways are downright scary. And if they aren't scary they are so dirty and unpleasant nobody would use them anyway.
- ❖ **Make the stairway environment more pleasant through music and art.** More attractive stairways might encourage people to give them a second look.

Try creating a stairway environment where people want to be, not just a place where they think they should be.

Strategy 88. Reduce the Price of Healthy Items
People will naturally eat more of a healthy food if it is cheaper.

Price matters. In one study, a 50% price reduction on food items increased food consumption by a whopping 93%. That's a big difference!

In my personal experience, price matters a lot. At one place I worked, apples were a quarter a piece. I bought an apple almost every day. At another place apples were $1. I didn't eat as many apples there. The same for the salad bar. At one place the salad bar was stocked with a lot of great choices and was relatively inexpensive. At another place, the salad bar was at a premium price and most people turned to the cheaper fried foods instead.

People like and are attracted to value. Make healthy foods cheaper in vending machines and in your cafeteria and people will naturally be drawn to make healthier food choices. You won't need to preach or beg people to eat healthier. The marketplace will do the work.

Companies often subsidize cafeteria and vending machine items anyway. It's not that big a step to make healthier foods less expensive than not so healthy foods. Drastically reducing the price on healthier foods could make a difference in health costs.

This strategy isn't just limited to the workplace it makes sense in schools too.

Strategy 89. Use a Standing Workstation

Standing burns 30% more calories than sitting.

In *The Power of Rest Threat* we learned how researchers found that obese people tended to sit for 2.5 hours more per day than thinner people and this tendency to sit was innate. If you could somehow sit less you could burn up to 350 additional calories a day.

Our environment today is very chair friendly. Many people sit while driving to work, sit all day at work, sit while driving home, and then sit all night at home. So it makes sense to try and find a way of sitting less at work because we spend so much time there.

One way to sit less at work is to use a standing workstation. Traditionally, an office has a desk and a chair and you sit at your desk while working. What if you could stand while working instead of sitting? Wouldn't that burn a few extra calories?

Big changes have been happening in office design. You can now create offices where your desk can be easily raised and lowered. This allows you to raise your desk and stand for as long you want, and when you get tired you can lower the desk and sit for a while. Changing the desk height is easy and takes only a few seconds.

Originally, standing workstations were created for ergonomic reasons. Sitting in the same posture for long periods of time is very hard on your body. Being able to stand eases the stress. You can use the same workstation design for both weight loss and ergonomic reasons. Work with your corporate facilities people on changing your office setup to use a standing workstation.

To Learn More

❈ If a standing workstation isn't your style, you might like the *Geek-a-Cycle* at *http://www.slimgeek.com/*. It combines an exer-cycle with a work desk so you can burn calories by pedaling while using your computer.

Strategy 90. Offer Paid Vacation for Meeting Physical Fitness Goals

Creative thinking may pay off with big returns.

Some companies have had good results by offering paid vacation to employees who meet some simple physical fitness goals every 6 months. Employee absenteeism dropped by more than 50% at one company. Given the high cost of employee absenteeism, that's a large return on investment.

Even if your company doesn't adopt this specific policy, by thinking creatively workplace strategies may pay off with big returns.

Chapter 24

Create Your School Safe Zone
Strategies 91–94

Kids spend a lot of time at school, so making schools free of potential slip-ups is a worthy goal, especially with the stunning rise of childhood obesity.

Everything we have been talking about Safe Zones applies to schools as well: organize schools so kids have the best possible chance of eating healthy and exercising more while minimizing their chances of slipping up.

Over the years, schools have transformed into danger zones where kids have an increased chance of gaining weight. Physical education has often been cut. Lunches are often made less healthy so they are more readily accepted by the kids. Vending machines have been installed so junk food is available at all times.

Helping kids means changing their schools from danger zones into Safe Zones.

· ·

 Strategy 91. Turn Students into Cooks

Cooking at school is a good way for students to learn the practical skill of cooking.

One of the strategies in this book is to learn how to cook. Cooking at school is a perfect learning ground. Rotate students through the cafeteria so they can cook lunch for the school. Put students in charge of ordering supplies, scheduling, budgeting, etc., just like real life. All under adult supervision of course!

The next step is to have the kids grow some of their own food in their own school garden. The University City High School in Philadelphia harvests vegetables from their own large indoor and outdoor garden. The garden acts as a classroom and a link to the real world because they also grow crops to sell at a weekly Farmers' Market. Crops from the garden would also make a delicious addition to school lunches.

To Learn More

❖   The *Urban Nutrition Initiative* website at *http://www.urban nutrition.org/gardens.htm* has more information.

Strategy 92. Add Back PE—But Not Your Father's PE

Return PE to the school day so kids will always get some exercise during the day.

Many schools have cut PE for funding reasons. Even in schools with PE, many end up spending little time being active.

Add back PE so kids will always get some exercise during the day. But PE doesn't have to be like the old PE. That was built around teaching sports skills. We would learn how to play volleyball, basketball, and other sports. Another way to look at PE is to **teach health and wellness,** much like an adult health club would do.

A vision of the new PE was created by Daniel Latham at West Middle School in Downey, California. He created his school's Cyberobics Center, a state of the art gym in which kids ride specially equipped exer-cycles hooked to video games. A kid's character in the game is awarded power based on their fitness. The fitter the student, the more power the character has. It's not like exercise at all. Cyberobics combines the best of the active life and the video game culture kids have grown up with. Sure sounds fun to me!

A new generation of active video games may be the key to getting kids interested in being active. You may have seen a game in the mall called "Dance Dance Revolution" (DDR) made by Konami. DDR has a platform with four arrows: up, down, left, and right. On the screen you are shown which arrows to touch with your feet. The game plays like a dance. I've played a few times and I am terrible, but it's a great workout. There are versions of DDR available for Playstation and Xbox video game systems.

You may not believe me about the workout, but it's intense. You're moving your feet around at a blistering pace. Tanya Jessen started playing DDR at age 17 and 4 years later she has lost 95 pounds. She credits her weight loss success to DDR.

The Wii™ video game console from Nintendo is another contender in the fitness arena. Playing the boxing game, you can burn up to 125 calories in a 15-minute session. Several workout-related games, like Wii Health Pack, are in development and will probably be available by the time this book is published.

These types of games may be the future of exercise and West Virginia is joining the future. West Virginia officials announced a deal to provide DDR in all of the state's 765 public schools.

This type of innovative thinking can help both kids and adults become more fit.

To Learn More

* The *P.E.4 Life* website at *http://pe4life.com/* has information on how to set up physical education programs for all children.
* The *Get Up Move* website at *http://GetUpMove.com/* talks about how both kids and adults can use dance video games for fitness.
* To combine your favorite video games with exercise take a look at the *Gamerunner Exercise Controller* at *http://www.gamerunner.us*. You use your body to play games instead of just sitting and using your hands.

Strategy 93. Serve Healthy Lunches—With a Side of Nutritional Education

Fully fund school lunch programs and serve good tasting healthy food.

Sometimes I just don't understand how the world works. The lack of funding for good healthy nutritional lunches is one way the world works that makes no sense to me at all.

Many school lunch programs are required to fund themselves through the money they take in from lunch and concessions. Who buys the food? Students. What do students want? Junk food.

To make money, the people running school lunch programs are forced to sell junk food. I've listened to a number of heart-wrenching radio interviews with people who run school lunch programs. They feel trapped because they don't have any other options.

Full funding of school lunch programs is a must. This is completely obvious and thankfully many communities are starting to take back the food environment at school from the junk food sellers.

But the kids won't eat healthy food, a lot of people say. Kids like popular brand named food and shy away from eating anything else. So many school lunch programs have given up and serve junk for lunch.

But it's possible to reverse this trend and start serving good food. Healthy food doesn't have to taste bad.

Dr. Antonia Demas has a program called "Food is Elementary" in which kids learn about healthy foods using games, songs, science experiments and other hands-on activities. It turns out that kids will eat healthy food if they are educated about it. Education is just part of it. Good food can be made tasty too. "When food is made in a way that's fun and sensory-based, kids will eat anything that's nutritious," says Demas.

Do healthy lunches even make a difference? Yes. A long-running Swedish study found a combination of nutritious lunches and a ban on sweets reduced the relative number of overweight 6- to 10-year olds by 6%. That's a significant decrease.

▌ Tracking Your Kids' Lunch Using Meal Management

Parents have responsibility for their kids, but often they are not given the capability to exercise that responsibility. School lunches are one such tricky area where students aren't accountable to their parents. If a school lunch program offers poor food choices, a parent may not be able to figure out what their child is eating for lunch. If a parent asks what their child had for lunch, they may tell the truth, or they may not. How is a parent to know? And if a parent doesn't know, how is a parent to do anything about it?

Enter web based meal management and tracking solutions. These services allow a parent to pay for school lunches over the Internet so their child doesn't have to carry money to school to pay for lunches. The parent can also pull up a report on what their child is choosing to eat for lunch each day. Armed with information about what their child is actually eating, they can take any action they think necessary as a parent.

That's the idea anyway. Emotions run high on this system. Some people say if you don't trust your kid then they'll never learn responsibility. Some people say if you can't trust your kid to tell you what they had for lunch you have bigger problems. Other people ask what kind of parent wouldn't supervise what their children are eating? Any thinking person can see all sides have good solid points.

It might be better if only healthy food was served in the school cafeteria so it wouldn't be necessary to track food choices so closely. But in a situation where a school serves unhealthy food, this type of system may be a good option for both parents and schools, especially for younger children. Once children reach age 10 or 12, parents may not have a huge impact on teaching nutrition, but before that age they can make a big difference.

To Learn More

❖ The Food Studies Institute website at *http://www.foodstudies.org* teaches children "by providing a positive experience of food and food preparation that is fun, hands-on and sensory-based."

Strategy 94. Create Walking School Buses

Instead of taking the bus or cars, parents walk with their kids to school.

In grade school and in college I rode my bike to school. In 1969, 50% of all children walked to school. Today people are understandably worried about the safety of their kids, so riding or walking may not always be an option. In fact, only 25% of kids who live a mile or less from school regularly walk to school.

To revive the ancient and healthy art of walking to school, a group in England started what is called the Walking School Bus. A walking school bus is a group of children who walk to school with one or more adults instead of taking the bus. A fun variation is to ride bikes instead of walking.

The simple idea is taking off. It's good for the parents and good for the kids.

To Learn More

❖ The *Walking School Bus Information* website at *http://www.walkingschoolbus.org/* talks about how to create your own walking school bus.

Chapter 25

Weight-Proof Your
Community Safe Zone
Strategies 95–99

Weight-Proofing extends all the way up to your community. The same ideas apply. Make it easy and natural for people to be active and they will be. Make it hard and people won't. For many years now we have been making it hard.

 Strategy 95. Build Active Communities
Encourage walking as a natural part of life.

Communities have been making it hard to be naturally active. How? It's a combination of factors, which nobody really thought about, but the end result is we walk a lot less than people used to.

In the past many people lived close enough to town they could walk to the store. Most services, like the grocery store, the hardware store, and the clothing store, were within walking distance. When services are close people naturally walk more. Another benefit of having a grocery store close to your home is that you can easily walk to the store and buy fresh fruits and vegetables.

The popularity of the car changed everything. It's fascinating to think how quickly the car changed society. For the first time, because of the car's mobility, the average person could live in their own home far from the city center. Who wouldn't want that?

But building housing so far away from services had a downside that we have just begun to realize and take steps to change. People stopped walking because they had to drive everywhere. We've seen in *The Power of Rest Threat* that we won't exercise naturally, so moving to the suburbs removed one of the natural environmental reasons to walk: getting places.

Many suburbs are built without sidewalks so you simply can't walk places even if you wanted to. In many areas, safety concerns have forced both kids and adults inside. And the poor and minorities have been found to have less access to parks, pools and other exercise opportunities. All these invisible forces add up to make a big difference in our health. It doesn't take much of a reduction in activity to push us into obesity.

The end results were shown by a University of British Columbia study, which found that people who live where stores and other businesses are within easy walking distance are much less likely to be overweight. The key was, people walked as a natural part of their life.

A University of Maryland study found that people who live in the most sprawling counties are the most likely to be overweight. You don't walk when you have to drive everywhere.

Communities are starting to reconstruct themselves to naturally encourage more activity.

Joel Hirshorn, director of natural resources policy studies at the National Governors Association, estimates there are nearly 200 old-style neighborhoods either already built or under construction. By old-style I mean communities, like those in our past, that were mixed use. They combine housing, shopping, and business in a smaller, more walkable and more connected living place. In such a community you are naturally encouraged to walk more. Nobody is forcing you, you will just do it, and that is what Weight-Proofing is all about.

An example of one of these new old-style communities is Southern Village in Chapel Hill, North Carolina. It was designed to have a small town-feel with a gorgeous main street, lots of parks and trails, and a school kids can walk to from their home.

Before you start thinking all this community planning is just a plot by the UN to take over the world, keep in mind a couple of things. First, there's always a design to communities. Creating suburbs was a design, we just didn't think about it as such. So, anything we do is design and has consequences. It's reasonable to think about those consequences and see if we can make a better design. Second, this is a movement back to an older way of life, not something new. The old way of creating communities was better.

To Learn More

- ❖ The *Walkable Communities, Inc.* website at *http://www.walkable. org* shows you how to find and help build a walkable community.
- ❖ The *Active Living by Design* website at *http://www.activelivingby design.org* talks about how to increase physical activity through community design.
- ❖ The *Stapleton* development website at *http://www.stapleton denver.com* is an actively designed community.

Strategy 96. Turn Blight into Might

Communities can find opportunities to build more pools, parks, bike paths and walking paths.

In Cleveland they are turning abandoned rail lines into trails for cycling and walking. They are also turning old industrial sites into parks. Most communities can probably find similar opportunities to build more pools, parks, bike paths and walking paths.

To Learn More

- ❖ The *Rails-to-Trails Conservancy* at website *http://www.railtrails. org/* talks about creating a nationwide network of trails from former rail lines and connecting corridors to build healthier places for healthier people.

Strategy 97. Make Playing Safe

Safety is at the heart of getting people to move outside.

Staying inside makes sense if people are afraid to go outside. I wouldn't spend a lot of time outside either if I was afraid of getting mugged, or worse.

Safety is at the heart of getting people moving outside. Kids should be able to walk to school. People should be able to walk the streets and parks in safety. This is a community and law enforcement issue requiring cooperation on all sides.

To Learn More

- ❖ The *Safe Routes to Schools* website at *http://www.saferoutesto schools.org/* talks about ways to decrease traffic and pollution and increase the health of children and the community.

Strategy 98. Create Policy Incentives

Government at all levels can create incentives to create Safe Zones.

Government at all levels plays a big role in creating a community's environment both in the laws it passes and the laws it doesn't pass. How might government policy help to create a community's Safe Zone? Here are some examples:

- ❖ In Minnesota there was a proposal to make federal food stamps worthless for junk food.
- ❖ In another state, a $10 voucher was given to people redeemable for fruit and vegetables at the farmer's market.
- ❖ Congress has funded more money for PE in schools.
- ❖ Planning codes are another area to investigate. They determine what gets built in a community. If your codes allow housing subdivisions to be built without sidewalks and parks, you can help get them changed.

Government can't solve all problems, but it can certainly solve some and it should try not to make other problems worse.

Strategy 99. Label All Foods with Calorie Counts

Knowing how many calories all your food has would help you make better food decisions.

We learned how to estimate calories for any meal in the *Honest Calorie Estimation Method* strategy, but doesn't that seem like too much work to estimate calorie counts?

Most people simply won't estimate calories or watch portion sizes because it's too error prone and too hard. Yet to make informed decisions about their diet, people need calorie counts for everything they eat.

I try to stay away from the "we need a new law" approach to solving problems, but one useful law would be to have **every food item displayed with the calories** right next to the item on the menu or display board.

When you are at your favorite fast food restaurant, right next to the price on the display should be the number of calories the item has. Right next to the price of soda at your local convenience store should be the calorie count for the soda. The menu at every sit-down restaurant should include both the price and the number of calories in the dish. Everywhere you see a food price you should also see a calorie count.

You don't need to outlaw or tax certain foods if you make the information people need to make intelligent purchasing decisions easily and clearly available. It can be very easy to forget that a super giant soda has 800 calories. If the calorie count was right next to the price, you might think twice about choosing the soda. Or you may buy it anyway. In either case it's your decision, but if you have calorie counts available, you are making an informed decision.

Information is the key to making decisions. Without information you can't make rational choices. It does you no good to have nutritional information on a website or in a booklet that is never available. Put the calorie information next to the price and people can make better decisions and be accountable for those decisions.

Chapter 26

Conclusion

We've come a long way together in this book. A lot of ideas have been presented. Maybe not always in the best way possible, but I hope you'll take away something useful. I want to thank you for sticking with me to the end. If you are one of those people who reads the end of a book before the beginning, I hope it's good enough to read twice. ☺

We all wish we could just take a pill and then eat what we want, when we want, and never gain weight. Why isn't it that simple? My very unoriginal conclusion is this:

We really like food and that makes us eat too much of it.

Food is simply one of our greatest sources of pleasure and joy. To deny food is to deny a big part of what makes life worth living. Who is willing to do that?

We really like food for good and honest reasons. It's not because of a lack of willpower or moral weakness as we've always been told. We humans are stunningly successful survival machines. Our bodies want to eat because eating when food is available has historically been the key to survival. Our bodies want us to eat and gain weight. And because cheap, great tasting, high calorie food is now available everywhere it's just our nature as humans to oblige.

It's not likely science will create a single miracle pill that will solve the obesity problem. Our bodies have so many ways of making us eat that finding a pill to handle all those possibilities will be difficult. Unfortunately, unless you are naturally thin or lived a hundred years ago, weight control may always be a challenge for you.

I really meant it earlier when I said you are among the first generation with complete responsibility for maintaining your weight. If you want to exercise more, you must find a way to make it happen. If you want to eat the right amount, you must find a way to make it happen. You can't rely on your environment to make you exercise and you can't rely on your environment to limit the number of calories you eat.

Staying on your diet is now all on you and it's hard. It's hard and until now there's really been no reason for you to have figured out how to stay on a diet given how radically the world has changed.

The ideas, skills and techniques we shared in this book are an attempt to help you re-create your world so it helps you control your weight while still respecting the powerful place the joy of food has in life. What did you learn to help create your perfect Designer Diet?

You learned the surprising truth that your body plays the **survival game;** most people play the **lose weight** game, while you really want to play the **stay on a diet** game.

How can you stay on a diet? By creating your Designer Diet. A diet that responds to changes in your life and that helps you find ways to lose weight that takes advantage of your strengths while avoiding the destructive power of your weaknesses.

You learned how to create your Designer Diet using the Designer Principles. The key principles are: 1) Take responsibility, 2) Understand your three natures, 3) Identify the threats that sabotage your diet, 4) Discover your strategies for defeating the threats, and 5) Follow the Designer Way for continuously improving your diet.

Through the **threats** you learned how amazingly complicated we humans are and how our nature provides a stunningly large number of ways to gain weight. From your understanding of the threats, you learned how to develop effective **strategies** for defeating the threats.

After mastering the threats and strategies, you can then follow the Designer Way to control your weight in an ever-changing world. With the Designer Way, you continually learn which strategies work for you by using a feedback system of your own creation. And then you continually improve your diet by making changes to your strategies. You are unique in all the world and you need to find the strategies that work for you and your life. The end result is a diet created just for you that gives you the best chance of losing weight and keeping it off permanently.

And because staying on your diet requires a joyful vision of life, we learned about **Joyful Eating.** Joyful Eating helps you experience pleasure from food without needing to overeat. This is key because without joy you can't stick to a diet.

We also learned about creating **Safe Zones** in which you "baby proof" your life by systematically removing diet slip-up opportunities from all areas of your life. This is key because you gain weight one little slip-up at a time. Minimizing slip-ups maximizes your chances of staying on your diet for the rest of your life, and that's what this book is all about.

Some people ask me how I feel now that I've solved all my weight problems. I have to laugh when I hear that question. My weight problems will never be completely solved. Controlling my weight will always be a struggle. What is different now is that when I start gaining weight I'll notice before it's too late and I'll be able to do something about it before my weight spirals out of control.

I may not have solved all my weight problems, but I no longer fear my weight either. I feel like I am back in control. And I like that feeling.

You may feel like you'll never be in control of your weight again, but that's not true. It's never too late. You can take control. I am just like you and I have learned to stay on my diet, not by being strong, but by learning how to create my own Designer Diet. I know you can do it too.

If you still want more, please come visit us at *http://YourDesignerDiet.com*. We'll try to support each other, learn from each other, and have a bit of fun. See you there!

References

Normally what you would see in this section is a list of references to papers and books used to write this book. I am going to do something a little different. Instead of creating a long list of references almost nobody will read, I am putting the list on my website. It's searchable. If you stacked up all the references I used to write this book it would be taller than I am! That much information is not very useful. What would be useful is a searchable database of the materials I used so you can go take a look for yourself.

And that's just what you can do. Go to *http://YourDesignerDiet.com* and you'll find a master list of all the references used to write this book in a searchable format. Unfortunately, not all the source materials are on-line, but a lot of them are and it can be very interesting to read some of the actual studies used to create the threats and strategies presented in *Your Designer Diet.*

Index

Printed in the United States
200596BV00005B/7-9/A

9 780979 707100